T0290470

Infections in Older Adults

Editors

PUJA VAN EPPS
DAVID H. CANADAY

INFECTIOUS DISEASE CLINICS OF NORTH AMERICA

www.id.theclinics.com

Consulting Editor
HELEN W. BOUCHER

March 2023 • Volume 37 • Number 1

ELSEVIER

1600 John F. Kennedy Boulevard • Suite 1800 • Philadelphia, Pennsylvania, 19103-2899.
http://www.theclinics.com

INFECTIOUS DISEASE CLINICS OF NORTH AMERICA Volume 37, Number 1
March 2023 ISSN 0891-5520, ISBN-13: 978-0-443-18224-2

Editor: Kerry Holland
Developmental Editor: Hannah Almira Lopez

Infectious Disease Clinics of North America (ISSN 0891-5520) is published in March, June, September, and December by Elsevier Inc., 360 Park Avenue South, New York, NY 10010-1710. Periodicals postage paid at New York, NY and additional mailing offices. Subscription prices are $368.00 per year for US individuals, $806.00 per year for US institutions, $100.00 per year for US students, $420.00 per year for Canadian individuals, $1,007.00 per year for Canadian institutions, $458.00 per year for international individuals, $1,007.00 per year for international institutions, $100.00 per year for Canadian students, and $200.00 per year for international students. To receive student rate, orders must be accompanied by name of affiliated institution, date of term, and the *signature* of program/residency coordinator on institution letterhead. Orders will be billed at individual rate until proof of status is received. Foreign air speed delivery is included in all *Clinics* subscription prices. All prices are subject to change without notice. **POSTMASTER**: Send address changes to *Infectious Disease Clinics of North America,* Elsevier Health Sciences Division, Subcription Customer Service, 3251 Riverport Lane, Maryland Heights, MO 63043. **Customer Service: 1-800-654-2452 (US). From outside of the US and Canada, call 1-314-447-8871. Fax: 1-314-447-8029. E-mail: JournalsCustomerService-usa@elsevier.com (print support) or JournalsOnlineSupport-usa@elsevier.com (online support).**

Infectious Disease Clinics of North America is also published in Spanish by Editorial Inter-Médica, Junin 917, 1ᵉʳ A 1113, Buenos Aires, Argentina.

Reprints. For copies of 100 or more, of articles in this publication, please contact the Commercial Reprints Department, Elsevier Inc., 360 Park Avenue South, New York, New York 10010-1710. Tel. 212-633-3874, Fax: 212-633-3820, E-mail: reprints@elsevier.com.

Infectious Disease Clinics of North America is covered in *MEDLINE/PubMed (Index Medicus), Current Contents/ Clinical Medicine, Science Citation Alert, SCISEARCH,* and *Research Alert.*

Contributors

CONSULTING EDITOR

HELEN W. BOUCHER, MD, FIDSA, FACP
Dean ad interim and Professor, Tufts University School of Medicine, Chief Academic
Officer, Tufts Medicine, Boston, Massachusetts

EDITORS

PUJA VAN EPPS, MD
Associate Professor of Medicine, Case Western Reserve University School of Medicine,
Division of Infectious Diseases and Geriatric Research, Education, and Clinical Center, VA
Northeast Ohio Healthcare System, Louis Stokes Cleveland VA Medical Center,
Cleveland, Ohio

DAVID H. CANADAY, MD
Professor of Medicine, Case Western Reserve University School of Medicine, Division of
Infectious Diseases and Geriatric Research, Education, and Clinical Center, Louis Stokes
Cleveland VA Medical Center, Cleveland, Ohio

AUTHORS

YASIN ABUL, MD
Center of Innovation in Long Term Services and Supports, Providence VA Medical Center,
Division of Geriatric and Palliative Medicine, The Warren Alpert Medical School of Brown
University, Brown University School of Public Health Center for Gerontology and
Healthcare Research, Providence, Rhode Island

MAHA AL-JABRI, MD
Division of Infectious Diseases and HIV Medicine, University Hospitals Cleveland Medical
Center, Case Western Reserve University, Cleveland, Ohio

ANTHONY W. BAFFOE-BONNIE, MD
Associate Professor of Medicine, Division of Infectious Diseases, Virginia Tech Carilion
School of Medicine, Carilion Clinic, Roanoke, Virginia

WESTYN BRANCH-ELLIMAN, MD, MMSC, FSHEA
Department of Medicine, Section of Infectious Diseases, VA Boston Healthcare System,
West Roxbury, Massachusetts; Department of Medicine, Harvard Medical School,
Boston, Massachusetts

TYLER J. BREHM, MD
Internal Medicine Resident, Section of General Internal Medicine, Department of
Medicine, Baylor College of Medicine, Houston, Texas

DAVID H. CANADAY, MD
Professor of Medicine, Case Western Reserve University School of Medicine, Division of
Infectious Diseases and Geriatric Research, Education, and Clinical Center, Cleveland VA
Medical Center, Cleveland, Ohio

CURTIS J. DONSKEY, MD
Geriatric Research Education and Clinical Center, Louis Stokes Cleveland VA
Medical Center, Case Western Reserve University School of Medicine, Cleveland,
Ohio

GHINWA DUMYATI, MD
Professor,Department of Medicine, Division of Infectious Diseases University of
Rochester School of Medicine and DentistryRochester, New York, USA

JASON R. FAULHABER, MD
Assistant Professor of Medicine, Division of Infectious Diseases, Virginia Tech Carilion
School of Medicine, Carilion Clinic, Roanoke, Virginia

STEFAN GRAVENSTEIN, MD, MPH
Center of Innovation in Long Term Services and Supports, Providence VA Medical Center,
Division of Geriatric and Palliative Medicine, The Warren Alpert Medical School of Brown
University, Brown University School of Public Health Center for Gerontology and
Healthcare Research, Providence, Rhode Island

PRATHIT A. KULKARNI, MD
Assistant Professor and Assistant Chief of Medicine, Medical Care Line, Michael E.
DeBakey VA Medical Center, Infectious Diseases Section, Department of Medicine,
Baylor College of Medicine, Houston, Texas

CIERA LEEDER, MD, MPH
Center of Innovation in Long Term Services and Supports, Providence VA Medical Center,
Division of Geriatric and Palliative Medicine, The Warren Alpert Medical School of Brown
University, Providence, Rhode Island

JEFFREY LARNARD, MD
Division of Infectious Disease, Beth Israel Deaconess Medical Center, Harvard Medical
School, Boston, Massachusetts

CANDICE J. MCNEIL, MD, MPH
Department of Internal Medicine, Section on Infectious Diseases, Wake Forest School of
Medicine, Winston-Salem, North Carolina

LEWIS MUSOKE, MD
Division of Infectious Diseases, Geriatric Research Education and Clinical Center, VA
Northeast Ohio Healthcare System, Division of Infectious Diseases, Department of
Medicine, University Hospitals Cleveland Medical Center, Cleveland, Ohio

ELEFTHERIOS MYLONAKIS, MD, PhD
Infectious Diseases Division, The Miriam Hospital and Rhode Island Hospital, The Warren
Alpert Medical School of Brown University, Rhode Island Hospital, Providence, Rhode
Island

NORA T. OLIVER, MD, MPH
Section of Infectious Diseases, Atlanta VA Medical Center, Decatur, Georgia

KRISANN K. OURSLER, MD
Professor of Medicine, Virginia Tech Carilion School of Medicine, VA Salem Healthcare
System, Virginia

OLADAYO A. OYEBANJI, MBChB, MS
Case Western Reserve University School of Medicine, Cleveland, Ohio

CHRISTIAN ROSERO, MD
Division of Infectious Diseases and HIV Medicine, University Hospitals Cleveland Medical Center, Case Western Reserve University, Cleveland, Ohio

ELIE A. SAADE, MD, MPH
Division of Infectious Diseases and HIV Medicine, University Hospitals Cleveland Medical Center, Cleveland, Ohio

MARION J. SKALWEIT, MD, PhD
Department of Medicine and Biochemistry, Case Western Reserve University School of Medicine, Cleveland, Ohio

WENDY STEAD, MD
Division of Infectious Disease, Beth Israel Deaconess Medical Center, Harvard Medical School, Boston, Massachusetts

BRENDA L. TESINI, MD
Assistant Professor, Department of Medicine, Division of Infectious Diseases University of Rochester School of Medicine and Dentistry, Rochester, New York

BARBARA W. TRAUTNER, MD, PhD
Professor and Deputy Associate Chief of Staff for Clinical Research, Center for Innovations in Quality, Effectiveness and Safety (IQuESt), Michael E. DeBakey VA Medical Center, Section of Health Services Research, Department of Medicine, Baylor College of Medicine, Houston, Texas

PUJA VAN EPPS, MD
Associate Professor of Medicine, Case Western Reserve University School of Medicine, Division of Infectious Diseases and Geriatric Research, Education, and Clinical Center, VA Northeast Ohio Healthcare System, Louis Stokes Cleveland VA Medical Center, Cleveland, Ohio

SHIKHA S. VASUDEVA, MD
Assistant Professor of Medicine, Virginia Tech Carilion School of Medicine, VA Salem Healthcare System, Virginia

Contents

Severe acute respiratory syndrome coronavirus 2 (SARS-CoV-2) infection
remains asymptomatic in 33% to 90% of older adults depending on their
immune status from prior infection, vaccination, and circulating strain.
Older adults symptomatic with SARS-CoV-2 often both present atypically,
such as with a blunted fever response, and develop more severe disease.
Early and late reports showed that older adults have increased severity of
coronavirus disease 2019 (COVID-19) with higher case fatality rates and
higher intensive care needs compared with younger adults. Infection and
vaccine-induced antibody response and long-term effects of COVID-19
also differ in older adults.

Institutionalized and community-dwelling older adults have been greatly
impacted by the coronavirus disease 2019 (COVID-19) pandemic with
increased morbidity and mortality. The advent of vaccines and their widespread use in this population has brought about a dramatic turnaround in
COVID-19 outcomes. The immunogenicity and effectiveness of the various
vaccine options worldwide are discussed. Optimization of vaccine usage
will still be important to maximize protection due to reduced initial immunity, development of variant strains, and fading of immunity over time.
There are also lessons learned specific to older populations for future
pandemics of novel pathogens.

Sexually transmitted infections (STIs) have been increasing in older adults.
Sexual health remains an important part of overall health care at any age.
There are several barriers and facilitators to addressing sexual health in
this population. Changes attributable to normal physiologic aging as well
as sexual dysfunction can affect sexuality in older adults. When it comes
to preventing STIs, combination prevention strategies remain applicable
in older adults. Addressing sexual health using a tailored approach is critical to stem the tide of increasing STIs rates in older adults.

Health care-associated infections (HAIs) are a global public health threat, which disproportionately impact older adults. Host factors including aging-related changes, comorbidities, and geriatric syndromes, such as dementia and frailty, predispose older individuals to infection. The HAI risks from medical interventions such as device use, antibiotic use, and lapses in infection control follow older adults as they transfer among a network of interrelated acute and long-term care facilities. Long-term care facilities are caring for patients with increasingly complex needs, and the home-like communal environment of long-term care facilities creates distinct infection prevention challenges.

Clostridioides difficile is a common cause of community-associated and health care-associated infections. Older adults are disproportionately affected, and long-term care facilities (LTCFs) have borne a substantial proportion of the burden of C difficile infection (CDI). Recurrences of CDI are common in older adults and have substantial adverse effects on quality of life. Appropriate diagnostic testing and management is essential for older adults in the community and in LTCFs. This review focuses on current concepts related to the epidemiology, diagnosis, and management of CDI in older adults.

Older adults are at an increased risk of vaccine-preventable diseases partly because of physiologic changes in the immune and other body systems related to age and/or accumulating comorbidities that increase the vulnerability to infections and decrease the response to vaccines. Strategies to improve the response to vaccines include using a higher antigenic dose (such as in the high-dose inactivated influenza vaccines) as well as adding adjuvants (such as MF59 in the adjuvanted inactivated influenza vaccine).

Outpatient parenteral antimicrobial therapy (OPAT) for older adults is a complex process that involves multiple stakeholders and care coordination, but it is a useful and patient-centered tool with opportunities for the treatment of complicated infections, improved patient satisfaction, and reduced health-care costs. Older age should not be an exclusion for OPAT but rather prompt the OPAT provider to thoroughly evaluate candidacy and safety. Amid the on-going COVID-19 pandemic, innovations in OPAT are needed to shepherd OPAT care into a more patient-centered, thoughtful practice, whereas minimizing harm to older patients from unnecessary health-care exposure and thus health-care associated infections.

Antibiotic administration is often a part of end-of-life (EOL) care, including among patients who are not critically ill. Guideline-issuing bodies recommend that antimicrobial stewardship providers (ASPs) provide support to prescribers making decisions about whether or not to treat infections in this population. Relatively little is known about the rationale for antimicrobial prescribing during the EOL period in noncritical care settings, although patient and family preferences are often an influencing factor. The effectiveness of antimicrobials in improving quantity or quality of life in this population is unclear and likely context-specific.

Effective and consistent antiretroviral therapy has enabled people with human immunodeficiency virus (HIV) (PWH) to survive longer than previously encountered earlier in the epidemic. Consequently, PWH are subject to the struggles and clinical conditions typically associated with aging. However, the aging process in PWH is not the same as for those who do not have HIV. There is a complex interplay of molecular, microbiologic, and pharmacologic factors that leads to accelerated aging in PWH; this leads to increased risk for certain age-related comorbidities requiring greater vigilance and interventions in routine care.

Acute and chronic bacterial prostatitis are clinically significant entities that can be difficult to diagnose and appropriately treat. Herein, we review when to suspect these clinical conditions, how to diagnose them, and how to effectively treat them based on the extant literature. Our aim was to equip the practicing clinician with the ability to proficiently diagnose and manage acute and chronic bacterial prostatitis, particularly in older patients.

INFECTIOUS DISEASE CLINICS OF NORTH AMERICA

Preface

The Intersection of Age and Infections: Understanding the Impacts from Diagnosis to Management

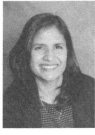 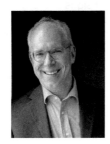

Puja Van Epps, MD   David H. Canaday, MD
Editors

According to the Pew Research Center,[1] by the year 2050, there are expected to be 81 million people over the age of 65 living in the United States, more than doubling their numbers from the start of the century. In fact, as a group, older adults are expected to expand faster than the general population, extending their representation to one in every four adults by the year 2060. With aging comes increasing likelihood of acute and chronic comorbid conditions, including infections. Given that over a third of all health care spending in the United States is for people 65 and older, in economic terms alone, this graying of the population is expected to have a significant impact.[2] For example, one study estimated that antibiotic-resistant pathogens among hospitalized older adults nationwide cost nearly $1.9 billion in a single year.[3] Beyond the economic implications, the fact remains that infections are a major source of morbidity and mortality in older individuals. According to the Centers for Disease Control and Prevention,[4] one-third of all deaths in people over the age of 65 are caused by infections.

Nothing has brought into focus the impact of aging on outcomes in infections more than the COVID-19 pandemic. In 2020, this infection alone was the third leading cause of death in older adults, with influenza and pneumonia being the 10th leading causes. Infections may even be a factor in other foremost causes of mortality in this age group, such as Alzheimer,[5] lower respiratory tract disease,[6] and diabetes.[7] Occasionally, infectious syndromes may also be implicated in thromboembolic events, such as cerebrovascular accidents and myocardial infarctions, which can be precipitated by prothrombotic states caused by infection, well documented in diseases such as pneumococcal pneumonia,[8] influenza,[9] and COVID-19.[10]

Infect Dis Clin N Am 37 (2023) xi–xiii
https://doi.org/10.1016/j.idc.2022.11.007
0891-5520/23/© 2022 Published by Elsevier Inc.

id.theclinics.com

Several biologic and structural factors not only work in synergy to make older adults more vulnerable to infection than their younger counterparts but also result in poorer outcomes when they do become infected. Many older adults are exposed to communal conditions, such as long-term care living facilities, making them more susceptible to the spread of infection. Age-associated changes in skin and mucosal barriers further result in conditions that make pathogen evasion more difficult.[11,12] Immunosenescence and "inflammaging" together make it more challenging for older adults to neutralize antigens and result in a heightened inflammatory response to infections.[13–15] To make matters worse, immunosenescence results in suboptimal vaccine responses in older adults, the singular best infection prevention tool we have.[16] Even diagnosis of infections can be a challenge in older adults. It is well documented that older adults may lack common presenting signs and symptoms of infection, such as fever, resulting in diagnostic delays. All these dynamics work together to create the perfect storm that leads to poor outcomes in infected older adults. In addition, due to issues related to polypharmacy, comorbid conditions, and structural barriers, age also has a profound impact on the management of infections.

In this issue of Infections in Older Adults, *Infectious Diseases Clinics of North America*, which serves as both an update and an extension to the 2017 issue, our goal is to give the readers a sense of the importance, scope, and complexities of infections in this population. Given the disproportionate impact of COVID-19 on older adults, we dedicate two articles exploring this important topic. We revisit some important perennial infections, such as *Clostridium difficile*, resistant gram-negative bacterial and nosocomial infections, and provide an update in these fields. Articles on bacterial prostatitis and outpatient parenteral antibiotic therapy highlight diagnostic and management dilemmas that are unique to older adults in the ambulatory setting. As we use more immunosuppressive therapies in older adults, opportunistic infections have become required reading for all infectious disease specialists. We hope the review on infectious complications of immunosuppressive therapy in older adults will serve as a relevant primer. A review on antibiotic stewardship at the end of life addresses the other end of the spectrum of infection management. Articles on vaccine-preventable infections and infection control in long-term care facilities serve as tools to prevent infections in this population. We also examine a crucial chronic viral infection, HIV, and its interaction with aging. And lastly, we present a review on an increasingly relevant subject in older adults, sexually transmitted infections.

We feel privileged to have worked with colleagues with such a breadth of expertise in infectious diseases and are truly grateful for their time and valuable contributions. Finally, we would like to thank the consulting editor for giving us the opportunity to curate this issue, and we thank the staff at *Infectious Disease Clinics of North America* for their patience as the COVID-19 pandemic continues to place extraordinary demands on our field.

Puja Van Epps, MD
10701 East Boulevard
Cleveland, OH 44106, USA

David H. Canaday, MD
10900 Euclid Avenue, BRB 1025
Cleveland, OH 44106-4984, USA

E-mail addresses:
PUJA.VANEPPS@VA.GOV (P. Van Epps)
dxc44@case.edu (D.H. Canaday)

REFERENCES

1. Pew Research Center. Demographic Projections. Available at: https://www.pewresearch.org/our-methods/demographic-projections/. Accessed November 15, 2022.
2. Centers for Medicare and Medicaid Services. National Health Expenditure Data. Available at: https://www.cms.gov/Research-Statistics-Data-and-Systems/Statistics-Trends-and-Reports/NationalHealthExpendData/NHE-Fact-Sheet. Accessed November 15, 2022.
3. Nelson RE, Hyun D, Jezek A, et al. Mortality, length of stay, and healthcare costs associated with multidrug-resistant bacterial infections among elderly hospitalized patients in the United States. Clin Infect Dis 2022;74(6):1070–80. https://doi.org/10.1093/cid/ciab696.
4. Centers for Disease Control and Prevention. Leading causes of death and injury. Available at: https://wisqars.cdc.gov/data/lcd/home. Accessed November 15, 2022.
5. Butler L, Walker KA. The role of chronic infection in Alzheimer's disease: instigators, co-conspirators, or bystanders? Curr Clin Microbiol Rep 2021;8(4):199–212. https://doi.org/10.1007/s40588-021-00168-6.
6. Sethi S. Infection as a comorbidity of COPD. Eur Respir J 2010;35(6):1209–15. https://doi.org/10.1183/09031936.00081409.
7. Casqueiro J, Casqueiro J, Alves C. Infections in patients with diabetes mellitus: a review of pathogenesis. Indian J Endocrinol Metab 2012;16(suppl 1):S27–36. https://doi.org/10.4103/2230-8210.94253.
8. Chen LF, Chen HP, Huang YS, et al. Pneumococcal pneumonia and the risk of stroke: a population-based follow-up study. PloS One 2012;7(12):e51452. https://doi.org/10.1371/journal.pone.0051452.
9. Kulick ER, Alvord T, Canning M, et al. Risk of stroke and myocardial infarction after influenza-like illness in New York State. BMC Public Health 2021;21(1):864. https://doi.org/10.1186/s12889-021-10916-4.
10. Kanner L, Glatt AE. Patients with COVID-19 had increased risk for acute MI and ischemic stroke at 14 d vs. matched controls. Ann Intern Med 2021;174(12):JC142. https://doi.org/10.7326/ACPJ202112210-142.
11. Chambers ES, Vukmanovic-Stejic M. Skin barrier immunity and ageing. Immunology 2020;160(2):116–25. https://doi.org/10.1111/imm.13152.
12. Sovran B, Hugenholtz F, Elderman M, et al. Age-associated impairment of the mucus barrier function is associated with profound changes in microbiota and immunity. Sci Rep 2019;9(1):1437. https://doi.org/10.1038/s41598-018-35228-3.
13. Oh SJ, Lee JK, Shin OS. Aging and the immune system: the impact of immunosenescence on viral infection, immunity and vaccine immunogenicity. Immune Netw 2019;19(6):e37. https://doi.org/10.4110/in.2019.19.e37.
14. Muller L, Di Benedetto S. How immunosenescence and inflammaging may contribute to hyperinflammatory syndrome in COVID-19. Int J Molec Sci 2021;22(22). https://doi.org/10.3390/ijms222212539.
15. Fulop T, Larbi A, Dupuis G, et al. Immunosenescence and inflamm-aging as two sides of the same coin: friends or foes? Front Immunol 2017;8:1960. https://doi.org/10.3389/fimmu.2017.01960.
16. Crooke SN, Ovsyannikova IG, Poland GA, et al. Immunosenescence and human vaccine immune responses. Immun Ageing 2019;16:25. https://doi.org/10.1186/s12979-019-0164-9.

Epidemiology and Clinical Presentation of COVID-19 in Older Adults

Yasin Abul, MD[a,b,c,*], Ciera Leeder, MD, MPH[a,b],
Stefan Gravenstein, MD, MPH[a,b,c]

KEYWORDS

• COVID-19 • Older adults • Epidemiology • Clinical presentation

KEY POINTS

• The range of presentation with severe acute respiratory syndrome coronavirus 2 (SARS-CoV-2) infection, from asymptomatic infection to critical illness, changes with age. Older adults will more commonly have an atypical clinical presentation, nonspecific symptoms, and blunted fever response to SARS-CoV-2 infection.

• Most coronavirus disease 2019 (COVID-19) hospitalization and mortality occur in older adults, with severity compounded by underlying illnesses.

• Although vaccination significantly reduces the risk of severe COVID-19 and mortality in older adults, it may take 3 or more exposures for the spike protein as antigen to develop an antibody repertoire that can neutralize a broader range of variants.

INTRODUCTION
History/Background

Coronaviruses, enveloped positive-stranded RNA viruses, infect both people and animals. In December 2019, the World Health Organization (WHO) identified a new coronavirus, reported first in Wuhan, China, as a cause of pneumonia in several countries including Thailand and Japan.[1,2] The International Committee on Virus Taxonomy named the new virus "severe acute respiratory syndrome coronavirus-2" (SARS-CoV-2).[3] WHO designated the disease it caused "COVID-19" (coronavirus disease 2019).[4] On January 21, 2020, the Centers for Disease Control and Prevention (CDC) reported the first confirmed travel-related case in the United States (US), in the state of Washington.[5] On January 31, 2020, WHO issued a Global Health Emergency. This was followed by a US public emergency declaration on February 3, 2020.[2]

[a] Center of Innovation in Long Term Services and Supports, Providence VA Medical Center, Providence, RI, USA; [b] Division of Geriatric and Palliative Medicine, Warren Alpert Medical School of Brown University, Providence, RI, USA; [c] Brown University, School of Public Health Center for Gerontology, Healthcare Research
* Corresponding author. Captain John H. Harwood Research Center at the VA Providence Health Care System, 373 Niagara Street., Providence, RI 02907.
E-mail address: yasin_abul@brown.edu

Infect Dis Clin N Am 37 (2023) 1–26
https://doi.org/10.1016/j.idc.2022.11.001
0891-5520/23/Published by Elsevier Inc.

id.theclinics.com

Abbreviations	
SARS-CoV-2	Severe Acute Respiratory Syndrome Coronavirus 2
ICU	Intensive Care Unit
CDC	Centers for Disease Control and Prevention
WHO	World Health Organization
CLIA	Clinical Laboratory Improvement Amendments
PPE	Personal Protective Equipment
PASC	Post-Acute Sequelae of COVID
COPD	Chronic Obstructive Pulmonary Disease

The similarity of SARS-CoV-2 coronavirus' RNA sequence to that of coronaviruses found in bats led scientists to consider bats as the primary reservoir of SARS-like coronaviruses[6] and the original source of the 2019 SARS-CoV-2 Wuhan strain.[7] SARS-CoV-2 binds to the human cell angiotensin-converting enzyme 2 host receptor as a primary mechanism to gain entrance.[8] SARS-CoV-2 continues to evolve over time, acquiring mutations that improve efficiency in infection and evasion of immunity in people. CDC's data projection tool, Nowcast, identifies and tracks emerging variants and predicts more recent proportions of circulating variants to inform appropriate public health action plans (**Fig. 1**).[9] The Omicron variant's added capacity to evade humoral immunity gives it a replication advantage over prior variants that can improve infectiousness and fuel its spread.[10–12]

Conservatively, in the US, SARS-CoV-2 has killed more than 1 million of the more than 90 million people infected by September, 2022.[13] Older adults suffered the greatest morbidity and mortality early in the COVID-19 pandemic.[14] Although adults aged older than 65 years represent only about 16% of the US population, they account for 31% of reported cases, 45% of hospitalizations, 53% of intensive care unit (ICU) admissions, and 80% of COVID-19–associated deaths.[15] CDC reports a considerably higher incidence of COVID-19 deaths per 100,000 population in those aged older than 65 years compared with younger individuals (**Fig. 2**).[16] In the subset living in nursing homes (NHs), SARS-CoV-2 infected more than 1 million, 13% of whom subsequently died by August, 2022.[17] This article will discuss epidemiology and different clinical presentations of COVID-19 in older adults.

Definitions

Centers for Disease Control and Prevention and World Health Organization definitions of coronavirus disease 2019 stages
Acute coronavirus disease 2019. (Table 1 and below)[18,19] Symptomatic SARS-CoV-2 infection with symptoms that last up to 4 weeks following illness onset.

Long COVID or postcoronavirus disease 2019 conditions. Some individuals infected with SARS-CoV-2 have persistent or new symptoms that last 2 to 3 months beyond their initial infection.[20–22] More formally known as postacute sequelae of COVID-19 (PASC), it is also called long COVID, long-haul COVID, postacute COVID-19, long-term effects of COVID-19, and chronic COVID-19.[23]

EPIDEMIOLOGY
Risk for Severe Acute Respiratory Syndrome Coronavirus 2 Infection in Older Adults

Immunosenescence and immunity in older adults with coronavirus disease 2019
Immunosenescence refers to a multifactorial process with aging that results in immune dysfunction.[24–26] Examples of consequences of immune senescence include

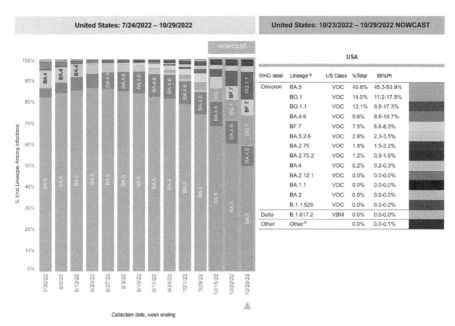

Fig. 1. Regional proportions from specimens collected week of October 29, 2022 in CDC page with a model that estimates more recent proportions of circulating variants. (From CDC Data Tracker: Monitoring Variant Proportions.) [a]Enumerated lineages are US VOC and lineages circulating above 1% nationally in at least one week period. "other" represents the aggregation of lineages which are circulating <1% nationally during all weeks displayed. [b]BA 1,BA 3 and their sublineages (except BA 1.1 and its sublineages) are aggregated with B.1.1.529. Except BA.2.12.1, BA.2.75.BA.2.75.2 and their sublineages, BA.2 sublineages are aggregated with BA.2.Except BA.4.6,sublineages of BA.4 are aggregated to BA.4. Except BF.7,BA.5.2.6,BQ.1 and BQ.1.1,sublineages of BA.5 are ggregated to BA.5.For all the lineages listed in the above table, their sublineages are aggregated to the listed parental lineages respectively. Previously, BA.5.2.6 were aggregated with BA.5. Lineages BA.2.75.2, BA.4.6,BF.5.2.6 and BQ.1.1 contain the spike substitution R346T. Available from: https://covid.cdc.gov/covid-data-tracker/?CDC_AA_refVal=https%3A%2F%2Fwww.cdc.gov%2Fcoronavirus%2F2019-ncov%2Fcases-updates%2Fvariant-proportions.html#circulatingVariants, Accessed on October 29, 2022).

alterations in inflammatory response, infection severity and recovery, and reduced vaccine response,[27] such as occurs with influenza and other causes of pneumonia.[20,28,29] Moreover, immune memory from prior infections and vaccination wanes over time, with a consequent increasing susceptibility to reinfection. For example, prior betacoronavirus infection that causes the common cold could offer some protection against SARS-CoV-2 by providing naturally acquired cross-protective immunity. Immunosenescence contributes to reduced initial vaccine response with age and also the more rapid decay in antibody levels following vaccination.[21,22,30] Poor or decreased capability to mount a cytokine response in the case of severe infection likely contributes to older adults' proneness to atypical presentations of severe COVID-19 infection, and lesser or delayed symptoms and blunted fever response.[31,32] Both cellular senescence, which leads to permanent cell growth arrest with aging, and decreased antibody response in older adults that occurs within immunosenescence, seem to play a significant role in SARS-CoV-2's impact on the host–pathogen

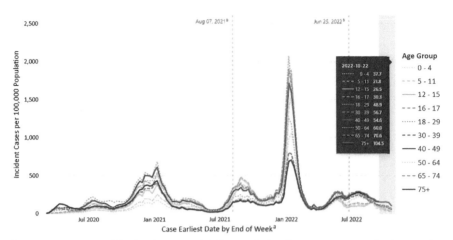

Fig. 2. COVID-19 weekly deaths per 100,000 population by age group, United States between March 01, 2020, and October 22, 2022. (*Adapted from* cdc data tracker: Monitoring variant proportions.) US: Includes data up to the week ending on October 22, 2022. Percentage of cases repoting age by date-99.91%. US territories are included in case and death counts but not in opulation counts. Potential six-week delay in case reporting to CDC denoted by gray bars. Weekly data with five or less cases have been suppressed. [a]Case Earliest Date is the earliest of the clinical date (related to illness or specimen collection and chosen by a defined hierarchy) and the Data Received by CDC. The date for the current week extends through Saturday. [b]Case rates for south dakota during the week ending Aug 07,2021,and Texas during the week ending Jun 25,2022, are reflective of a data reporting artifafct.Surveillance data are providional, and as additional clinical data becomes available,the case rates over time are subject to change. Available from: https://covid.cdc.gov/ covid-data-tracker/?CDC_AA_refVal=https%3A%2F%2Fwww.cdc.gov%2Fcoronavirus%2F 2019-ncov%2Fcases-updates%2Fvariant-proportions.html#circulatingVariants, Accessed October 22, 2022). Source: CDC COVID-19 Case line-level data, 2019 US census, HHS protect; visualization: Data analytics & visualization task force and CDC DEO situational awareness public health science team.

interaction.[32–34] Natural killer (NK) cells, participants in innate immunity, serve as first-line defenders against viral infections in the human body.[35,36] The phenotype and function of NK cells change and decay during aging by way of transformed surface molecules, which reduces their capacity to bind to virally infected cells.[35] SARS-CoV-2 also exhausts NK cell phenotypes. This may potentiate the severity of disease by allowing the virus to escape from the NK cells' first-line cellular antiviral reactivity.[37–39] Therefore, both aging and SARS-CoV-2 impair functioning of the antiviral cytotoxic NK cells in a way that can increase the severity of COVID-19 in older adults.[32]

Aging also impairs T cell receptor (TCR) diversity, an essential mechanism that facilitates the immune system's ability to detect foreign antigens. TCR diversity, driven by thymic stimulation of T cells in the first decades of life, persists with the homeostatic proliferation of naïve T cells.[40]

Progressive regression in thymic size and senescence of certain T cell clones results in a declining output of new naïve T cells and reduces TCR diversity.[41] COVID-19 patients have significantly less TCR diversity compared with healthy controls, a feature compounding the reduced diversity resulting from aging. Thus, the COVID-19 pathophysiology seen in older adults seems to relate to the impairment in TCR diversity.[42,43]

Table 1
Definitions

Term	Definition	
SARS-CoV-2	Severe acute respiratory syndrome coronavirus-2SARS-CoV-2 named by the International Committee on Virus Taxonomy is the virus that causes COVID-19[3]	
COVID-19	Coronavirus disease 2019 is an infectious disease, designated by WHO as COVID-19, which is caused by SARS-CoV-2, a coronavirus discovered in 2019[4]	
Asymptomatic infection	Infection while having no symptoms. Includes both presymptomatic individuals and individuals who will never develop symptoms	
Presymptomatic infection	Infection before inevitable development of symptoms	
Transmission[144]	Presymptomatic	An index has no symptoms during the exposure period of their closed contacts but later develops symptoms
	Asymptomatic	An index case never develops symptoms or signs of infection
	Postsymptomatic	An index case has no symptoms during the exposure period of their close contacts, but previously had symptoms
Criteria of suspected cases of SARS-CoV-2 infection[101,145] When suspicious: new onset fever and/or respiratory symptoms (eg, sore throat, cough, nasal congestion, rhinorrhea, shortness of breath). Other common nonrespiratory symptoms: new changes in taste or smell, diarrhea, chills, anorexia, headache, and muscle pain	Clinical criteria Epidemiologic criteria	Acute onset of fever and cough OR Acute onset of any 3 or more of the following signs or symptoms: fever, cough, general weakness/fatigue, headache, myalgia, sore throat, coryza, dyspnea, nausea, diarrhea, and anorexia Contact of a probable or confirmed case or linked to a COVID-19 cluster
	Illness	Severe acute respiratory illness
	Testing	No clinical signs or symptoms, nor meeting epidemiologic criteria, with a positive professional use or self-test SARS-CoV-2 antigen-RDT
Clinical criteria in the absence of a more likely diagnosis (CDC)[146] (Organ systems and associated symptoms and signs by all ages and older adults are summarized in **Fig. 3**. As discussed later in this article, older adults may present differently.)	Acute onset or worsening of at least 2 symptoms or signs OR Acute onset or worsening of at least one symptoms or sign	Fever (measured or subjective), chills, rigors, myalgia, headache, sore throat, nausea or vomiting, diarrhea, fatigue, congestion, and runny nose Cough; shortness of breath; difficulty breathing; olfactory disorder; taste

(continued on next page)

Table 1 (continued)		
Term		**Definition**
		disorder; confusion or change in mental status; persistent pain or pressure in the chest; pale, gray, or blue-colored skin, lips, or nail beds, depending on skin tone; inability to wake or stay awake
	OR Severe respiratory illness with at least	Clinical or radiographic evidence of pneumonia, or acute respiratory distress syndrome
Laboratory criteria (CDC)[146,147] Laboratory evidence using methods approved or authorized by the US Food and Drug Administration (FDA) or designated authority	Confirmatory laboratory evidence	Detection of SARS-CoV-2 ribonucleic acid (RNA) in a postmortem respiratory swab or clinical specimen using a diagnostic molecular amplification test performed by a Clinical Laboratory Improvement Amendments (CLIA)-certified provider *OR* Detection of SARS-CoV-2 by genomic sequencing
	Presumptive laboratory evidence	Detection of SARS-CoV-2–specific antigen in a postmortem obtained respiratory swab or clinical specimen using a diagnostic test performed by a CLIA-certified provider
	Supportive laboratory evidence	Detection of antibody in serum, plasma, or whole blood specific to natural infection with SARS-CoV-2 (antibody to nucleocapsid protein) *OR* Detection of SARS-CoV-2–specific antigen by immunocytochemistry in an autopsy specimen *OR* Detection of SARS-CoV-2 RNA or specific antigen using a test performed without CLIA oversight

(continued on next page)

Table 1
(continued)

Term		Definition
Epidemiologic linkage[146]	One or both of the following exposures in the prior 14 d (CDC)	Close contact[a] with a confirmed or probable case of COVID-19 disease *OR* Member of an exposed risk cohort as defined by public health authorities during an outbreak or high transmission
	Probable case (WHO)[145]	An individual who meets clinical criteria of suspected case *and* is a contact of a probable or confirmed case, *or* is linked to a COVID-19 cluster
	Confirmed case (WHO)[145]	An individual with a positive nucleic acid amplification test (NAAT), regardless of clinical criteria or epidemiologic criteria *OR* A person meeting clinical criteria and/or epidemiologic criteria with a positive professional use or self-test SARS-CoV-2 antigen-RDT
	Symptomatic case (WHO)[145]	An individual who is infected with SARS-CoV-2 and has symptoms
Case classification (CDC)[146]	Suspect	Meets supportive laboratory evidence with no prior history of being a confirmed or probable case
	Probable	Meets clinical criteria and epidemiologic linkage with no confirmatory or presumptive laboratory evidence for SARS-CoV-2 *OR* Meets presumptive laboratory evidence *OR* Meets vital records criteria with no confirmatory laboratory evidence for SARS-CoV-2
	Confirmed	Meets confirmatory laboratory evidence

(continued on next page)

Table 1 (continued)		
Term		**Definition**
Testing	Positive test	A positive test indicates likelihood of present or past SARS-CoV-2 infection whether symptomatic or recovered
	Types of tests[148–151]	Direct detection of SARS-CoV-2 RNA by NAATs or reverse-transcription polymerase chain reaction from the upper respiratory tract)
		Serologic tests detecting antibodies to the virus in the blood. Usually used to detect previous infection or response to vaccine
		Antigen tests detecting SARS-CoV-2 antigen with nasal swab or saliva sample
		Breathalyzer that uses gas chromatography-mass spectrometry to detect exhaled volatile organic compounds specific to SARS-CoV-2 infection
		Interferon-gamma release assay
Definition of COVID stages (CDC and WHO)[18,19]	Acute COVID-19	Symptoms of COVID-19, up to 4 wk following the onset of illness
	Long COVID or Post-COVID Conditions (PCC)	(See text for details) (Also called long-haul COVID, postacute COVID-19, postacute sequelae of SARS CoV-2 infection (PASC), long-term effects of COVID, chronic COVID)[23]

[a] Close contact is generally defined as being within 6 feet for a cumulative period of at least 15 min during a 24-h period. However, this depends on several exposure and setting variables (eg, in the setting of an aerosol-generating procedure in a health-care setting without proper PPE, it may be "any period of time."

Aging lymphocytes have lower capacity of proliferation in defense against viral infections, and higher proportions of B and T lymphocytes become apoptotic with aging.[44] Adults aged 65 years or older have impaired coordination of SARS-CoV-2 antigen-specific immune responses, and aging and poor COVID-19 outcomes are associated with paucity of naïve T cells.[45]

Vaccination in older adults with coronavirus disease 2019
Four manufacturers produce COVID-19 vaccines for the US. For the initial vaccination series, available vaccines include 2 mRNA vaccines, BNT162b2 (Pfizer-BioNTech, Michigan, USA) and mRNA-1273 (Moderna, Massachusetts, USA), an adjuvant

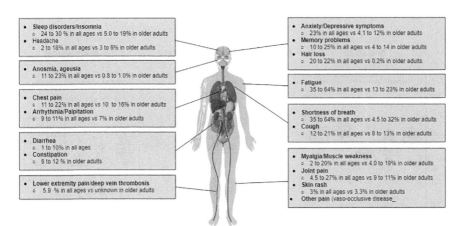

Fig. 3. Organ and systems which are affected by SARS-CoV-2 in the long term with symptoms and signs of COVID-19.[121,127,136–143] (Figure was adapted from Designed by Freepik from www.freepik.com).

recombinant protein vaccine, NVX-CoV2373 (Novavax, Maryland, USA), and an adenoviral vector vaccine, Ad26.COV2 (Janssen/Johnson & Johnson, Indiana, USA).[46–50] The mRNA vaccines also have been used to boost the initial series until September, 2022, when the booster doses were replaced by bivalent mRNA vaccines that include code for both the ancestral strain used in the original series and the then circulating Omicron BA.4 and BA.5 strains. For individuals unvaccinated against COVID-19, infection provides only fleeting or partial protection from recurrent infection and disease.[51] Older individuals vaccinated with BNT162b2 mRNA vaccine without prior SARS-CoV-2 infection (infection naïve) have significantly lower antibody levels than infection naïve younger adults. Unsurprisingly, the negative correlation between age and antibody levels after vaccination with SARS-CoV-2 vaccination also occurs with other vaccines.[22,30] This lower antibody response in older adults likely signifies less absolute and less durable protection from infection, with shorter intervals of protective titers and increased likelihood of breakthrough infection.[30] Antibody decline occurs from 2 weeks to 6 months after administration of the initial pair of BNT162b2 mRNA vaccine in NH residents. NH residents experienced a more than 81% drop of antispike, receptor-binding domain (RBD), and neutralizing antibody level regardless of prior COVID-19 infection status during these 6 months (**Fig. 4** and **Fig. 5**).[21,30] Although antibody levels may wane, booster doses seem to improve clinical protection in NH residents.[52] Future boosting strategies, particularly for older adults, need to address the relative drop in antibody levels and other measures of immunity following vaccination to their relevance for clinical protection, especially in the context of their relevance to the evolving virus.

Aging (affecting clearing of virus)
Mucociliary clearance, a first line of defense against lower respiratory tract infections, functions by sweeping mucus, particles, and microorganisms up and out of the lungs. Both aging and SARS-CoV-2 impair mucociliary clearance and affect older adults' ability to clear the virus.[53–55] This reduced clearance of microorganisms can also increase the risk of coinfection with age. In Hong Kong, the risk of hospitalization with dual infection increases with age, where less than 35% of hospitalizations with dual infection occur in the group of individuals aged younger than 65 years, and 65%

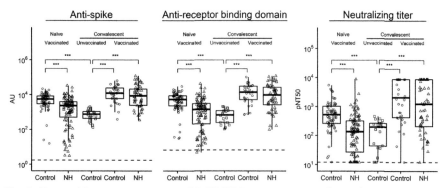

Fig. 4. Humoral immune assessment of BNT162b2 messenger RNA (mRNA) vaccine vaccination in NH residents. Postvaccination anti-spike, anti-receptor-binding domain (RBD) and serum neutralization titers are shown.Control: vaccinated younger healthcare workers or unvaccinated SARS-CoV-2-convalescent individuals. The dotted lines: median preimmunization value in the SARS-CoV-2-naive subjects. Abbreviations: AU, antibody unit; NH, nursing home; pNT50, pseudovirus neutralization titer.[30]

occurs in older adults who represent only 19% of the overall population.[56,57] SARS-CoV-2 infection introduces the possibility of dual infections and thereby worse outcomes.[58] As older adults experience worse outcomes overall with SARS-CoV-2 infection, the association of coinfection with COVID-19 severity may have an amplified risk in older adults.

Hearing and visual changes with age
Sensory changes with age can indirectly affect SARS-CoV-2 infection risk. For example, presbycusis may lead individuals to shout or lower their masks to facilitate communication for those with the most hearing impairment, increasing the risk for more efficient virus aerosolization and thereby transmission.[59–61] Potential and frequent SARS-CoV-2 transmission can also occur via ocular droplet deposition, a feature that remains considerably underestimated as a mode of transmission.[62] However, because visual impairment also occurs more commonly with advanced age, the consequent increased use of eyeglasses[63] could offer a modicum of protection against SARS-CoV-2 inoculation.[64,65]

Multiple Morbidities (Affecting Immune Competence, Clearance of Virus)
COVID-19 severity, defined as hospitalization due to COVID-19, intensive care unit admission, need for intubation/mechanical ventilation, and COVID-19–related mortality, depends in part, on underlying conditions and morbidities. Severe COVID-19 occurs more often with the following risk factors that we also see more commonly in older adults[66–70]:

- Cancer
- Cerebrovascular diseases
- Chronic kidney disease
- Chronic lung diseases (including COPD, interstitial lung diseases, bronchiectasis, pulmonary embolism, and pulmonary hypertension)
- Chronic liver diseases (including cirrhosis, alcoholic hepatitis, alcoholic liver disease, and nonalcoholic fatty liver disease)

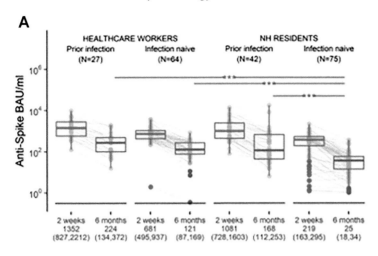

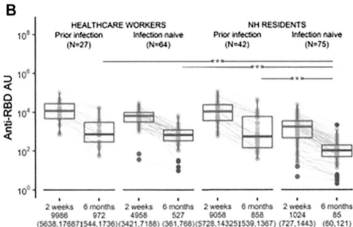

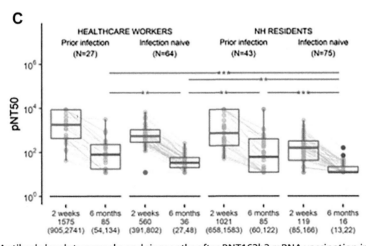

Fig. 5. Antibody levels two weeks and six months after BNT162b2 mRNA vaccination in healthcare workers (HCWs) and NH residents with and without SARS-CoV-2 infection prior to vaccination. Abbreviations: AU, arbitrary unit; BAU, binding arbitrary unit; NH, nursing home; pNT50, pseudovirus neutralization; RBD, receptor-binding domain.[21] (Designed by Freepik).

- Type-2 diabetes mellitus
- Disabilities
- Congestive heart failure, coronary artery disease, and other cardiomyopathies
- Dementia
- Obesity (body mass index [BMI] $\geq$30 kg/m^2)
- Physical inactivity
- Smoking history
- Use of immunosuppressive medications including steroids

Underlying morbidities in older adults have added significance, given the synergies of aging and morbidities on COVID-19 severity. The February 28 and March 18, 2020, long-term care facility SARS-CoV-2 outbreaks in Washington State offer an example of this. The hospitalization rate of 55% and fatality rate of 34% occurred in a group with a median age of 83 years (n = 101) and with 94% having an underlying chronic condition.[71] State and territorial jurisdiction cases reported through July 21, 2022, show a 330-times higher rate of death in individuals aged older than 85 years, compared with individuals aged 18 to 29 years.[68] Even vaccination does not entirely overcome the more severe age-associated outcomes in late life. Risk for a severe COVID-19 outcome after primary vaccination was higher in individuals aged older than 65 years and in individuals with at least one underlying condition.[72]

Exposure and Transmissibility

Older adults in long-term care settings endure common and uncommon respiratory disease outbreaks.[73–75] SARS-CoV-2 spreads by direct contact and respiratory droplets or secretions. Transmission occurs through fomites from contaminated hands or by contact with contaminated surfaces before self-inoculation, such as through touching the eyes, nose, or mouth.[76] Frequent and close contact between health-care staff and nursing residents with functional impairments increase the risk of COVID-19 transmission.[77–79] Some patients with cognitive impairment cannot maintain social distance or use personal protective devices, affecting their risk for getting infected or infecting others once infected, thus increasing the transmission risk in the long-term care setting. Cognitive impairment and delirium can complicate proper use of personal protective equipment (PPE), and thereby could result in higher rates of transmission.[80] The long-term care workforce has many challenges that can leave it unprepared to manage infectious outbreaks, from adequate PPE resources to high turnover that affects the ability to keep staff trained, increased use of per diem staff, and the risk of unexpected vectors of infection.[81–87] Frail older adults with functional impairment, particularly those in long-term care settings, are at significantly higher risk of SARS-CoV-2 infection, such as when they receive close, hands-on care from asymptomatic health-care workers who could unwittingly inoculate them.[77,88]

Data from 44,672 confirmed cases of COVID-19 during the first COVID-19 transmission surge in China showed that an initial overall case-fatality rate of 2.3% increased to 8.0% among older adults aged 70 to 79 years, and 14.8% for those aged 80 years and older.[89] Older individuals not only experience higher fatality rates but also seem more likely to spread infection.[90] The higher old-age dependency ratio (the number of individuals aged older than 64 years relative to the number of working-age individuals [15–64 year old]), suggests a higher level of transmission among the older population. This conceivably could influence both the severity and longevity of COVID-19 symptoms in older adults. Those with sustained increased risk of close contact transmission (higher inoculum) may have asymmetrically greater risk for infection and more severe outcomes. This risk could occur especially in situations where individuals live in close quarters or share bedrooms, bathrooms, and dining areas.[91]

Reinfection and Breakthrough Infection in Older Adults

Reinfection with SARS-CoV-2 that causes COVID-19 occurs when a SARS-CoV-2–infected individual recovers, and later becomes reinfected.[92] Breakthrough infection, or vaccine breakthrough infection, occurs after an individual is vaccinated against SARS-CoV-2 and nevertheless becomes infected and symptomatic with SARS-CoV-2.[93] Before the Omicron variant wave of infections, risk for reinfection was less. Apparently, the level of added protection reduced the risk of reinfection for pre-Omicron variants by around 80%, lasting 6 to 9 months.[94,95] However, the reduced reinfection risk did not pertain to infection with Omicron, a feature attributed to Omicron's immune evasion characteristics.[10–12]

Clinical Characteristics of Coronavirus Disease 2019 in Older Adults

Multimorbidity, frailty, and immunosenescence combine to increase the vulnerability to COVID-19 with advanced age.[96] SARS-CoV-2 infection often remains asymptomatic, a likelihood that changes with underlying immunity from infection, such as acquired from infection with its betacoronavirus cousins and vaccination.[97–100]

When SARS-CoV-2 infection produces symptoms, that is, COVID-19, they may include any combination of fever, cough, fatigue, shortness of breath, myalgia, anorexia, sore throat, headache, chills, and loss of taste and smell sensation[101] (**Fig. 5**). During the early surge of COVID-19, shortness of breath occurred more frequently among adults aged older than 60 years (12%), compared with younger adults (3%).[102] A research collaboration of 86 emergency departments (EDs) in 27 US states used the RECOVER Network registry for a multicenter cohort study. Older adults in this study had more atypical presentations: neurologic symptoms, especially confusion and altered mental status, and more malaise and dyspnea compared with younger individuals.[96] Additionally, clinicians may miss shortness of breath in older adults when it presents as functional decline with impaired mobility or frequent falls, rather than a more obvious respiratory symptom that occurs with SARS-CoV-2 infection.[103]

Changes with advanced age can blunt fever response, dyspnea, and cough with COVID-19.[96,104] A study of Veterans living in 134 community living centers (CLCs) operated by the Veterans Administration evaluated temperatures through the course of SARS-CoV-2 infection. One-fourth of them did not have meaningful temperature elevations over baseline. Moreover, the temperature for 75% of these NH residents with SARS-CoV-2 infection never exceeded 38°C at any time during the 2 weeks before and after their maximum temperature (**Fig. 6**).[104] Thus, in older adults, particularly those in NH settings where SARS-CoV-2 may be circulating, using a lower temperature threshold to 37.2°C will alert staff to consider early testing and will improve sensitivity for screening by temperature for SARS-CoV-2 infection.[105] A second elevated reading improves specificity for infection. CDC suggests that isolation and further evaluation for COVID-19 should be triggered by more than 2 temperatures greater than 37.2°C, especially with the presence of atypical symptoms of worsening malaise, new dizziness, or diarrhea[106] but temperature elevation alone should be enough to trigger isolation and further evaluation for COVID-19 if there is an index of suspicion from known contact.

As noted above, older adults can remain asymptomatic with SARS-CoV-2 infection or develop symptoms more slowly. At a long-term care skilled facility in King County, Washington, 56% of residents with SARS-CoV-2 infection had no symptoms at the

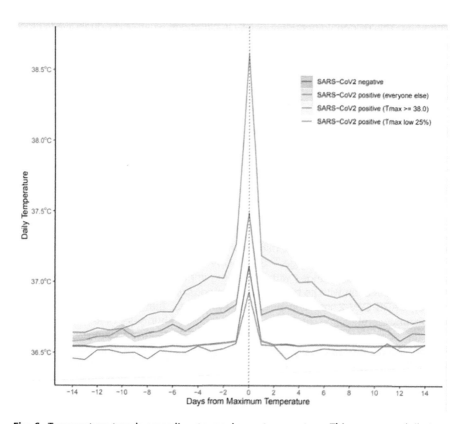

Fig. 6. Temperature trends according to maximum temperature. This compares daily temperatures relative to the maximum temperature. The shaded area denotes the 95% confidence intervals, and T0 refers the testing date for SARS-CoV-2. (*Adapted from* Rudolph, J.L., et al., Temperature in Nursing Home Residents Systematically Tested for SARS-CoV-2. J Am Med Dir Assoc, 2020. 21(7): p. 895–899.e1; with permission).

time of testing, whereas 77% were presymptomatic at time of testing. Screening by fever and symptom-based criteria would have missed half of these cases.[107]

Coronavirus disease 2019 complications

COVID-19 can lead to many complications. In a retrospective cohort study, individuals aged 65 years and older who were continuously enrolled in a Medicare Advantage plan with prescription drug coverage from January, 2019, to the date of SARS-CoV-2 diagnosis had higher the risk of complications that include respiratory failure, fatigue, hypertension, memory problems, kidney injury, mental health problems, hypercoagulopathy, and cardiac rhythm problems, compared with matched comparison groups without COVID-19.[108] A nationwide study from Sweden reported higher incidence of deep vein thrombosis and pulmonary embolism in older adults with highest rate of pulmonary embolism in the age group 50 to 70 years. The increase in incidence rate ratio with age specific to deep vein thrombosis during 1 to 90 days after SARS-CoV-2 infection was greatest for the first compared with the second and third pandemic waves in Sweden.[109]

Severity of coronavirus disease 2019

National Institute of Health (NIH) guidelines define individuals with severe COVID-19 as having ".SpO2 <94% on room air at sea level, a ratio of arterial partial pressure of oxygen to fraction of inspired oxygen (Pao_2/Fio_2) <300 mm Hg, a respiratory rate >30 breaths/min, or lung infiltrates >50%." NIH defines individuals with critical COVID-19 as having ".respiratory failure, septic shock, and/or multiple organ dysfunction." Underlying morbidity modulates the risk for severe COVID-19 in older adults such as cardiopulmonary disease, diabetes, cancer, obesity, or chronic kidney disease.[67] Although COVID-19 vaccination reduces the risk of severe illness, vaccine immunogenicity and efficacy to BNT162b2 mRNA declines with advanced age leaving some people vulnerable to a breakthrough infection that can result in severe illness.[21,110]

Coronavirus disease 2019 in older adults: risk stratification, risk factors, and prevention

Initial Chinese, United Kingdom (UK), and US COVID-19 cohorts show that among all the risk factors, age dominates as the most important determinant of severity.[15,89,111] Individuals aged 70 to 79 years and older than 80 years had hospitalization and case fatality rates at least 4-fold that among the entire Chinese cohort.[89] Among adults aged older than 80 years in a UK cohort, the risk of mortality was 20-fold that among adults aged 50 to 59 years.[111] In the US cohort, individuals aged older than 65 years accounted for 80% of total deaths.[15] In older adults, comorbidity burden also contributes to the risk for severe COVID-19. Individuals with both advanced age and a high comorbidity burden commonly experience severe COVID-19. Individuals with one reported underlying condition have a 6-fold higher hospitalization rate and 12-fold higher mortality rate than those with no underlying conditions (45.4% vs 7.6% and 19.5% vs 1.6%, respectively).[112]

Primary prevention offers the best approach to counter introduction and spread of COVID-19 and has proven especially effective in the long-term care setting. In NHs, implementation of basic and fundamental prevention methods begins with setting policy, education, and adherence to and monitoring of best practices. Best practices address vaccination, surveillance, and other policies. Staff should seek to maximize and track resident and staff vaccination rates while keeping vaccines up-to-date. Routine symptom screening can directly trigger testing for SARS-CoV-2 or other infections. When a test result identifies a SARS-CoV-2 infection, it should trigger contact tracing if not broader testing of other residents on the ward or in the facility. Staff also should model and promote appropriate use of masks and restrict visitors according to prevailing CDC or local health department guidelines. As a sole strategy to determine who to isolate or mask, symptom-screening alone will fail to prevent the transmission of SARS-CoV-2 in NHs because symptom screening alone will fail to detect 40% or more of SARS-CoV-2 infections.[113,114] These findings remind us that more than 50% of NH residents infected with SARS-CoV-2 were asymptomatic or presymptomatic at time of testing. Moreover, given that some have nondiagnostic tests followed by a diagnostic test day,[115] which means neither symptoms nor testing fully discriminate those infected with SARS-CoV-2 infection from those who are not at a given moment. Considered together, these point to a very important contributory factor of the transmission of SARS-CoV-2 in this population, that is, the failure to recognize the limitations to our approach to surveillance, and consequent premature relaxation of policies that limit transmission.

Successful masking strategies in NH residents and health-care professionals can critically limit the opportunity for SARS-CoV-2 transmission. N-95 respirators offer better protection for care activities with NH residents than surgical masks. However, masking, along with distancing and hand washing, reducing time in shared air spaces (reduced ventilation), high efficiency air filtration, and other strategies collectively can reduce the likelihood of transmission.[114] However, NH residents can be infected with low inoculum viral load and may stay asymptomatic despite of all those precautions.[91]

Atypical clinical presentation of coronavirus disease 2019 in older adults

Older adults with COVID-19 present to the ED with more atypical symptoms. Health-care providers should consider COVID-19 in differential diagnosis in the ED and/or NH settings when faced with older adults with nonspecific symptoms such as falls, confusion, delirium, and worsening of functional impairment, especially when SARS-CoV-2 is known to be circulating in the community.[96,103,116] Gastrointestinal symptoms are less commonly reported in older adults compared with younger adults, and older adults more commonly present to the ED with neurologic symptoms including altered mental status and confusion. Older adults presenting to the ED more often have abnormal laboratory findings, including elevated troponin and leukocyte levels, compared with younger individuals presenting to the ED.[96] Radiological differences are also noted between younger and older individuals with COVID-19; older adults with COVID-19 also more often have extensive lung involvement, and subpleural line and pleural thickening,[117] with one study showing that in older adults with COVID-19, pleural effusion can be used as a distinctive prognostic marker.[118] In NHs and other settings with older adults, awareness of these atypical findings and clinical presentations can help identify additional indications for early screening and other preventive measurements to support infection control efforts and improve patient outcomes.[116]

Long COVID or postacute sequelae of coronavirus disease 2019 older adults

The risk for Long COVID, formally called PASC, in older adults differs depending on the data sources. Reportedly, 1 in 4 older adults experience at least one potential PASC condition compared with 1 in 5 younger adults.[119] However, new data from the US Household Pulse Survey performed by the National Center for Health Statistics indicate older adults less often reported PASC conditions than younger adults, with approximately 3 times as many adults aged 50 to 59 years having Long COVID relative to individuals aged older than 80 years.[120] In data on Veterans living in CLCs where daily symptom surveillance and trigger and sweep testing protocols are in place to optimally detect COVID, data suggests that around 1 in 5 of these older Veterans has one or more new PASC symptoms more than 2 months from their initial diagnosis.[121] This rate exceeds that of the observational study and underlines the limitations in surveying older adults for PASC, where a variety of reasons can lead to their nonparticipation and undercounting, from issues that relate to privacy, illness, ability to respond through technology or telephone.[120] As such, the relative risk for PASC with age remains uncertain. A recent study suggests that nearly 55% of patients have at least 1 post-COVID sequelae 2 years after SARS-CoV-2 infection.[122] Another study suggests that risk for this outcome increases with each additional infection. Those with Long COVID symptoms at 2 years scored lower on quality-of-life metrics had worse exercise capacity, more mental health abnormalities, and increased health-care use after discharge, compared with survivors without Long COVID symptoms.[122–125]

A universally acceptable definition will need to wait until we know more about the symptoms, cause, and risk factors of PASC.[126] Some of the physical and mental symptoms of PASC include fatigue, muscle weakness, shortness of breath, chest pain, cough, anxiety, depression, posttraumatic stress disorder, poor memory, sleep disturbances, and concentration deficiency.[127,128] Depression, insomnia, dyspnea, myalgias, anxiety, cognitive impairment, and fatigue are the most common PASC symptoms, in descending order among older Veterans living in CLCs.[121] Risk factors for developing PASC include increased age, number of acute phase symptoms (>5), BMI, and female sex.[129] Notably, severity of illness in the initial infection has not correlated with the risk of developing PASC, although initial reports of PASC after hospitalization seem to indicate greater susceptibility to outcomes of PASC for hospitalized patients. Evidence linking the development of PASC to elevated inflammatory markers such as red cell distribution width, erythrocyte sedimentation rate, and C-reactive protein remains inconclusive.[130]

PASC in older adults compared with those aged younger than 65 years, as extracted from the CERNER electronic health record database, more often includes renal failure, thromboembolic events, cerebrovascular disease, type 2 diabetes, muscle disorders, neurologic conditions, and mental health conditions (including mood disorders, anxiety, other mental conditions, and substance-related disorders).[119] Persistent impaired cognitive functions in older adults have been reported for up to 1 year after acute COVID-19.[131]

FUTURE DIRECTIONS

- COVID-19 vaccine frequency and acceptance to optimize immunologic response and clinical effectiveness need further studies that emphasize outcomes in older adults.
- The refinement of definitions for PASC, its epidemiology, impact, and approaches to management will evolve as new data become available.
- We need to better understand what drives the severity of SARS-CoV-2 infection in older adults, especially because it relates to frailty, immune senescence, and inflammation.

CLINICS CARE POINTS

- Older adults with COVID-19 have higher hospitalization and case fatality rates than younger adults.[132]

- SARS-CoV-2 infection remains asymptomatic from 33% to 90% of older adults, depending on underlying immune status from prior infection, vaccination, and circulating strain.[133]

- The high frequency of asymptomatic SARS-CoV-2 infection makes symptom-based testing ineffective as a sole means for early outbreak detection of SARS-CoV-2 in NH populations.[113]

- Fever response is blunted in older adults with COVID-19; setting a lower threshold for triggering SARS-CoV-2 testing in older adults in NH settings improves sensitivity and can alert staff to consider the need to test for SARS-CoV-2 days earlier.[104,105]

- Older adults with underlying morbidities disproportionately suffer the most severe COVID-19 outcomes.[134,135]

- Health-care providers should consider adding COVID-19 to the differential diagnosis of clinical presentations such as falls, confusion, delirium, and worsening of functional impairment. This should drive SARS-CoV-2 testing, treatment, and measures to reduce spread (eg, distancing, masking, isolation).[116]

- Older adults more often experience any of a broad range of sequelae of respiratory failure, fatigue, hypertension, memory problems, kidney injury, mental health problems, hypercoagulopathy, cardiac dysrhythmias, deep vein thrombosis, pulmonary embolism, and bleeding after COVID-19.[108,109]

- In older adults, vaccination reduces SARS-CoV-2 incident infection and subsequent severity,[134,135] effects bolstered by booster vaccines.[52]

- N-95 respirators provide superior protection to other masks and can protect users from getting infection when caring for or visiting those infected with SARS-CoV-2.[114] In conjunction with social distancing, minimizing time in rooms with infected individuals, frequent hand washing, and proper use of other PPE, individuals can avoid becoming infected. Absent N-95 respirator availability, other masks still can offer some protection. The use of masks should follow the greater standard of personal preference of health department guidelines.

DISCLOSURE

Y. Abul: Received support from the Veterans Affairs Office of Academic Affiliations during the preparation of this article. C. Leeder: None to declare. S. Gravenstein (SG): SG reports potential conflicts with vaccine manufacturers Sanofi, Seqirus, Pfizer, related to grants, consulting, and speaking engagements. S G also consults with other pharmaceutical companies such as Langevoron, Genentec, Janssen, Novavax, Moderna, and Merck and has grants with Sunovion, and Essity.

ACKNOWLEDGMENT

The authors thank Margo Katz for providing editorial assistance for this article.

REFERENCES

1. AJMC. What we're reading: roots of chinese illness discovered. Available at: https://www.ajmc.com/view/what-were-reading-roots-of-chinese-illness-discovered-birth-costs-soar-public-health-emergency-in-puerto-rico. Accessed on July 20, 2022.
2. AJMC. A timeline of COVID-19 developments in 2020. Available at: https://www.ajmc.com/view/a-timeline-of-covid19-developments-in-2020. Accessed on July 20, 2022.
3. The species Severe acute respiratory syndrome-related coronavirus: classifying 2019-nCoV and naming it SARS-CoV-2. Nat Microbiol 2020;5(4):536–44.
4. WHO Director-General's remarks at the media briefing on 2019-nCoV on 11 February 2020. Available at: https://www.who.int/director-general/speeches/detail/who-director-general-s-remarks-at-the-media-briefing-on-2019-ncov-on-11-february-2020. Accessed on July 20, 2022.
5. CDC. First travel-related case of 2019 novel coronavirus detected in United States. Available at: https://www.cdc.gov/media/releases/2020/p0121-novel-coronavirus-travel-case.html. Accessed on July 20, 2022.
6. Li W, Shi Z, Yu M, et al. Bats are natural reservoirs of SARS-like coronaviruses. Science 2005;310(5748):676–9.
7. Shang J, Ye G, Shi K, et al. Structural basis of receptor recognition by SARS-CoV-2. Nature 2020;581(7807):221–4.
8. Zhou P, Yang L, Wang XG, et al. A pneumonia outbreak associated with a new coronavirus of probable bat origin. Nature 2020;579(7798):270–3.
9. CDC Data Tracker. Monitoring Variant Proportions. Available at: https://covid.cdc.gov/covid-data-tracker/?CDC_AA_refVal=https%3A%2F%2Fwww.cdc.gov%2Fcoronavirus%2F2019-ncov%2Fcases-updates%2Fvariant-proportions.html#circulatingVariants. Accessed on October 29, 2022.
10. CDC. New SARS-CoV-2 Variant of Concern Identified: Omicron (B.1.1.529) Variant. Available at: https://emergency.cdc.gov/han/2021/han00459.asp. Accessed on July 24, 2022.

11. Tegally H, Moir M, Everatt M, et al. Emergence of SARS-CoV-2 Omicron lineages BA.4 and BA.5 in South Africa. Nat Med 2022;28(9):1785–90.
12. Pulliam JRC, et al. Increased risk of SARS-CoV-2 reinfection associated with emergence of Omicron in South Africa. Science 2022;376(6593):eabn4947.
13. CDC: COVID Data Tracker. Available at: https://covid.cdc.gov/covid-data-tracker/#datatracker-home. Accessed on July 20, 2022.
14. Wang D, Hu C, Zhu X, et al. Clinical Characteristics of 138 Hospitalized Patients With 2019 Novel Coronavirus-Infected Pneumonia in Wuhan, China. Jama 2020; 323(11):1061–9.
15. Severe Outcomes Among Patients with Coronavirus Disease 2019 (COVID-19) - United States, February 12-March 16, 2020. MMWR Morb Mortal Wkly Rep 2020;69(12):343–6.
16. CDC Data Tracker. COVID-19 weekly cases and deaths per 100,000 population by age, race/ethnicity, and sex. Available at: https://covid.cdc.gov/covid-data-tracker/#demographicsovertime. Acessed October 22, 2022.
17. Centers for Medicare&Medicaid Services. COVID-19 Nursing Home Data. Available at: https://data.cms.gov/covid-19/covid-19-nursing-home-data. Accessed July 7, 2022.
18. Soriano JB, Murthy S, Marshall JC, et al. A clinical case definition of post-COVID-19 condition by a Delphi consensus. Lancet Infect Dis 2022;22(4): e102–7.
19. CDC. Post-COVID conditions: information for healthcare providers. Available at: https://www.cdc.gov/coronavirus/2019-ncov/hcp/clinical-care/post-covid-conditions.html. Accessed on July 28, 2022.
20. CDC. Leading Causes of Death and Injury. Available at: https://www.cdc.gov/injury/wisqars/LeadingCauses.html. Accessed on July 29, 2022.
21. Canaday DH, Oyebanji OA, Keresztesy D, et al. Significant reduction in vaccine-induced antibody levels and neutralization activity among healthcare workers and nursing home residents 6 months following coronavirus disease 2019 BNT162b2 mRNA vaccination. Clin Infect Dis 2021;75(1):e884–7.
22. Bates TA, Leier HC, Lyski ZL, et al. Age-Dependent Neutralization of SARS-CoV-2 and P.1 Variant by Vaccine Immune Serum Samples. Jama 2021;326(9): 868–9.
23. CDC. Long COVID or Post-COVID Conditions. Available at: https://www.cdc.gov/coronavirus/2019-ncov/long-term-effects/index.html. Accessed on July 28, 2022.
24. Walford RL. The immunologic theory of aging. Gerontologist 1964;4:195–7.
25. Effros RB. Roy Walford and the immunologic theory of aging. Immun Ageing 2005;2(1):7.
26. Azar A, Ballas ZK. Immune function in older adults. In: UpToDate, Marsh R (Ed), UpToDate, Waltham, MA, Accessed on July 29, 2022.
27. Gustafson CE, Kim C, Weyand CM, et al. Influence of immune aging on vaccine responses. J Allergy Clin Immunol 2020;145(5):1309–21.
28. Gravenstein S, Davidson HE, Taljaard M, et al. Comparative effectiveness of high-dose versus standard-dose influenza vaccination on numbers of US nursing home residents admitted to hospital: a cluster-randomised trial. Lancet Respir Med 2017;5(9):738–46.
29. Keilich SR, Bartley JM, Haynes L. Diminished immune responses with aging predispose older adults to common and uncommon influenza complications. Cell Immunol 2019;345:103992.

30. Canaday DH, Carias L, Oyebanji OA, et al. Reduced BNT162b2 messenger RNA vaccine response in severe acute respiratory syndrome coronavirus 2 (SARS-CoV-2)-naive nursing home residents. Clin Infect Dis 2021;73(11): 2112–5.
31. Norman DC. Fever in the elderly. Clin Infect Dis 2000;31(1):148–51.
32. Witkowski JM, Fulop T, Bryl E. Immunosenescence and COVID-19. Mech Ageing Dev 2022;204:111672.
33. Gatza C HG, Moore L, Dumble M, et al. p53 and Cellular Senescence. In: Masoro E AS, editor. Handbook of the biology of aging. Burlington (MA): Academic Press is an imprint of Elsevier; 2006. p. 151–4.
34. Salminen A. Increased immunosuppression impairs tissue homeostasis with aging and age-related diseases. J Mol Med (Berl) 2021;99(1):1–20.
35. Hazeldine J, Lord JM. The impact of ageing on natural killer cell function and potential consequences for health in older adults. Ageing Res Rev 2013; 12(4):1069–78.
36. Lodoen MB, Lanier LL. Natural killer cells as an initial defense against pathogens. Curr Opin Immunol 2006;18(4):391–8.
37. Yoo JS, Sasaki M, Cho SX, et al. SARS-CoV-2 inhibits induction of the MHC class I pathway by targeting the STAT1-IRF1-NLRC5 axis. Nat Commun 2021;12(1): 6602.
38. Cunningham L, Kimber I, Basketter D, et al. Perforin, COVID-19 and a possible pathogenic auto-inflammatory feedback loop. Scand J Immunol 2021;94(5): e13102.
39. Zheng M, Gao Y, Wang G, et al. Functional exhaustion of antiviral lymphocytes in COVID-19 patients. Cell Mol Immunol 2020;17(5):533–5.
40. Qi Q, Liu Y, Cheng Y, et al. Diversity and clonal selection in the human T-cell repertoire. Proc Natl Acad Sci U S A 2014;111(36):13139–44.
41. Naylor K, Li G, Vallejo AN, et al. The influence of age on T cell generation and TCR diversity. J Immunol 2005;174(11):7446–52.
42. Wang W, Thomas R, Oh J, et al. Thymic Aging May Be Associated with COVID-19 Pathophysiology in the Elderly. Cells 2021;10(3).
43. Hou X, Wang G, Fan W, et al. T-cell receptor repertoires as potential diagnostic markers for patients with COVID-19. Int J Infect Dis 2021;113:308–17.
44. Bryl E, Witkowski JM. Decreased proliferative capability of CD4(+) cells of elderly people is associated with faster loss of activation-related antigens and accumulation of regulatory T cells. Exp Gerontol 2004;39(4):587–95.
45. Rydyznski Moderbacher C, Ramirez SI, Dan JM, et al. Antigen-specific adaptive immunity to SARS-CoV-2 in acute covid-19 and associations with age and disease severity. Cell 2020;183(4):996–1012.e19.
46. Hahn WO, Wiley Z. COVID-19 Vaccines. Infect Dis Clin North Am 2022;36(2): 481–94.
47. US Food and Drug Administration. Pfizer-BioNTech Fact Sheets (English) and FAQs. Available at: https://www.fda.gov/emergency-preparedness-and-response/coronavirus-disease-2019-covid-19/comirnaty-and-pfizer-biontech-covid-19-vaccine#additional. Accessed on August 03, 2022.
48. US Food and Drug Administration. Spikevax and Moderna COVID-19 Vaccine. Available at: https://www.fda.gov/emergency-preparedness-and-response/coronavirus-disease-2019-covid-19/spikevax-and-moderna-covid-19-vaccine. Accessed on August 03, 2022.

49. Emergency Use Authorization (EUA) of the Novavax COVID-19 vaccine, adjuvanted to prevent coronavirus disease 2019 (COVID-19). Available at: https://www.fda.gov/media/159897/download. Accessed on August 03, 2022.
50. US Food and Drug Administration. Emergency use authorization (EUA) of the Janssen COVID-19 vaccine to prevent coronavirus disease 2019 (COVID-19). Available at: https://www.fda.gov/media/146304/download. Accessed on August 03, 2022.
51. Cavanaugh AM, Spicer KB, Thoroughman D, et al. Reduced Risk of Reinfection with SARS-CoV-2 After COVID-19 Vaccination - Kentucky, May-June 2021. MMWR Morb Mortal Wkly Rep 2021;70(32):1081–3.
52. McConeghy KW, White EM, Blackman C, et al. Effectiveness of a Second COVID-19 Vaccine Booster Dose Against Infection, Hospitalization, or Death Among Nursing Home Residents - 19 States, March 29-July 25, 2022. MMWR Morb Mortal Wkly Rep 2022;71(39):1235–8.
53. Roth Y, Aharonson EF, Teichtahl H, et al. Human in vitro nasal and tracheal ciliary beat frequencies: comparison of sampling sites, combined effect of medication, and demographic relationships. Ann Otol Rhinol Laryngol 1991;100(5 Pt 1):378–84.
54. Bailey KL, Kharbanda KK, Katafiasz DM, et al. Oxidative stress associated with aging activates protein kinase Cε, leading to cilia slowing. Am J Physiol Lung Cell Mol Physiol 2018;315(5):L882–90.
55. Robinot R, Hubert M, de Melo GD, et al. SARS-CoV-2 infection induces the dedifferentiation of multiciliated cells and impairs mucociliary clearance. Nat Commun 2021;12(1):4354.
56. Liu Y, Ling L, Wong SH, et al. Outcomes of respiratory viral-bacterial co-infection in adult hospitalized patients. EClinicalMedicine 2021;37:100955.
57. Hong Kong: Age distribution from 2011 to 2021. Available at: https://www.statista.com/. Accessed on September 13, 2022.
58. Feldman C, Anderson R. The role of co-infections and secondary infections in patients with COVID-19. Pneumonia (Nathan) 2021;13(1):5.
59. Mürbe D, Kriegel M, Lange J, et al. Aerosol emission of adolescents voices during speaking, singing and shouting. PLoS One 2021;16(2):e0246819.
60. Asadi S, Wexler AS, Cappa CD, et al. Aerosol emission and superemission during human speech increase with voice loudness. Sci Rep 2019;9(1):2348.
61. Barreda S, Asadi Sima, Cappa Christopher D, et al. The impact of vocalization loudness on COVID-19 transmission in indoor spaces. arXiv 2009;04060:2020, preprint arXiv.
62. Coroneo MT, Collignon PJ. SARS-CoV-2: eye protection might be the missing key. Lancet Microbe 2021;2(5):e173–4.
63. Carter TL. Age-related vision changes: a primary care guide. Geriatrics 1994;49(9):37–42, 45; quiz 46-7.
64. Zeng W, Wang X, Li J, et al. Association of Daily Wear of Eyeglasses With Susceptibility to Coronavirus Disease 2019 Infection. JAMA Ophthalmol 2020;138(11):1196–9.
65. Lehrer S, Rheinstein P. Eyeglasses Reduce Risk of COVID-19 Infection. Vivo 2021;35(3):1581–2.
66. Centers for Disease Control and Prevention. Underlying medical conditions associated with high risk for severe COVID-19: Information for healthcare providers. Available at: https://www.cdc.gov/coronavirus/2019-ncov/hcp/clinical-care/underlyingconditions.html. Accessed on August 3, 2022.

67. Centers for Disease Control and Prevention. Science brief: Evidence used to up-date the list of underlying medical conditions that increase a person's risk of se-vere illness from COVID-19. Available at: https://www.cdc.gov/coronavirus/2019-ncov/hcp/clinical-care/underlying-evidence-table.html. Accessed on August 3, 2022.

68. Centers for Disease Control and Prevention. Risk for COVID-19 infection, hospi-talization, and death by age group. Available at: https://www.cdc.gov/coronavirus/2019-ncov/covid-data/investigations-discovery/hospitalization-death-by-age.html. Accessed on August 3, 2022.

69. Gold JAW, Rossen LM, Ahmad FB, et al. Race, Ethnicity, and Age Trends in Per-sons Who Died from COVID-19 - United States, May-August 2020. MMWR Morb Mortal Wkly Rep 2020;69(42):1517–21.

70. Kenneth M, H.K. COVID-19: Clinical features. In: UpToDate, Hirsch M (Ed), Up-ToDate, Waltham, MA, Accessed on July 28, 2022. Published by UpToDate in Waltham, MA.

71. McMichael TM, Currie DW, Clark S, et al. Epidemiology of Covid-19 in a long-term care facility in king county, washington. N Engl J Med 2020;382(21):2005–11.

72. Yek C, Warner S, Wiltz JL, et al. Risk factors for severe COVID-19 outcomes among persons aged ≥18 years who completed a primary COVID-19 vaccina-tion series - 465 health care facilities, United States, december 2020-October 2021. MMWR Morb Mortal Wkly Rep 2022;71(1):19 25.

73. Uyeki TM, Bernstein HH, Bradley JS, et al. Clinical Practice Guidelines by the Infectious Diseases Society of America: 2018 Update on Diagnosis, Treatment, Chemoprophylaxis, and Institutional Outbreak Management of Seasonal Influen-zaa. Clin Infect Dis 2019;68(6):895–902.

74. Lansbury LE, Brown CS, Nguyen-Van-Tam JS. Influenza in long-term care facil-ities. Influenza Other Respir Viruses 2017;11(5):356–66.

75. Hand J, Rose EB, Salinas A, et al. Severe Respiratory Illness Outbreak Associ-ated with Human Coronavirus NL63 in a Long-Term Care Facility. Emerg Infect Dis 2018;24(10):1964–6.

76. CDC. How COVID-19 Spreads. Available at: https://www.cdc.gov/coronavirus/2019-ncov/prevent-getting-sick/how-covid-spreads.html. Accessed on July 28, 2022.

77. Dosa D, Jump RL, LaPlante K, et al. Long-term care facilities and the coronavi-rus epidemic: practical guidelines for a population at highest risk. J Am Med Dir Assoc 2020;21(5):569–71.

78. CDC guidance for living in close quarters. Available at: https://www.salisbury.edu/coronavirus/_files/CDC-GuidanceCloseQuarters.pdf. Accessed on July 29, 2022.

79. Bayer TA, DeVone F, McConeghy K, et al. Dementia prevalence, a contextual factor associated with SARS-CoV-2 in veterans affairs community living centers. J Am Geriatr Soc 2022;70(10):2973–9.

80. Emmerton D, Abdelhafiz A. Delirium in older people with COVID-19: clinical sce-nario and literature review. SN Compr Clin Med 2020;2(10):1790–7.

81. Fisman DN, Bogoch I, Lapointe-Shaw L, et al. Risk Factors Associated With Mor-tality Among Residents With Coronavirus Disease 2019 (COVID-19) in Long-term Care Facilities in Ontario, Canada. JAMA Netw Open 2020;3(7):e2015957.

82. American Geriatrics Society (AGS). Policy Brief: COVID-19 and Assisted Living Facilities. J Am Geriatr Soc 2020;68(6):1131–5.

83. Meis-Pinheiro U, Lopez-Segui F, Walsh S, et al. Clinical characteristics of COVID-19 in older adults. A retrospective study in long-term nursing homes in Catalonia. PLoS One 2021;16(7):e0255141.

84. Amore S, Puppo E, Melera J, et al. Impact of COVID-19 on older adults and role of long-term care facilities during early stages of epidemic in Italy. Sci Rep 2021;11(1):12530.

85. McGarry BE, Grabowski DC, Barnett ML. Severe Staffing And Personal Protective Equipment Shortages Faced By Nursing Homes During The COVID-19 Pandemic. Health Aff (Millwood) 2020;39(10):1812–21.

86. Gravenstein S, McConeghy K, Saade E, et al. Adjuvanted Influenza Vaccine and Influenza Outbreaks in US Nursing Homes: Results From a Pragmatic Cluster-Randomized Clinical Trial. Clin Infect Dis 2021;73(11):e4229–36.

87. Shallcross L, Burke D, Abbott O, et al. Factors associated with SARS-CoV-2 infection and outbreaks in long-term care facilities in England: a national cross-sectional survey. Lancet Healthy Longev 2021;2(3):e129–42.

88. Nanda A, Vura N, Gravenstein S. COVID-19 in older adults. Aging Clin Exp Res 2020;32(7):1199–202.

89. Wu Z, McGoogan JM. Characteristics of and Important Lessons From the Coronavirus Disease 2019 (COVID-19) Outbreak in China: Summary of a Report of 72 314 cases from the chinese center for disease control and prevention. JAMA 2020;323(13):1239–42.

90. Notari A, Torrieri G. COVID-19 transmission risk factors. Pathog Glob Health 2022;116(3):146–77.

91. Guallar MP, Meiriño R, Donat-Vargas C, et al. Inoculum at the time of SARS-CoV-2 exposure and risk of disease severity. Int J Infect Dis 2020;97:290–2.

92. CDC. Reinfections and COVID-19. Available at: https://www.cdc.gov/coronavirus/2019-ncov/your-health/reinfection.html. Accessed on Aug 02, 2022.

93. COVID-19 after Vaccination: Possible Breakthrough Infection. Available at: https://www.cdc.gov/coronavirus/2019-ncov/vaccines/effectiveness/why-measure-effectiveness/breakthrough-cases.html. Accessed Aug 02, 2022.

94. Helfand M, Fiordalisi C, Wiedrick J, et al. Risk for reinfection after SARS-CoV-2: a living, rapid review for american college of physicians practice points on the role of the antibody response in conferring immunity following sars-CoV-2 infection. Ann Intern Med 2022;175(4):547–55.

95. Sheehan MM, Reddy AJ, Rothberg MB. Reinfection Rates Among Patients Who Previously Tested Positive for Coronavirus Disease 2019: A Retrospective Cohort Study. Clin Infect Dis 2021;73(10):1882–6.

96. Goldberg EM, Southerland LT, Meltzer AC, et al. Age-related differences in symptoms in older emergency department patients with COVID-19: Prevalence and outcomes in a multicenter cohort. J Am Geriatr Soc 2022;70(7):1918–30.

97. Boyton RJ, Altmann DM. The immunology of asymptomatic SARS-CoV-2 infection: what are the key questions? Nat Rev Immunol 2021;21(12):762–8.

98. Townsend JP, Hassler HB, Wang Z, et al. The durability of immunity against reinfection by SARS-CoV-2: a comparative evolutionary study. Lancet Microbe 2021;2(12):e666–75.

99. North CM, Barczak A, Goldstein RH, et al. Determining the Incidence of Asymptomatic SARS-CoV-2 Among Early Recipients of COVID-19 Vaccines (DISCOVER-COVID-19): a prospective cohort study of healthcare workers before, during and after vaccination. Clin Infect Dis 2022;74(7):1275–8.

100. Tang L, Hijano DR, Gaur AH, et al. Asymptomatic and Symptomatic SARS-CoV-2 Infections After BNT162b2 Vaccination in a Routinely Screened Workforce. JAMA 2021;325(24):2500–2.
101. CDC. Symptoms of COVID-19. Available at: https://www.cdc.gov/coronavirus/2019-ncov/symptoms-testing/symptoms.html. Accessed on July 27, 2022.
102. Lian J, Jin X, Hao S, et al. Analysis of epidemiological and clinical features in older patients with coronavirus disease 2019 (COVID-19) outside Wuhan. Clin Infect Dis 2020;71(15):740–7.
103. Nikolich-Zugich J, Knox KS, Rios CT, et al. SARS-CoV-2 and COVID-19 in older adults: what we may expect regarding pathogenesis, immune responses, and outcomes. Geroscience 2020;42(2):505–14.
104. Rudolph JL, Halladay CW, Barber M, et al. Temperature in nursing home residents systematically tested for SARS-CoV-2. J Am Med Dir Assoc 2020;21(7):895–9.e1.
105. Elhamamsy S, DeVone F, Bayer T, et al. Can we use temperature measurements to identify pre-symptomatic SARS-CoV-2 infection in nursing home residents? J Am Geriatr Soc 2022.
106. Interim Infection Prevention and Control Recommendations to Prevent SARS-CoV-2 Spread in Nursing Homes. Available at: https://www.cdc.gov/coronavirus/2019-ncov/hcp/long-term-care.html. Accessed August 04, 2022.
107. Kimball A, Hatfield KM, Arons M, et al. Asymptomatic and Presymptomatic SARS-CoV-2 Infections in Residents of a Long-Term Care Skilled Nursing Facility - King County, Washington, March 2020. MMWR Morb Mortal Wkly Rep 2020;69(13):377–81.
108. Cohen K, Ren S, Heath K, et al. Risk of persistent and new clinical sequelae among adults aged 65 years and older during the post-acute phase of SARS-CoV-2 infection: retrospective cohort study. Bmj 2022;376:e068414.
109. Katsoularis I, Fonseca-Rodríguez O, Farrington P, et al. Risks of deep vein thrombosis, pulmonary embolism, and bleeding after covid-19: nationwide self-controlled cases series and matched cohort study. Bmj 2022;377:e069590.
110. Levin EG, Lustig Y, Cohen C, et al. Waning Immune Humoral Response to BNT162b2 Covid-19 Vaccine over 6 Months. N Engl J Med 2021;385(24):e84.
111. Williamson EJ, Walker AJ, Bhaskaran K, et al. Factors associated with COVID-19-related death using OpenSAFELY. Nature 2020;584(7821):430–6.
112. Stokes EK, Zambrano LD, Anderson KN, et al. Coronavirus Disease 2019 Case Surveillance - United States, January 22-May 30, 2020. MMWR Morb Mortal Wkly Rep 2020;69(24):759–65.
113. Arons MM, Hatfield KM, Reddy SC, et al. Presymptomatic SARS-CoV-2 Infections and Transmission in a Skilled Nursing Facility. N Engl J Med 2020;382(22):2081–90.
114. Chu DK, Akl EA, Duda S, et al. Physical distancing, face masks, and eye protection to prevent person-to-person transmission of SARS-CoV-2 and COVID-19: a systematic review and meta-analysis. Lancet 2020;395(10242):1973–87.
115. Recker A, White EM, Yang X, et al. Factors Affecting SARS-CoV-2 test discordance in skilled nursing facilities. J Am Med Dir Assoc 2022;23(8):1279–82.
116. Ohuabunwa U, Turner J, Johnson T. Atypical presentations among older adults with COVID-19 disease: a need for broadening the differential diagnosis. Gerontol Geriatr Med 2021;7. 2333721421999313.
117. Zhu T, Wang Y, Zhou S, et al. A Comparative Study of Chest Computed Tomography Features in Young and Older Adults With Corona Virus Disease (COVID-19). J Thorac Imaging 2020;35(4):W97–101.

118. Okoye C, Finamore P, Bellelli G, et al. Computed tomography findings and prognosis in older COVID-19 patients. BMC Geriatr 2022;22(1):166.
119. Otterson LB BS, Saydah S, Boehmer T, et al. Post–COVID Conditions Among Adult COVID-19 Survivors Aged 18–64 and ≥65 Years — United States, March 2020–November 2021. Morbidity Mortality Weekly Rep (Mmwr) 2022;71(21): 713–7.
120. CDC. Nearly One in Five American Adults Who Have Had COVID-19 Still Have "Long COVID". Available at: https://www.cdc.gov/nchs/pressroom/nchs_press_releases/2022/20220622.htm#:~:text=Nearly%20three%20times%20as%20many,5.5%5%25 https://www.cdc.gov/nchs/covid19/pulse/long-covid.htm. Accessed on August 02, 2022.
121. Leeder C. Long-COVID symptoms among veterans. J Am Geriatr Soc April 2022;70:S195.
122. Huang L, Li X, Gu X, et al. Health outcomes in people 2 years after surviving hospitalisation with COVID-19: a longitudinal cohort study. Lancet Respir Med 2022;10(9):863–76.
123. Groff D, Sun A, Ssentongo AE, et al. Short-term and Long-term Rates of Postacute Sequelae of SARS-CoV-2 Infection: A Systematic Review. JAMA Netw Open 2021;4(10):e2128568.
124. Chopra V, Flanders SA, O'Malley M, et al. Sixty-Day Outcomes Among Patients Hospitalized With COVID-19. Ann Intern Med 2021;174(4):576–8.
125. Ayoubkhani D, Bermingham C, Pouwels KB, et al. Trajectory of long covid symptoms after covid-19 vaccination: community based cohort study. BMJ 2022;377: e069676.
126. Rando HM, Bennett TD, Byrd JB, et al. Challenges in defining long COVID: striking differences across literature, electronic health records, and patient-reported information. medRxiv 2021.
127. Huang C, Huang L, Wang Y, et al. 6-month consequences of COVID-19 in patients discharged from hospital: a cohort study. Lancet 2021;397(10270): 220–32.
128. Lopez-Leon S, Wegman-Ostrosky T, Perelman C, et al. More than 50 long-term effects of COVID-19: a systematic review and meta-analysis. Sci Rep 2021; 11(1):16144.
129. Mendelson M, Nel J, Blumberg L, et al. Long-COVID: An evolving problem with an extensive impact. S Afr Med J 2020;111(1):10–2.
130. Sneller MC, Liang CJ, Marques AR, et al. A longitudinal study of COVID-19 sequelae and immunity: baseline findings. Ann Intern Med 2022;175(7):969–79.
131. Mueller AL, McNamara MS, Sinclair DA. Why does COVID-19 disproportionately affect older people? Aging (Albany NY) 2020;12(10):9959–81.
132. Nyberg T, Ferguson NM, Nash SG, et al. Comparative analysis of the risks of hospitalisation and death associated with SARS-CoV-2 omicron (B.1.1.529) and delta (B.1.617.2) variants in England: a cohort study. Lancet 2022; 399(10332):1303–12.
133. Oran DP, Topol EJ. The proportion of SARS-CoV-2 infections that are asymptomatic : a systematic review. Ann Intern Med 2021;174(5):655–62.
134. Steele MK, Couture A, Reed C, et al. Estimated number of COVID-19 infections, hospitalizations, and deaths prevented among vaccinated persons in the US, december 2020 to september 2021. JAMA Netw Open 2022;5(7):e2220385.
135. White EM, Yang X, Blackman C, et al. Incident SARS-CoV-2 Infection among mRNA-vaccinated and unvaccinated nursing home residents. N Engl J Med 2021;385(5):474–6.

136. Nalbandian A, Sehgal K, Gupta A, et al. Post-acute COVID-19 syndrome. Nat Med 2021;27(4):601–15.
137. Carfi A, Bernabei R, Landi F. Persistent Symptoms in Patients After Acute COVID-19. JAMA 2020;324(6):603–5.
138. Carvalho-Schneider C, Laurent E, Lemaignen A, et al. Follow-up of adults with noncritical COVID-19 two months after symptom onset. Clin Microbiol Infect 2021;27(2):258–63.
139. Arnold DT, Hamilton FW, Milne A, et al. Patient outcomes after hospitalisation with COVID-19 and implications for follow-up: results from a prospective UK cohort. Thorax 2021;76(4):399–401.
140. Moreno-Pérez O, et al. Post-acute COVID-19 syndrome. Incidence and risk factors: A Mediterranean cohort study. J Infect 2021;82(3):378–83.
141. Halpin SJ, McIvor C, Whyatt G, et al. Postdischarge symptoms and rehabilitation needs in survivors of COVID-19 infection: A cross-sectional evaluation. J Med Virol 2021;93(2):1013–22.
142. Garrigues E, Janvier P, Kherabi Y, et al. Post-discharge persistent symptoms and health-related quality of life after hospitalization for COVID-19. J Infect 2020;81(6):e4–6.
143. Xie Y, Bowe B, Al-Aly Z. Burdens of post-acute sequelae of COVID-19 by severity of acute infection, demographics and health status. Nat Commun 2021;12(1):6571.
144. Mugglestone MA, Ratnaraja NV, Bak A, et al. Presymptomatic, asymptomatic and post-symptomatic transmission of SARS-CoV-2: joint British Infection Association (BIA), Healthcare Infection Society (HIS), Infection Prevention Society (IPS) and Royal College of Pathologists (RCPath) guidance. BMC Infect Dis 2022;22(1):453.
145. WHO Covid-19 Case Definition. Available at: WHO/2019-nCoV/Surveillance_Case_Definition/2022.1. Accessed on July 27, 2022.
146. CDC. Coronavirus Disease 2019 (COVID-19) 2021 Case Definition. Available at: https://ndc.services.cdc.gov/case-definitions/coronavirus-disease-2019-2021/. Accessed on July 28, 2022.
147. FDA Emergency Use Authorizations. Available at: https://www.fda.gov/medical-devices/emergency-situations-medical-devices/emergency-use-authorizations https://www.fda.gov/medical-devices/emergency-situations-medical-devices/faqs-testing-sars-cov-2#nolonger. Accessed on July 28, 2022.
148. Fang FC, Naccache SN, Greninger AL. The Laboratory Diagnosis of Coronavirus Disease 2019- Frequently Asked Questions. Clin Infect Dis 2020;71(11):2996–3001.
149. Caliendo AM, Hanson KE. COVID-19: Diagnosis. In: UpToDate, Hirsch M (Ed), UpToDate, Waltham, MA, Accessed on July 28, 2022.
150. US FDA. Coronavirus (COVID-19) Update: FDA Authorizes First COVID-19 Diagnostic Test Using Breath Samples. Available at: https://www.fda.gov/news-events/press-announcements/coronavirus-covid-19-update-fda-authorizes-first-covid-19-diagnostic-test-using-breath-samples. Accessed on July 27, 2022.
151. Murugesan K, Agannathan P, Pham TD, et al. Interferon-γ release assay for accurate detection of severe acute respiratory syndrome coronavirus 2 t-cell response. Clin Infect Dis 2021;73(9):e3130–2.

Vaccines for the Prevention of Coronavirus Disease 2019 in Older Adults

Oladayo A. Oyebanji, MBChB, MS[a], Eleftherios Mylonakis, MD, PhD[b], David H. Canaday, MD[a,c],*

KEYWORDS

- COVID-19 vaccine • Aging • Vaccine effectiveness • Immunogenicity • Geriatric
- Older adults

KEY POINTS

- Immunosenescence, inflammaging, and frailty are associated with the suboptimal immunogenicity of vaccines in older adults.
- Immunogenicity is reduced in older individuals for both vaccine-specific antibody and T-cell levels.
- Vaccine effectiveness to the current COVID-19 vaccines, however, is preserved in the older population despite reduced immunogenicity.
- Being a vulnerable population, vaccination campaigns should continue to prioritize older adults for optimal protection against COVID-19.

INTRODUCTION

Institutionalized and community-dwelling older adults have been greatly impacted by the coronavirus disease 2019 (COVID-19) pandemic.[1] Older adults have a higher incidence of hospitalizations and death compared with younger populations. Older adults, especially those with comorbidities, are specifically prone to having the severe disease when infected with severe acute respiratory syndrome coronavirus 2 (SARS-CoV-2), the virus that causes COVID-19.[2,3] Thus, they are a population of utmost concern amid the pandemic, which has often led to their prioritization in vaccine recommendations.[4,5] Despite the advent of vaccines, this group has experienced increased breakthrough infections.[6,7] Whether this is due to inadequate vaccine coverage or vaccine ineffectiveness is unclear. Vaccination remains the most feasible

[a] Case Western Reserve University, School of Medicine, 10900 Euclid Ave, BRB 1025, Cleveland, OH 44106-4984, USA; [b] Infectious Diseases Division, The Miriam Hospital and Rhode Island Hospital, Warren Alpert Medical School of Brown University, Rhode Island Hospital, 593 Eddy Street, POB, 3rd Floor, Suite 328/330, Providence, RI 02903, USA; [c] Geriatric Research, Education and Clinical Center, Cleveland Veterans Affairs Medical Center, 10900 Euclid Ave, BRB 1025, Cleveland, OH 44106-4984, USA
* Corresponding author.
E-mail address: dxc44@case.edu

Infect Dis Clin N Am 37 (2023) 27–45
https://doi.org/10.1016/j.idc.2022.11.002
0891-5520/23/Published by Elsevier Inc.
id.theclinics.com

and easily accessible preventive measure used for protection against COVID-19 among older adults. Thus, there is a significant need to optimize current vaccination measures to protect these populations against COVID-19.

IMMUNE CHANGES IN OLDER ADULTS: CLINICAL IMPLICATIONS FOR VACCINATION

Older adults generate suboptimal immune responses to virtually all vaccines when compared with the younger adult population.[8] Vaccines such as those for influenza, pneumococcus, and hepatitis B are less immunogenic and effective in adults older than 65 years.[9] In addition, vaccine-induced antibodies tend to be more short-lived among this population.[10]

Immunosenescence and inflammaging are two established phenomena associated with the suboptimal immunogenicity of vaccines in older adults. In *immunosenescence*, the aging immune system is plagued with a progressive functional decline, which reduces its ability to mount an adequate response to new or previously encountered antigens in the form of vaccines or infections.[11] This decline in cellular and humoral immunity is marked by reduced production of naive B and T cells, an increase in dysfunctional memory cells, and the involution of primary lymphoid organs such as the thymus.[12] These physiologic changes make older adults more susceptible to infections as they continue to age.[13] Furthermore, a characteristic reduction in the production of lymphocytes (lymphopoiesis) results in the impairment of the adaptive and innate immune response,[14] which is also marked by the increased production of autoantibodies and low-affinity antibodies.[10] Changes within the bone marrow, such as myelofibrosis, result in the production of short-lived and apoptosis-prone immune cells, with a shift toward myeloid precursor cells.[15] These cumulative changes create "immune system fatigue" and dampen the ability of the immune system in older adults to be appropriately stimulated by neoantigens and previously encountered antigens alike.

Inflammaging is a progressive state of chronic, sterile low-grade inflammation that contributes to developing disease conditions associated with aging.[16] Inflammaging is characterized by increased production of proinflammatory cytokines (such as interleukin [IL]-1, IL-6, and tumor necrosis factor [TNF] α) with an increase in the ratio of Th17 cells, a proinflammatory subset of $CD4^+$ T cells, to regulatory T cells. There is also the production of highly inflammatory late memory B cells with reduced telomerase activity, and reduced neutrophilic, monocytic, and dendritic cell functions such as chemotaxis, phagocytosis, signaling pathways, and intracellular killing via free radical production.[11] Furthermore, elevated levels of TNF-α characteristic of inflammaging exist in the serum and resting B cells.[17] As a result, inflammaging causes impairment in B cell function, and it has been reported that these systemically abundant proinflammatory cytokines tend to prevent optimal response to vaccines.[18] This propensity toward a heightened anti-inflammatory response to low-grade chronic inflammation and suppression of acute inflammatory processes has clinical implications in the form of reduced reactions to vaccines observed in older adults.[16]

Frailty further contributes to the severity of complications suffered from disease and infections. This multifactorial syndrome is marked by a decline in physiologic function and increased susceptibility to environmental stressors,[19,20] and it is a summation of an individual's functional status, mortality risk, and chronic medical conditions.[21] The Frailty Index, an objective measure of frailty using key clinical and laboratory markers is often used to assess overall health status and risk stratification for serious disease complications among older adults.[22] Generally, frailty is associated with aging and thus, predominantly occurs among older adults. Notably, a higher degree of frailty is associated with immune function decline, and consequently, the inability to mount an appropriate response to antigenic stimulation by either an infection or vaccine.

These resultant effects of aging on the immune system have diverse ramifications on response to vaccination among this age group. Consequences such as the ability of antigens from vaccines and infections to elicit an appropriate immune response (immunogenicity) and side effects of vaccines (reactogenicity) among these subjects differ from other age groups. These immunologic realities in this age group demonstrate the critical need for studies to best deploy available vaccines and/or engineer better ones.

Immune correlates of protection. Antibodies generally confer protection against infections, and specific antibody levels are often correlated with protection from such infections. Having an immune correlate of protection is very helpful for vaccine development and approval, allowing more rapid and less costly approvals for new vaccines or variations on current vaccines. Although specific correlates of protection from SARS-CoV-2 infection are yet to be established,[23–26] seroprotective levels of neutralizing and non-neutralizing antibodies are widely accepted as surrogates for protection in other viruses such as varicella zoster and hepatitis B virus.[27] The discordance between immunogenicity and efficacy findings for older adults often observed in COVID-19 vaccine trials underscores the difficulty in defining specific immunologic correlates of clinical protection. Emerging variant strains pose an additional challenge because immune correlate may vary depending on the variant. All this taken together suggests that a well-defined immune correlate of protection across age and strain might not exist for COVID-19 vaccines.

EFFICACY OF CURRENT CORONAVIRUS DISEASE 2019 VACCINES AMONG OLDER ADULTS

The rapid development of COVID-19 vaccines has helped mitigate the pandemic's devastating effects across all eligible age groups, especially among vulnerable groups including older adults. The World Health Organization (WHO) registry contains more than 300 vaccines in development at different phases of clinical trials of which 11 have been approved for emergency use worldwide.[28] These approved vaccines use different technologies (**Fig. 1**); they include the novel messenger RNA (mRNA) vaccines (Pfizer–BioNTech's Comirnaty BNT162b2 and Moderna's Spikevax mRNA-1273) and the non-mRNA vaccines such as adenovirus vector-based vaccines (Johnson & Johnson–Janssen's Jcovden Ad26.COV2.S, CanSino's Convidecia AD5-nCOV, and AstraZeneca's Covishield and Vaxzevria AZD1222; ChAdOx1), adjuvanted protein vaccines (Novavax's Covovax and Nuvaxovid NVX-CoV2373), and inactivated virus vaccines (Sinopharm's Covilo, Sinovac's CoronaVac, and Bharat Biotech's Covaxin). These vaccines and the recently approved bivalent boosters have varying acceptance and usage in different parts of the world but have all remained effective in reducing morbidity and mortality among older adults, as well as other populations.[29]

As is typical of vaccine development, initial safety and immunogenicity studies of many of these vaccines focused on middle-aged adults with much less older adult representation. The phase 3 approval trials, however, had better older adult representation with about 25% to 40% of subjects in an older age group category from greater than 55, 60, 65, or 70 years depending on the study (**Table 1**). This is a reasonable representation in the phase 3 trials. Results from these trials show that most COVID-19 vaccines did not have a significant initial difference in efficacy across the adult age spectrum (see **Table 1**). This observation suggests independence of vaccine efficacy (VE) from age as it applies to the COVID-19 vaccines in use. Rather than age, frailty may be a better predictor of the efficacy of certain COVID-19 vaccines.[30] As explained

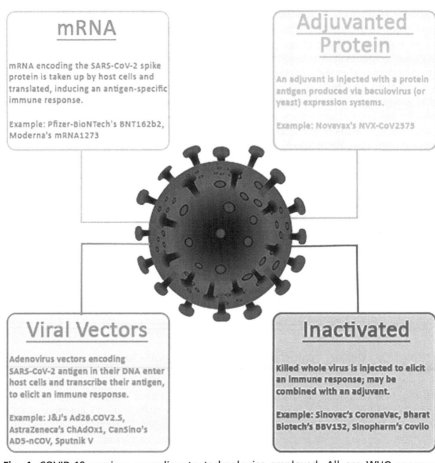

mRNA

mRNA encoding the SARS-CoV-2 spike protein is taken up by host cells and translated, inducing an antigen-specific immune response.

Example: Pfizer-BioNTech's BNT162b2, Moderna's mRNA1273

Adjuvanted Protein

An adjuvant is injected with a protein antigen produced via baculovirus (or yeast) expression systems.

Example: Novavax's NVX-CoV2373

Viral Vectors

Adenovirus vectors encoding SARS-CoV-2 antigen in their DNA enter host cells and transcribe their antigen, to elicit an immune response.

Example: J&J's Ad26.COV2.S, AstraZeneca's ChAdOx1, CanSino's AD5-nCOV, Sputnik V

Inactivated

Killed whole virus is injected to elicit an immune response; may be combined with an adjuvant.

Example: Sinovac's CoronaVac, Bharat Biotech's BBV152, Sinopharm's Covilo

Fig. 1. COVID-19 vaccines according to technologies employed. All are WHO-approved except the viral vector sputnik V vaccine. mRNA, Messenger Ribonucleic Acid; SARS-CoV-2, Severe Acute Respiratory Syndrome Coronavirus 2; J&J, Johnson and Johnson.

earlier, immunosenescence has implications for the durability of vaccine-induced antibodies in older adults. Consequently, age and frailty are negatively associated with the durability of antibodies postvaccination, whereas a prior infection with SARS-CoV-2 increases durability regardless of age and frailty.[31–34]

Like previous vaccines, the COVID-19 vaccines generated reduced cellular and humoral response when compared with the younger population.[35,36] However, this initial reduction in immunogenicity does not necessarily translate into reduced protection for this population because exact immune correlates of protection are yet to be defined. More so, both real-world and trial-reported VE among these older adult populations compares impressively with those reported among other age groups further downplaying the effect of the disparity in observed immunogenicity. Although females have been reported to generate better immune responses to vaccines in general,[37,38] such disparities have not been reported with the COVID vaccines currently in use.[39,40] Of note, the authors caution that a head-to-head comparison of vaccine trials is not ideal due to variables, such as differences in trial settings and participants, symptomatic illness criteria, and predominant variants at the time trials were conducted.[41]

Table 1
Summary of older age-specific vaccine efficacy data in phase 3 coronavirus disease 2019 vaccine trials

Vaccine	Type	Number of Older Adult Participants (% of Total Participants) Age Cutoff	VE in Older Adults % (95% CI)	Overall Efficacy (95% CI)	Median Follow-Up (in days)[a]
BNT162b2 (Pfizer)	mRNA vaccine encoding spike glycoprotein	15,921 (42.2) >55 y	93.7 (80.6–98.8)	95.0 (90.0–97.9)	60
mRNA-1273 (Moderna)	mRNA vaccine encoding spike glycoprotein	7512 (25.8) ≥65 y	86.4 (61.4–95.2)	94.1 (89.3–96.8)	63
NVX-CoV2373 (NVX; Novavax)	Nanoparticle vaccine containing purified spike glycoprotein and adjuvant	3910 (27.9) >65 y	88.9 (20.2–99.7)	89.7 (80.2–94.6)	56
ChAdOx-nCov19 (ChAd; AZD1222, AstraZeneca)	Replication-deficient chimpanzee adenovirus-vectored vaccine, expressing spike glycoprotein	7238 (22.4) ≥65 y	83.5 (54.2–94.1)	74.0 (65.3–80.5)	61
Ad26.COV2.S (Ad26; Janssen)	Replication-deficient adenovirus vector vaccine constructed to encode a spike glycoprotein	14,672 (33.5) ≥60 y	66.2 (36.7–83.0)	66.1 (55.0–74.8)	58
rAd26 and rAd5 vector-based (Sputnik V, Gam-COVID-Vac)	Heterologous rAd-based vaccine encoding spike glycoprotein	2144 (10.8%) >60 y	91.8 (67.1–98.3)	91·6 (85.6–95.2)	21 d after first dose
Inactivated whole virus vaccine (CoronaVac, Sinovac Biotech)	Inactivated whole SARS-CoV-2	43,774 (100%) ≥70 y	55.4 (46.5–62.8)	Same	Not stated
BBV152 (Covaxin, Bharat Biotech Intl.)	Inactivated whole SARS-CoV-2 with Toll-like receptor 7/8 adjuvant adsorbed to alum	1858 (10.9%) ≥60 y	67.8 (8·0–90.0).	77.8 (65·2–86.4)	99

Nine of 11 WHO-approved COVID-19 vaccines shown as well as the Sputnik V vaccine.
Abbreviations: CI, confidence interval; rAd, recombinant adenovirus; VE, vaccine efficacy.
[a] Median follow-up is counted after the second dose unless otherwise specified.

Effectiveness and Immunogenicity of the mRNA Vaccines in Older Adults

The mRNA vaccines, such as those manufactured by Pfizer (BNT162b2) and Moderna (mRNA-1273), were the earliest vaccines approved for emergency use in the United States and are the most widely used vaccines, especially in developed countries with cost, transport, and storage logistics being a major factor limiting their use in developing countries.

The BNT162b2 mRNA vaccine is a lipid nanoparticle-formulated, nucleoside-modified RNA vaccine that encodes a membrane-anchored SARS-CoV-2 full-length spike, stabilized in the prefusion conformation.[42] This vaccine is administered in a 2-dose regimen 21 days apart. The early phase 2 trial that included 45 healthy adults aged 65 to 85 years reported a decline in immunogenicity with increasing age; however, this response exceeded that of convalescent subjects suggesting the superiority of vaccine-induced immunity over that of natural infection among this age group.[42] Phase 3 trials reported an overall efficacy of 95.0% (90.0–97.9) after a median follow-up of 2 months with subgroup analysis revealing a consistent but slightly lower VE of 93.7% (80.6–98.8) among adults older than 55 years, 94.7% (66.7–99.9) among adults older than 65 years, and 100.0% (−13.1–100.0) in adults older than 75 years.[43] The lower immunogenicity trend of the BNT1652b2 primary series observed among older adults seems to be reversed with the booster doses where they were reported to have mounted better responses.[44] Phase 1 trial of the third dose of the Pfizer vaccine showed a better neutralization capacity in older adults compared with younger adults. Evaluating twelve 65- to 85-year-old participants over 1 month, the geometric mean ratio of neutralizing antibodies was consistently higher between the second and third dose for these older adults than their younger counterparts, underlining the efficacy of an additional dose in this population of older adults.[44]

The mRNA-1273 vaccine is a lipid nanoparticle-encapsulated mRNA-based vaccine that encodes the prefusion-stabilized full-length spike protein of the SARS-CoV-2 virus; it is administered in 2 doses, 28 days apart. A phase 2 open-label trial of the mRNA-1273 vaccine in adults aged 56 years and older showed a dose- and time-dependent robust immune response among these older adults.[45] Measured binding and neutralizing antibodies were not dependent on age and were commensurate with levels earlier reported among adults aged 18 to 55 years.[46] In phase 3 randomized, observer-blinded, placebo-controlled trial conducted at 99 centers across the United States, adults aged 65 years or older had a reported VE of 86.4% (61.4–95.2) against an overall VE of 94.1% (89.3–96.8).[47]

Although the Pfizer and Moderna trials were not designed to measure the impact on transmission explicitly, real-world studies have shown associated vaccine benefits in reducing incidences of SARS-CoV-2 infections. In a metadata study of 280 nursing homes (NH) across 21 states in the United States, Mor and colleagues[48] used resident-level data to compare the rate of new resident infections as well as hospital transfers and/or deaths in facilities with early versus later vaccination clinics, adjusting for infection rates in each facility. Among early recipients of 2 doses of the mRNA vaccines, the investigators reported a magnitude of 5.2 fewer cases per 100 at-risk NH residents and an average cumulative reduction in hospitalization or death of 5 events per 100 infected residents per day up to 7 weeks.[48] Similarly, in a large study involving residents of long-term care facilities in Israel, Muhsen and colleagues[49] reported significantly lower rates of SARS-CoV-2 infection and hospitalization for severe COVID-19. Following up with residents up to 6 weeks after receiving a third dose of the BNT162b2 mRNA vaccine, the investigators observed an incidence ratio of 0.29

for overall infection and 0.20 for hospitalization, which corresponded to a relative rate reduction of 71% and 80%, respectively.[50]

Looking at real-world data, McConeghy and colleagues[51] studied the additional role a fourth vaccine dose plays in reducing morbidity and mortality from COVID-19. Comparing a single mRNA COVID-19 vaccine booster dose, with a second booster dose, they found that a second booster dose provided additional protection against COVID-19-associated severe outcomes among NH residents during the Omicron period. Other smaller studies have reported similar protection among NH residents who have received the fourth vaccine dose to date.[49,52]

It is not clear what exact role and magnitude T cells play in protection from SARS-CoV-2, but they play a role in other viral infections in disease mitigation once infected. Owing to the prevailing realities of immunosenescence and inflammaging, older adults tend to have impaired vaccine-specific T-cell responses. Following 2 doses of the BNT162b2 mRNA vaccine, the frequencies of vaccine-specific IFNγ$^+$ and IFNγ$^+$IL-2$^+$TNFα$^+$ CD4+ and the frequency of specific CD8$^+$ T cells were lower in COVID-19-naive older adults than in COVID-19-naive young adults.[53] T-cell responses were the same in the older and younger populations that were vaccinated after prior COVID-19. Several studies specifically address issues related to immunosenescence and inflammaging. Palacios-Pedrero et al observed lower vaccine-specific responses in the older group, and interestingly found a correlation between naive CD4+ cells and reduced vaccine-induced CD4 cells. This finding supports a major component of immunosenescence: poorer response in the aged is due to loss of naive cells.[54] Vitallé and colleagues[55] demonstrated that older persons display less frequency and poly-functionality of vaccine-induced T cells. Potentially demonstrating elements of both immunosenescence and inflammaging, they found that aging-related lower thymic function, altered T-cell homeostasis, proinflammatory monocyte profile, and altered dendritic cell features and function were associated with these reduced responses.

Effectiveness and Immunogenicity of the Non-mRNA Vaccines in Older Adults

The Novavax NVX-CoV2373 is a recombinant nanoparticle vaccine against SARS-CoV-2 that contains the full-length spike glycoprotein (S-protein) of the prototype strain plus Matrix-M adjuvant that is administered in 2-dose primary series 21 days apart. In a phase 3 randomized placebo-controlled trial conducted in the United Kingdom that included 1953 older adults aged between 65 and 84 years, the NVX-CoV2373 recorded a VE of 88.9% (20.2–99.7) followed up for a median of 56 days after the second dose. This VE compares impressively with the 89.8% VE reported for participants younger than 65 years.[56] A similar phase 3 trial conducted in the United States and Mexico for a median follow-up of 64 days after the second dose reported a VE of 91% in participants at overall high risk for COVID-19, defined as subjects aged 65 years or older and those of any age with chronic health conditions or an increased risk for COVID-19 due to elevated exposure.[57]

Among older adults, in a phase 2 immunogenicity trial, a homologous booster dose of the NVX-CoV2373 vaccine administered approximately 6 months following the primary 2-dose series resulted in a significantly enhanced immunogenicity producing S-protein IgG and neutralization titers that were 4-fold higher than after the primary 2-dose series. Subgroup analysis for the ancestral Wuhan-Hu-1 strain showed slightly lower antibody responses in older adults (aged 60–84 years) than in those in younger adults (aged 18–59 years).[58]

The Jansen's Ad26.COV2.S vaccine is a recombinant, replication-incompetent human adenovirus type 26 vector encoding full-length SARS-CoV-2 S-protein in a prefusion-stabilized conformation administered as a single-dose primary vaccination.

In the initial phase 3 trial, participants aged 60 years or older had a VE of 76.3% (61.6–86.0) against moderate to severe-critical COVID-19 and a VE of 74.5% (57.9–84.3) against severity-adjusted symptomatic COVID-19, both higher than the overall VE reported in all age groups.[59] Remarkably, although estimates of VE differed between older adults with or without coexisting conditions at short-term follow-up, they became similar with a longer follow-up time. The final analysis of the trial reported a VE of 55.0% (42.9–64.7) after 14 days of follow-up, which dropped to 46.6% (30.7–59.0) beyond 28 days among participants older than 60 years.[60] This drop in efficacy between the primary and final analysis is believed to be due to more virulent circulating variants of SARS-CoV-2 that emerged after the primary analysis was carried out. In a double-blinded phase 3 randomized trial in which a homologous Ad26.COV2.S booster was administered 2 months after the primary series, efficacy against moderate to severe-critical COVID-19 among participants older than 60 years was 66.2% (−14.0–92.2) lower than the overall efficacy of 75.2% (54.6–87.3).[61] However, the development of vaccine-induced thrombotic thrombocytopenia has limited the continued use of the Ad26.COV2.S vaccine either as a primary series or a booster[62] and thus limited its further use among older adults; many of whom have comorbid conditions that predispose them to thrombotic events.

The ChAdOx1 nCoV-19 (AZD1222) is a replication-defective adenovirus-vectored vaccine expressing the full-length SARS-CoV-2 spike glycoprotein gene. The vaccine is administered in a prime-boost regimen 4 weeks apart and has been shown to have similar immunogenicity across age groups.[63] After 15 days or more follow-up in a double-blind, randomized placebo-controlled phase 3 trial, older adults had an estimated VE of 83.5% (54.2–94.1) that was better than the overall 74.0% (65.3–80.5) observed for all age groups.[64] A homologous booster dose of ChAdOx1 nCoV-19 given 6 to 8 months after completion of the primary series produced similar levels of boosting effect on anti-spike IgG and cellular responses after 28 days between older adults aged 70 years or older and adults aged between 18 and 69 years.[65]

The Gam-COVID-Vac (Sputnik V) is a recombinant adenovirus (rAd)-based vaccine that contains the full-length SARS-CoV-2 glycoprotein S gene. The vaccine is administered in a prime(rAd26)-boost(rAd5) regimen, 21 days apart. Despite the halt in its emergency use and approval by the WHO,[66] the Sputnik V vaccine showed good efficacy among older adults. Although the initial safety and immunogenicity trial did not include adults older than 60 years,[39] the phase 3 trials conducted in Russia had 2144 adults older than 60 years completing the study. At a median follow-up time of 48 days after the first dose, VE among this older age group was reported to be 91.8% (67.1–98.3), slightly higher than the overall efficacy of 91.6% (85.6–95.2).[67]

The CoronaVac (Sinovac Life Sciences) is an inactivated whole virus vaccine that has been shown to have immunogenicity and efficacy against COVID-19. CoronaVac, when administered in the standard 2-dose regimen 28 days apart, produces immunogenicity in adults aged 60 years and older, which is similar to adults aged 18 to 59 years, in a dose-dependent manner.[68,69] A phase 3 trial of adults aged 70 years and older in Brazil found adjusted VE against hospital admissions was 55.5% (46.5% to 62.9%) and against deaths was 61.2% (48.9% to 70.5%) at greater than equal to 14 days after the second dose.[70] A decline in effectiveness particularly in those older than 80 years was also reported. CoronaVac-induced antibodies tend to wane at a faster rate in older adults after the primary series but tend to be more durable after the third dose. For instance, older adults (aged 60 years or older) in a single-center phase 2 trial had an approximate decline of 10.7-fold in neutralizing antibodies 6 months after the second dose of the CoronaVac vaccine versus 6.8-fold observed for adults between 18 and 59 years. However, the rate of decline after a third dose given 8 months after the second dose was 2.5-fold among older adults versus 4.1-fold in the 18 to 59-year-old cohort over the same period.[71]

Although Covaxin (BBV152, Bharat Biotech International) does not seem to be currently in production or distribution, it was overwhelmingly the predominant vaccine initially used in India. The BBV152 is a whole-virion inactivated SARS-CoV-2 vaccine formulated with a Toll-like receptor 7/8 agonist molecule adsorbed to alum (Algel-IMDG) administered in a 2-dose regimen 4 weeks apart.[72] A total of 1858 older participants aged 60 years or older participated in the phase 3 trial and were found to have a modestly reduced VE to symptomatic disease of 67.8% (8.0–90.0) after a median follow-up of 99 days compared with 79.4% (66.0–88.2) VE in those younger than age 60 years.[73]

Hybrid Immunity from Vaccine and Infection

Hybrid immunity has been shown to confer some additional protection against SARS-CoV-2, even against the immune-escaping Omicron variants.[74–76] Vaccination following a previous SARS-CoV-2 infection increases all SARS-CoV-2-specific immunologic parameters due to the activation of immunologic memory generated from prior exposure.[77] This prior antigenic exposure has direct beneficial quantitative and qualitative effects on vaccine response in older adults. Vaccine-induced neutralizing and non-neutralizing antibodies are markedly increased among NH residents who had recovered from prior infection to the levels comparable to the younger comparator group[36] and had more durable antibodies than their naive counterparts.[78,79]

This enhanced response seems to be even better with extended intervals between infection and vaccination. Fedele and colleagues[80] found that a longer interval between previous SARS-CoV-2 infection and vaccination results in a higher antibody response 2 and 6 months postvaccination among NH residents. This finding is consistent with studies that observed an enhanced humoral response using a 2-dose SARS-CoV-2 regimen with extended intervals.[81–83] Considering the initial reduced immune response documented among this aging population,[36] it is thus interesting to note that an appropriate dosing interval, especially in convalescent elderly vaccinees, may overcome this initial diminished immune response to produce a robust response.[81]

CHALLENGES OF VACCINATION IN OLDER ADULTS
Vaccine Uptake Among Older Adults

Despite the difficulties in achieving adequate vaccine compliance,[84] older adults remain the target for vaccination policies.[5] Early in the pandemic, age was associated with a lower willingness to receive a COVID-19 vaccine in the United States.[85] However, there has been a dramatic turnaround in this trend with the older adult population accounting for the largest percentage of vaccinated individuals in the United States at the time of writing this review.[86]

Factors such as lower life expectancy, concerns about side effects, and efficacy historically influence vaccine uptake in this population. For COVID-19 vaccines, safety was the primary concern reported among unwilling older adults followed by doubts about their effectiveness and misinformation.[87] Notable misinformation included the belief of long-lasting immunity once infected with SARS-CoV-2, protection by certain blood group types, and erroneous belief of magnets or chips implanted in vaccines among others.[88] In a certain adult population aged 65 years and older in the United States, Nikolovski and colleagues[89] reported a significant unwillingness to receive the COVID-19 vaccines among female subjects and African American subjects. These subjects were, however, willing to discuss this uncertainty/unwillingness with their healthcare providers, suggesting an essential rolehealthcare providers may play in the battle against vaccine hesitancy.[90] In a community-based multidisciplinary study of more than 20,000 adults older than 60 years in Singapore, direct contact and clarity in communication using mutually understood languages as well as direct access and consultation with allergists were found to significantly increase the willingness of unvaccinated enrollees to receive the COVID-19 vaccine after a 3-month follow-up.[88]

Older adults who were willing to take the vaccine were likely to do so to protect themselves and others as well as contribute to ending the pandemic.[90] Furthermore, influenza vaccination or a willingness to receive the vaccine was strongly associated with a willingness to receive COVID-19 vaccines among older adults.[87] Thus, approaches that have been used in improving the uptake of influenza vaccines may be beneficial in increasing COVID-19 vaccine coverage among older adults.[91]

Reactogenicity in Older Adults

Generally, older adults tolerate vaccines better than younger adults.[11,92] Considering that reactions result from immune system activation, it is not so surprising that older adults do not have as many side effects from vaccines because they generate less robust responses.[12] In addition, reactions such as injection site pain, headache, and muscle pain may be more tolerable by older adults and as such, may be underreported among this age group.[93,94] Accordingly, the COVID-19 vaccines currently in use have all demonstrated good safety profiles among older adults with reactogenicity mostly mild to moderate.[63,95] For instance, there are fewer local and systemic reactions reported among older adults (aged $\geq$65 years) following the 2-dose mRNA-based COVID-19 vaccines compared with younger adults (aged <65 years).[96]

This reduced reactogenicity is consistent with findings among older adults who received the inactivated vaccines.[97] A third dose of the BNT162b2 mRNA vaccine had mild to moderate side effects among participants aged 65 to 85 years in the Pfizer trials, like that of the second dose with no unsolicited adverse event.[44] The Novavax trials reported a lower incidence of local and systemic reactions among participants older than 65 years compared with younger participants.[56] Owing to the negative relationship between age, reactogenicity, and immunogenicity, it has often been hypothesized that reactogenicity could be related to immunogenicity. Certain groups found somewhat modest relationships between these 2 immunologic phenomena concerning the COVID-19 vaccines,[93,98–100] whereas others did not observe any appreciable link between them.[33,101] Differences in the study setting, analytical model, and manner of soliciting for vaccine reactions may have contributed to the differences in these findings. Nevertheless, older adults are known to report fewer postvaccination side effects and achieve lower antibody production compared with younger adults. This association needs further exploration through larger studies.

PROPOSED STRATEGIES TO OPTIMIZE VACCINES FOR OLDER ADULTS

With the attendant reality of immunosenescence and inflammaging, a focused vaccine strategy that considers these immunologic effects could be helpful for older adults. A challenging feature of SARS-CoV-2 is its mutation ability leading to the production of more infectious and immune-escaping variants of concern. Although monovalent vaccines have some cross-variant activity,[102,103] the bivalent vaccines recently approved for use have shown better neutralizing capacities and could provide better protection against the immune-evasive Omicron family.[104] The initial bivalent vaccine approved by the European Union authorities adds the early Omicron BA1 strain to the Wuhan-containing current vaccine, and the version approved in the United States adds the more recent Omicron BA4/5. Chalkias and colleagues[105] studied the immunogenicity of the bivalent BA1 vaccine in a population that had 40% of subjects aged 65 years or older. The investigators found superior anti-omicron neutralization compared with the monovalent vaccine.[105] These data would suggest that the bivalent vaccine might be effective, but the clinical efficacy data of the bivalent vaccine are not yet available.

Overall, it is imperative that older adults are up to date with vaccinations because progressively significant benefits have been established with each extra dose administered in this age group.[106] In a study of NH residents and healthcare workers, the authors observed that a booster dose is needed to achieve significant Omicron neutralization activity among this population even if they had an infection before the Omicron era.[102] This observation is consistent with findings reported among younger adults.[103] In the current Omicron era, this is essential to protect this age group from the possible devastating effects of infection with the immune-escaping Omicron variants. This additional dose was also shown to reduce transmission among NH residents compared with the primary vaccine series alone.[107] Although the benefits of an extra dose on antibody levels abound among NH residents,[79] cellular immunity seems to be impacted to a lesser degree among this population.[108,109]

Like the timing of vaccination after infection with SARS-CoV-2 as discussed earlier, modifications in the intervals between doses may help boost vaccine-induced immunity. Older adults 80 years or older receiving the 2-dose BNT162b2 mRNA vaccine at an extended interval of 11 to 12 weeks were found to produce a peak antibody response 3.5 times those that received the standard regimen 3 weeks apart. However, peak cellular responses were lower[81]; this is similar to findings in a younger healthcare worker cohort receiving the BNT162b2 vaccine.[82] In like manner, an extended-interval protocol for the adenovirus-based ChAdOx1 vaccine has increased spike-specific antibody responses by 2.3-fold and improved VE across all age groups.[110] Although this carries the risk of extending the period of partial vaccination, a single dose of the BNT162b2 vaccine produces favorable immunogenicity and clinical efficacy[29,110–112] and is durable.[113] Thus, the timing of subsequent doses could be targeted appropriately using the half-life of vaccine-induced antibodies.

An initial 3-dose series could be considered in this setting where the vaccine is a neoantigen vaccine because it is not boosting prior immunity but rather must generate a response from naive cells. A 3-dose series could allow several benefits as observed by our data and those of others. One benefit is the increased breadth of response that particularly occurs with the third dose providing better anti-Omicron immunity. The other benefit is that the third dose boosted antibody levels among the hyporesponders to the primary series; this is a subset of the older multimorbid NH resident population that produced negligible or very low vaccine-induced antibodies similar to the levels observed in immunocompromised individuals. Previously, immunocompromised adults received a Centers for Disease Control and Prevention recommendation for a 3-dose series.[114] Thus, adopting a 3-dose vaccination schedule may be beneficial for this population of hyporesponders, and by extension, older adults; this would particularly apply to neoantigen vaccines. Alternatively, screening this population for possible hyporesponsiveness can help identify those who would need extra doses and thus, optimize protection for these adults.[109,115,116]

Moreover, heterologous boosting, which involves the administration of booster doses from a platform other than that of the primary series, has shown some effectiveness in enhancing protection against COVID-19. This strategy helps to maximize the quantity and breadth of vaccine-induced antibodies.[117–119] This carries the potential for antibody diversity owing to the subtle differences that have been described between the 2 mRNA vaccines currently in use[120] and even more, vaccines across different platforms.[35,121] In a large cohort study among veterans, the incidence of infection and moderate-to-severe disease was significantly reduced among those who had been primed with an adenoviral vaccine and were boosted with an mRNA vaccine compared with those who had homologous vaccination with either the adenoviral or mRNA vaccines.[122] More investigation is clearly needed in the older population to determine the optimal primary series, booster schedules, and booster vaccine products that could apply to both COVID-19 and new pathogen outbreaks.

SUMMARY

Vaccination remains a key tool in protecting older adults against severe outcomes of COVID-19. Thus, this population should remain of high priority for vaccination campaigns and must be kept up to date on additional doses for optimal protection. Vaccine protocols and formulations could be adapted to cater to the attendant immune changes in this population. Considering the high likelihood of hyporesponders to vaccination in this group, appropriate screening measures should be put in place. Finally, vaccination protocols should be tailored to maximize the benefits in this population and, with the robust benefits of a third dose among older adults, a 3-dose regimen with modified intervals should be considered, as well as heterologous boosting.

CLINICS CARE POINTS

- Due to the high risk of SARS-CoV-2 infection in the older population, they should remain a high priority for vaccination campaigns and must be kept up to date on additional doses for optimal protection.
- A 3-dose primary series enhances antibody production and breadth significantly providing better cross-variant protection and could be considered.
- Older adults who report no vaccine side effects and/or have never been infected with SARS-CoV-2 should be prioritized when screening for vaccine responsiveness.

ACKNOWLEDGEMENT

This work was supported by NIH AI129709-03S1, U01 CA260539-01, and CDC 200-2016-91773.

REFERENCES

1. COVID-19 nursing home data - centers for Medicare & Medicaid Services data. 2022. https://data.cms.gov/covid-19/covid-19-nursing-home-data. Accessed October 25, 2022.
2. Onder G, Rezza G, Brusaferro S. Case-fatality rate and characteristics of patients dying in relation to COVID-19 in Italy. JAMA 2020;323(18):1775–6.
3. Remelli F, Volpato S, Trevisan C. Clinical Features of SARS-CoV-2 Infection in Older Adults. Clin Geriatr Med 2022;38(3):483–500.
4. COVID-19 vaccination Program Operational Guidance | CDC. 2022. https://www.cdc.gov/vaccines/covid-19/covid19-vaccination-guidance.html. Accessed September 15, 2022.
5. Dooling K, McClung N, Chamberland M, et al. The Advisory Committee on Immunization Practices' Interim Recommendation for Allocating Initial Supplies of

COVID-19 Vaccine — United States, 2020. MMWR Morb Mortal Wkly Rep 2020; 69(49):1857–9.

6. Williams C, Al-Bargash D, MacAlintal C, et al. Coronavirus Disease 2019 (COVID-19) Outbreak Associated With Severe Acute Respiratory Syndrome Coronavirus 2 (SARS-CoV-2) P.1 Lineage in a Long-Term Care Home After Implementation of a Vaccination Program—Ontario, Canada, April–May 2021. Clin Infect Dis 2022;74(6):1085–8.

7. Lafuente-Lafuente C, Rainone A, Guérin O, et al. COVID-19 Outbreaks in Nursing Homes Despite Full Vaccination with BNT162b2 of a Majority of Residents. Gerontology 2022;1–9.

8. Weinberger B. Vaccines for the elderly: Current use and future challenges. Immun Ageing 2018;15(1):1–8.

9. Osterholm MT, Kelley NS, Sommer A, et al. Efficacy and effectiveness of influenza vaccines: A systematic review and meta-analysis. Lancet Infect Dis 2012;12(1):36–44.

10. Siegrist CA, Aspinall R. B-cell responses to vaccination at the extremes of age. Nat Rev Immunol 2009;9(3):185–94.

11. Ciabattini A, Nardini C, Santoro F, et al. Vaccination in the elderly: The challenge of immune changes with aging. Semin Immunol 2018;40:83–94.

12. Crooke SN, Ovsyannikova IG, Poland GA, et al. Immunosenescence and human vaccine immune responses. Immun Ageing 2019;16(1):1–16.

13. Pawelec G. Age and immunity: What is "immunosenescence". Exp Gerontol 2018;105:4–9.

14. Linton PJ, Dorshkind K. Age-related changes in lymphocyte development and function. Nat Immunol 2004;5(2):133–9.

15. Kirkland JL, Tchkonia T, Pirtskhalava T, et al. Adipogenesis and aging: does aging make fat go MAD? Exp Gerontol 2002;37(6):757–67.

16. Franceschi C, Garagnani P, Parini P, et al. Inflammaging: a new immune–metabolic viewpoint for age-related diseases. Nat Rev Endocrinol 2018; 14(10):576–90.

17. Frasca D, Diaz A, Romero M, et al. High TNF-α levels in resting B cells negatively correlate with their response. Exp Gerontol 2014;54:116–22.

18. McElhaney JE, Kuchel GA, Zhou X, et al. T-cell immunity to influenza in older adults: A pathophysiological framework for development of more effective vaccines. Front Immunol 2016;7(FEB):41.

19. Bergman H, Ferrucci L, Guralnik J, et al. Frailty: An Emerging Research and Clinical Paradigm—Issues and Controversies. Journals Gerontol Ser A 2007; 62(7):731–7.

20. Strandberg TE, Pitkälä KH. Frailty in elderly people. Lancet 2007;369(9570): 1328–9.

21. Fried LP, Ferrucci L, Darer J, et al. Untangling the Concepts of Disability, Frailty, and Comorbidity: Implications for Improved Targeting and Care. Journals Gerontol Ser A 2004;59(3):M255–63.

22. Rockwood K, Song X, MacKnight C, et al. A global clinical measure of fitness and frailty in elderly people. CMAJ 2005;173(5):489–95.

23. Earle KA, Ambrosino DM, Fiore-Gartland A, et al. Evidence for antibody as a protective correlate for COVID-19 vaccines. Vaccine 2021;39(32):4423–8.

24. Khoury DS, Cromer D, Reynaldi A, et al. Neutralizing antibody levels are highly predictive of immune protection from symptomatic SARS-CoV-2 infection. Nat Med 2021;27(7):1205–11.

25. Krammer F. Correlates of protection from SARS-CoV-2 infection. Lancet 2021; 397(10283):1421–3.
26. Asamoah-Boaheng M, Goldfarb DM, Karim ME, et al. The Relationship Between Anti-Spike SARS-CoV-2 Antibody Levels and Risk of Breakthrough COVID-19 Among Fully Vaccinated Adults. J Infect Dis 2022. https://doi.org/10.1093/INFDIS/JIAC403. In press.
27. Plotkin SA. Correlates of Protection Induced by Vaccination. Clin Vaccin Immunol 2010;17(7):1055–65.
28. WHO – COVID19 Vaccine Tracker. https://covid19.trackvaccines.org/agency/who/. Accessed October 20, 2022.
29. Bernal JL, Andrews N, Gower C, et al. Effectiveness of the Pfizer-BioNTech and Oxford-AstraZeneca vaccines on covid-19 related symptoms, hospital admissions, and mortality in older adults in England: test negative case-control study. BMJ 2021;373. https://doi.org/10.1136/BMJ.N1088.
30. Semelka CT, Partnership C-19 CR, DeWitt ME, et al. Frailty and COVID-19 mRNA Vaccine Antibody Response in the COVID-19 Community Research Partnership. Journals Gerontol Ser A 2022;77(7):1366–70.
31. Dyer AH, Noonan C, McElheron M, et al. Previous SARS-CoV-2 Infection, Age, and Frailty Are Associated With 6-Month Vaccine-Induced Anti-Spike Antibody Titer in Nursing Home Residents. J Am Med Dir Assoc 2022;23(3):434–9.
32. Søgaard OS, Reekie J, Johansen IS, et al. Characteristics associated with serological COVID-19 vaccine response and durability in an older population with significant comorbidity: the Danish Nationwide ENFORCE Study. Clin Microbiol Infect 2022;28(8):1126–33.
33. Müller L, Andrée M, Moskorz W, et al. Age-dependent immune response to the Biontech/Pfizer BNT162b2 COVID-19 vaccination. Clin Infect Dis 2021;73(11): 2065–72. https://doi.org/10.1101/2021.03.03.21251066.
34. Canaday DH, Oyebanji OA, Keresztesy D, et al. Significant Reduction in Vaccine-Induced Antibody Levels and Neutralization Activity Among Healthcare Workers and Nursing Home Residents 6 Months Following Coronavirus Disease 2019 BNT162b2 mRNA Vaccination. Clin Infect Dis 2022;75(1):e884–7.
35. Medeiros GX, Sasahara GL, Magawa JY, et al. Reduced T cell and antibody responses to inactivated coronavirus vaccine among individuals above 55 years old. Front Immunol 2022;13:666.
36. Canaday DH, Carias L, Oyebanji OA, et al. Reduced BNT162b2 Messenger RNA Vaccine Response in Severe Acute Respiratory Syndrome Coronavirus 2 (SARS-CoV-2)–Naive Nursing Home Residents. Clin Infect Dis 2021;73(11): 2112–5.
37. Kleina SL, Marriott I, Fish EN. Sex-based differences in immune function and responses to vaccination. Trans R Soc Trop Med Hyg 2015;109(1):9–15.
38. Voigt EA, Ovsyannikova IG, Kennedy RB, et al. Sex differences in older adults' immune responses to seasonal influenza vaccination. Front Immunol 2019; 10:180.
39. Logunov DY, Dolzhikova IV, Zubkova OV, et al. Safety and immunogenicity of an rAd26 and rAd5 vector-based heterologous prime-boost COVID-19 vaccine in two formulations: two open, non-randomised phase 1/2 studies from Russia. Lancet 2020;396(10255):887–97.
40. Jabal KA, Ben-Amram H, Beiruti K, et al. Impact of age, ethnicity, sex and prior infection status on immunogenicity following a single dose of the BNT162b2 MRNA COVID-19 vaccine: Real-world evidence from healthcare workers, Israel, December 2020 to January 2021. Eurosurveillance 2021;26(6):2100096.

41. Rapaka RR, Hammershaimb EA, Neuzil KM. Are Some COVID-19 Vaccines Better Than Others? Interpreting and Comparing Estimates of Efficacy in Vaccine Trials. Clin Infect Dis 2022;74(2):352–8.

42. Walsh EE, Frenck RW, Falsey AR, et al. Safety and Immunogenicity of Two RNA-Based Covid-19 Vaccine Candidates. N Engl J Med 2020;383(25):2439–50.

43. Polack FP, Thomas SJ, Kitchin N, et al. Safety and Efficacy of the BNT162b2 mRNA Covid-19 Vaccine. N Engl J Med 2020;383(27):2603–15.

44. Falsey AR, Frenck RW, Walsh EE, et al. SARS-CoV-2 Neutralization with BNT162b2 Vaccine Dose 3. N Engl J Med 2021;385(17):1627–9.

45. Anderson EJ, Rouphael NG, Widge AT, et al. Safety and Immunogenicity of SARS-CoV-2 mRNA-1273 Vaccine in Older Adults. N Engl J Med 2020; 383(25):2427–38.

46. Jackson LA, Anderson EJ, Rouphael NG, et al. An mRNA Vaccine against SARS-CoV-2 — Preliminary Report. N Engl J Med 2020;383(20):1920–31.

47. Baden LR, Sahly HM El, Essink B, et al. Efficacy and Safety of the mRNA-1273 SARS-CoV-2 Vaccine. N Engl J Med 2021;384(5):403–16.

48. Mor V, Gutman R, Yang X, et al. Short-term impact of nursing home SARS-CoV-2 vaccinations on new infections, hospitalizations, and deaths. J Am Geriatr Soc 2021;69(8):2063 9.

49. Muhsen K, Maimon N, Mizrahi AY, et al. Association of Receipt of the Fourth BNT162b2 Dose With Omicron Infection and COVID-19 Hospitalizations Among Residents of Long-term Care Facilities. JAMA Intern Med 2022;182(8):859–67.

50. Muhsen K, Maimon N, Mizrahi A, et al. Effects of BNT162b2 Covid-19 Vaccine Booster in Long-Term Care Facilities in Israel. N Engl J Med 2022;386(4): 399–401.

51. McConeghy KW, White EM, Blackman C, et al. Effectiveness of a Second COVID-19 Vaccine Booster Dose Against Infection, Hospitalization, or Death Among Nursing Home Residents — 19 States, March 29–July 25, 2022. MMWR Morb Mortal Wkly Rep 2022;71(39):1235–8.

52. Grewal R, Kitchen SA, Nguyen L, et al. Effectiveness of a fourth dose of covid-19 mRNA vaccine against the omicron variant among long term care residents in Ontario, Canada: test negative design study. BMJ 2022;378. https://doi.org/ 10.1136/BMJ-2022-071502.

53. Demaret J, Corroyer-Simovic B, Alidjinou EK, et al. Impaired Functional T-Cell Response to SARS-CoV-2 After Two Doses of BNT162b2 mRNA Vaccine in Older People. Front Immunol 2021;12:4639.

54. Palacios-Pedrero MÁ, Jansen JM, Blume C, et al. Signs of immunosenescence correlate with poor outcome of mRNA COVID-19 vaccination in older adults. Nat Aging 2022;2(10):896–905.

55. Vitallé J, Pérez-Gómez A, Ostos FJ, et al. Immune defects associated with lower SARS-CoV-2 BNT162b2 mRNA vaccine response in aged people. JCI Insight 2022;7(17). https://doi.org/10.1172/JCI.INSIGHT.161045.

56. Heath PT, Galiza EP, Baxter DN, et al. Safety and Efficacy of NVX-CoV2373 Covid-19 Vaccine. N Engl J Med 2021;385(13):1172–83.

57. Dunkle LM, Kotloff KL, Gay CL, et al. Efficacy and Safety of NVX-CoV2373 in Adults in the United States and Mexico. N Engl J Med 2022;386(6):531–43.

58. Mallory RM, Formica N, Pfeiffer S, et al. Safety and immunogenicity following a homologous booster dose of a SARS-CoV-2 recombinant spike protein vaccine (NVX-CoV2373): a secondary analysis of a randomised, placebo-controlled, phase 2 trial. Lancet Infect Dis 2022;22(11):1565–76.

59. Sadoff J, Gray G, Vandebosch A, et al. Safety and Efficacy of Single-Dose Ad26.COV2.S Vaccine against Covid-19. N Engl J Med 2021;384(23):2187–201.

60. Sadoff J, Gray G, Vandebosch A, et al. Final Analysis of Efficacy and Safety of Single-Dose Ad26.COV2.S. N Engl J Med 2022;386(9):847–60.

61. Hardt K, Vandebosch A, Sadoff J, et al. Efficacy, safety, and immunogenicity of a booster regimen of Ad26.COV2.S vaccine against COVID-19 (ENSEMBLE2): results of a randomised, double-blind, placebo-controlled, phase 3 trial. Lancet Infect Dis 2022;0(0). https://doi.org/10.1016/s1473-3099(22)00506-0.

62. Coronavirus (COVID-19) Update: FDA Limits Use of Janssen COVID-19 vaccine to certain individuals | FDA. 2022. https://www.fda.gov/news-events/press-announcements/coronavirus-covid-19-update-fda-limits-use-janssen-covid-19-vaccine-certain-individuals. Accessed October 20, 2022.

63. Ramasamy MN, Minassian AM, Ewer KJ, et al. Safety and immunogenicity of ChAdOx1 nCoV-19 vaccine administered in a prime-boost regimen in young and old adults (COV002): a single-blind, randomised, controlled, phase 2/3 trial. Lancet 2020;396(10267):1979–93.

64. Falsey AR, Sobieszczyk ME, Hirsch I, et al. Phase 3 Safety and Efficacy of AZD1222 (ChAdOx1 nCoV-19) Covid-19 Vaccine. N Engl J Med 2021; 385(25):2348–60.

65. Munro APS, Janani L, Cornelius V, et al. Safety and immunogenicity of seven COVID-19 vaccines as a third dose (booster) following two doses of ChAdOx1 nCov-19 or BNT162b2 in the UK (COV-BOOST): a blinded, multicentre, randomised, controlled, phase 2 trial. Lancet 2021;398(10318):2258–76.

66. Webster P. Russian COVID-19 vaccine in jeopardy after Ukraine invasion. Nat Med 2022. https://doi.org/10.1038/d41591-022-00042-y. Accessed September 20, 2022.

67. Logunov DY, Dolzhikova IV, Shcheblyakov DV, et al. Safety and efficacy of an rAd26 and rAd5 vector-based heterologous prime-boost COVID-19 vaccine: an interim analysis of a randomised controlled phase 3 trial in Russia. Lancet 2021;397(10275):671–81.

68. Wu Z, Hu Y, Xu M, et al. Safety, tolerability, and immunogenicity of an inactivated SARS-CoV-2 vaccine (CoronaVac) in healthy adults aged 60 years and older: a randomised, double-blind, placebo-controlled, phase 1/2 clinical trial. Lancet Infect Dis 2021;21(6):803–12.

69. Zhang Y, Zeng G, Pan H, et al. Safety, tolerability, and immunogenicity of an inactivated SARS-CoV-2 vaccine in healthy adults aged 18–59 years: a randomised, double-blind, placebo-controlled, phase 1/2 clinical trial. Lancet Infect Dis 2021;21(2):181–92.

70. Ranzani OT, Hitchings MDT, Dorion M, et al. Effectiveness of the CoronaVac vaccine in older adults during a gamma variant associated epidemic of covid-19 in Brazil: test negative case-control study. BMJ 2021;374:2015.

71. Xin Q, Wu Q, Chen X, et al. Six-month follow-up of a booster dose of CoronaVac in two single-centre phase 2 clinical trials. Nat Commun 2022;13(1):1–7.

72. Ella R, Vadrevu KM, Jogdand H, et al. Safety and immunogenicity of an inactivated SARS-CoV-2 vaccine, BBV152: a double-blind, randomised, phase 1 trial. Lancet Infect Dis 2021;21(5):637–46.

73. Ella R, Reddy S, Blackwelder W, et al. Efficacy, safety, and lot-to-lot immunogenicity of an inactivated SARS-CoV-2 vaccine (BBV152): interim results of a randomised, double-blind, controlled, phase 3 trial. Lancet 2021;398(10317): 2173–84.

74. Hui DS. Hybrid immunity and strategies for COVID-19 vaccination. Lancet Infect Dis 2022;0(0). https://doi.org/10.1016/s1473-3099(22)00640-5.

75. Carazo S, Skowronski DM, Brisson M, et al. Protection against omicron (B.1.1.529) BA.2 reinfection conferred by primary omicron BA.1 or pre-omicron SARS-CoV-2 infection among health-care workers with and without mRNA vaccination: a test-negative case-control study. Lancet Infect Dis 2022; 0(0). https://doi.org/10.1016/s1473-3099(22)00578-3.

76. Malato J, Ribeiro RM, Leite PP, et al. Risk of BA.5 Infection among Persons Exposed to Previous SARS-CoV-2 Variants. N Engl J Med 2022;387(10):953–4.

77. Crotty S. Hybrid immunity. Science (80-) 2021;372(6549):1392–3.

78. Katz MJ, Heaney CD, Pisanic N, et al. Evaluating immunity to SARS-CoV-2 in nursing home residents using saliva IgG. J Am Geriatr Soc 2022;70(3):659–68.

79. Vanshylla K, Tober-Lau P, Gruell H, et al. Durability of omicron-neutralising serum activity after mRNA booster immunisation in older adults. Lancet Infect Dis 2022;22(4):445–6.

80. Fedele G, Palmieri A, Damiano C, et al. Humoral immunity induced by mRNA COVID-19 vaccines in Nursing Home Residents previously infected with SARS-CoV-2. Aging Clin Exp Res 2022;1–8.

81. Parry H, Bruton R, Stephens C, et al. Extended interval BNT162b2 vaccination enhances peak antibody generation. npj Vaccin 2022;7(1):1–5.

82. Payne RP, Longet S, Austin JA, et al. Immunogenicity of standard and extended dosing intervals of BNT162b2 mRNA vaccine. Cell 2021;184(23):5699–714.e11.

83. Tauzin A, Gong SY, Beaudoin-Bussières G, et al. Strong humoral immune responses against SARS-CoV-2 Spike after BNT162b2 mRNA vaccination with a 16-week interval between doses. Cell Host Microbe 2022;30(1):97–109.e5.

84. Bridges CB, Hurley LP, Williams WW, et al. Meeting the Challenges of Immunizing Adults. Vaccine 2015;33:D114–20.

85. Kreps S, Prasad S, Brownstein JS, et al. Factors Associated With US Adults' Likelihood of Accepting COVID-19 Vaccination. JAMA Netw Open 2020;3(10): e2025594.

86. COVID-19 vaccination coverage and vaccine Confidence among adults | CDC. 2021. https://www.cdc.gov/vaccines/imz-managers/coverage/covidvaxview/ interactive/adults.html. Accessed September 15, 2022.

87. Basta NE, Sohel N, Sulis G, et al. Factors Associated With Willingness to Receive a COVID-19 Vaccine Among 23,819 Adults Aged 50 Years or Older: An Analysis of the Canadian Longitudinal Study on Aging. Am J Epidemiol 2022;191(6):987–98.

88. Moosa AS, Wee YMS, Jaw MH, et al. A multidisciplinary effort to increase COVID-19 vaccination among the older adults. Front Public Heal 2022;10:2526.

89. Nikolovski J, Koldijk M, Weverling GJ, et al. Factors indicating intention to vaccinate with a COVID-19 vaccine among older U.S. adults. PLoS One 2021;16(5): e0251963.

90. Nichol KL, Zimmerman R. Generalist and Subspecialist Physicians' Knowledge, Attitudes, and Practices Regarding Influenza and Pneumococcal Vaccinations for Elderly and Other High-Risk Patients: A Nationwide Survey. Arch Intern Med 2001;161(22):2702–8.

91. Malosh R, Ohmit SE, Petrie JG, et al. Factors associated with influenza vaccine receipt in community dwelling adults and their children. Vaccine 2014;32(16): 1841–7.

92. Hervé C, Laupèze B, Giudice G Del, et al. The how's and what's of vaccine reactogenicity. NPJ Vaccin 2019;4(1):1–11.

93. Oyebanji OA, Wilson B, Keresztesy D, et al. Does a lack of vaccine side effects correlate with reduced BNT162b2 mRNA vaccine response among healthcare workers and nursing home residents? Aging Clin Exp Res 2021;33(11):3151–60.

94. King A, Daniels J, Lim J, et al. Time to listen: a review of methods to solicit patient reports of adverse events. BMJ Qual Saf 2010;19(2):148–57.

95. Mathioudakis AG, Ghrew M, Ustianowski A, et al. Self-Reported Real-World Safety and Reactogenicity of COVID-19 Vaccines: A Vaccine Recipient Survey. Life 2021;11(3):249.

96. Chapin-Bardales J, Gee J, Myers T. Reactogenicity following Receipt of mRNA-Based COVID-19 Vaccines. JAMA - J Am Med Assoc 2021;325(21):2201–2. https://doi.org/10.1001/jama.2021.5374.

97. Wan EYF, Wang Y, Chui CSL, et al. Safety of an inactivated, whole-virion COVID-19 vaccine (CoronaVac) in people aged 60 years or older in Hong Kong: a modified self-controlled case series. Lancet Heal Longev 2022;3(7):e491–500.

98. Braun E, Horowitz NA, Leiba R, et al. Association between IgG antibody levels and adverse events after first and second Bnt162b2 mRNA vaccine doses. Clin Microbiol Infect 2022;0(0). https://doi.org/10.1016/j.cmi.2022.07.002.

99. Hermann EA, Lee B, Balte PP, et al. Association of Symptoms After COVID-19 Vaccination With Anti–SARS-CoV-2 Antibody Response in the Framingham Heart Study. JAMA Netw Open 2022;5(10):e2237908.

100. Held J, Esse J, Tascilar K, et al. Reactogenicity Correlates Only Weakly with Humoral Immunogenicity after COVID-19 Vaccination with BNT162b2 mRNA (Comirnaty®). Vaccines 2021;9(10):1063.

101. Hwang YH, Song KH, Choi Y, et al. Can reactogenicity predict immunogenicity after COVID-19 vaccination? Korean J Intern Med 2021;36(6):1486–91.

102. Canaday DH, Oyebanji OA, White E, et al. COVID-19 vaccine booster dose needed to achieve Omicron-specific neutralisation in nursing home residents. eBioMedicine 2022;80. https://doi.org/10.1016/j.ebiom.2022.104066.

103. Garcia-Beltran WF, Denis KJ St, Hoelzemer A, et al. mRNA-based COVID-19 vaccine boosters induce neutralizing immunity against SARS-CoV-2 Omicron variant. Cell 2022;185(3):457–66.e4.

104. Chalkias S, Harper C, Vrbicky K, et al. A Bivalent Omicron-Containing Booster Vaccine against Covid-19. N Engl J Med 2022;387(14):1279–91. https://doi.org/10.1056/NEJMOA2208343.

105. Chalkias S, Eder F, Essink B, et al. Safety, immunogenicity and antibody Persistence of a bivalent Beta-containing booster vaccine. Nat Med 2022. https://doi.org/10.21203/RS.3.RS-1555201/V1.

106. Blain H, Tuaillon E, Gamon L, et al. Strong Decay of SARS-CoV-2 Spike Antibodies after 2 BNT162b2 Vaccine Doses and High Antibody Response to a Third Dose in Nursing Home Residents. J Am Med Dir Assoc 2022;23(5):750–3.

107. Prasad N, Derado G, Nanduri SA, et al. Effectiveness of a COVID-19 Additional Primary or Booster Vaccine Dose in Preventing SARS-CoV-2 Infection Among Nursing Home Residents During Widespread Circulation of the Omicron Variant — United States, February 14–March 27, 2022. MMWR Morb Mortal Wkly Rep 2022;71(18):633–7.

108. Giménez E, Albert E, Zulaica J, et al. Severe Acute Respiratory Syndrome Coronavirus 2 Adaptive Immunity in Nursing Home Residents Following a Third Dose of the Comirnaty Coronavirus Disease 2019 Vaccine. Clin Infect Dis 2022;75(1):e865–8.

109. Praet JT Van, Vandecasteele S, Roo A De, et al. Dynamics of the Cellular and Humoral Immune Response After BNT162b2 Messenger Ribonucleic Acid

Coronavirus Disease 2019 (COVID-19) Vaccination in COVID-19-Naive Nursing Home Residents. J Infect Dis 2021;224(10):1690–3.

110. Voysey M, Clemens SAC, Madhi SA, et al. Single-dose administration and the influence of the timing of the booster dose on immunogenicity and efficacy of ChAdOx1 nCoV-19 (AZD1222) vaccine: a pooled analysis of four randomised trials. Lancet 2021;397(10277):881–91.

111. Hall VJ, Foulkes S, Saei A, et al. COVID-19 vaccine coverage in health-care workers in England and effectiveness of BNT162b2 mRNA vaccine against infection (SIREN): a prospective, multicentre, cohort study. Lancet 2021; 397(10286):1725–35.

112. Skowronski DM, De Serres G. Safety and Efficacy of the BNT162b2 mRNA Covid-19 Vaccine. N Engl J Med 2021;384(16):1576–8.

113. Doria-Rose N, Suthar MS, Makowski M, et al. Antibody Persistence through 6 Months after the Second Dose of mRNA-1273 Vaccine for Covid-19. N Engl J Med 2021;384(23):2259–61.

114. Clinical Guidance for COVID-19 vaccination | CDC. 2022. https://www.cdc.gov/vaccines/covid-19/clinical-considerations/interim-considerations-us.html. Accessed October 25, 2022.

115. Witkowski W, Gerlo S, Smet E De, et al. Humoral and Cellular Responses to COVID-19 Vaccination Indicate the Need for Post-Vaccination Testing in Frail Population. Vaccines 2022;10(2):260. *Page 260.*

116. Castro MC, Singer B. Prioritizing COVID-19 vaccination by age. Proc Natl Acad Sci U S A 2021;118(15):e2103700118.

117. Mok CKP, Chen C, Yiu K, et al. A Randomized Clinical Trial Using CoronaVac or BNT162b2 Vaccine as a Third Dose in Adults Vaccinated with Two Doses of CoronaVac. Am J Respir Crit Care Med 2022;205(7):844–7.

118. Cheng SMS, Mok CKP, Leung YWY, et al. Neutralizing antibodies against the SARS-CoV-2 Omicron variant BA.1 following homologous and heterologous CoronaVac or BNT162b2 vaccination. Nat Med 2022;28(3):486–9.

119. Takano T, Sato T, Kotaki R, et al. Heterologous booster immunization with SARS-CoV-2 spike protein after mRNA vaccine elicits durable and broad antibody responses. Research Square 2022. https://doi.org/10.21203/RS.3.RS-2014078/V1.

120. Kaplonek P, Cizmeci D, Fischinger S, et al. mRNA-1273 and BNT162b2 COVID-19 vaccines elicit antibodies with differences in Fc-mediated effector functions. Sci Transl Med 2022;14(645):2311.

121. Clemens SAC, Weckx L, Clemens R, et al. Heterologous versus homologous COVID-19 booster vaccination in previous recipients of two doses of CoronaVac COVID-19 vaccine in Brazil (RHH-001): a phase 4, non-inferiority, single blind, randomised study. Lancet 2022;399(10324):521–9.

122. Mayr FB, Talisa VB, Shaikh O, et al. Effectiveness of Homologous or Heterologous Covid-19 Boosters in Veterans. N Engl J Med 2022;386(14):1375–7.

Sexually Transmitted Infections in Older Adults

Increasing Tide and How to Stem It

Puja Van Epps, MD[a,*], Lewis Musoke, MD[b,c],
Candice J. McNeil, MD, MPH[d]

KEYWORDS

- Sexually transmitted infections • Older adults • Prevention • Sexual health

KEY POINTS

- As the general population, sexually transmitted infections (STIs) are increasing in older adults.
- Sexuality remains a key part of a healthy adult life; all the while factors related to aging may make older adults especially vulnerable to STIs.
- Barriers may make older adults uniquely disadvantaged when it comes to addressing their sexual health.
- Combination prevention remains the cornerstone to decreasing STIs in older adults.
- There are unique challenges when it comes to treatment of STIs in older adults.

INTRODUCTION

Over the past decade, there has been an alarming increase in sexually transmitted infections (STIs) among all age groups in the United States (US), reaching meteoric proportions in the last few years. In 2019, according to the US Centers for Disease Control and Prevention (CDC), there were more than 2.5 million reported cases of chlamydia, gonorrhea, and syphilis alone, reaching record highs for a sixth consecutive year.[1] Although the increase in STIs is not as dramatic as their younger counterparts, older adults have not been spared of this troubling trend. Surveillance data reported through

[a] Division of Infectious Diseases, Geriatric Research Education and Clinical Center, VA Northeast Ohio Healthcare System, Louis Stokes Cleveland VA Medical Center, 10701 East Boulevard, Cleveland, OH, USA; [b] Division of Infectious Diseases, Geriatric Research Education and Clinical Center, VA Northeast Ohio Healthcare System; [c] Division of Infectious Diseases, Department of Medicine, University Hospitals Cleveland Medical Center, Cleveland, OH, USA; [d] Department of Internal Medicine, Section on Infectious Diseases, Wake Forest School of Medicine, Medical Center Boulevard, Winston-Salem, NC 27157, USA
* Corresponding author. VA Northeast Ohio Healthcare System, Louis Stokes Cleveland VA Medical Center, 10701 East Boulevard, Cleveland, OH.
E-mail address: puja.vanepps@va.gov

Infect Dis Clin N Am 37 (2023) 47–63
https://doi.org/10.1016/j.idc.2022.11.003
0891-5520/23/Published by Elsevier Inc.

id.theclinics.com

the CDC Atlas Plus system comparing STI rates between 2009 and 2019 lay bare this phenomenon, with data showing a 5-fold increase in rates of syphilis and more than a 2-fold increase in gonorrhea and chlamydia rates in persons older than 65 years.[2] Similar to other age groups, older Black men and women have borne a disproportionate burden of STIs. For example, in 2019 although Black men and women made up only 9% of the US population older than 65 years, they represented more than 28% of syphilis and gonorrhea cases in this age group older than 65 years.[2] Even when we consider human immunodeficiency virus (HIV), an STI where rates have been consistently declining, older adults remain an important constituency, both in terms of incidence and prevalence.[3] Although STI incidence and prevalence are much lower in older adults compared with younger individuals, these trends and inequities remain of concern.

Yet, when it comes to sexual health of older adults, there remains a mismatch between these epidemiologic realities and perceptions among health care providers (HCPs) and general public alike. Although notable proportions of older adults remain sexually active, sexual health of older adults is deprioritized in the health care system and public health policies.[4–6] Here in, the authors explore specific STI epidemiologic trends in older adults and examine the intersection of sexuality and aging; within the context of barriers and facilitators, they provide a roadmap for clinicians to address sexual health in this population.

EPIDEMIOLOGY OF SEXUALLY TRANSMITTED INFECTIONS IN OLDER ADULTS

Chlamydia, the most commonly reported bacterial STI in the US, saw 1,579,885 (494.7 cases per 100,000) cases in 2020 with more than two-thirds of cases in adolescents and young adults and disproportionate representation in Black persons.[2] In 2020, less than 1% of chlamydia cases were reported in older persons predominantly occurring in men. In 2020, a total of 677,769 (206.5 cases per 100,000) cases of gonorrhea were reported in the US, representing a 111% increase since an all-time low in 2009.[2] Approximately 2.5% of these cases were among older persons, whereas most cases were among young adults and adolescents in 2020. Disproportionally, the burden of gonorrhea in the US has been among Black men. However, reviewing reported cases by age and race/ethnicity, older Black and non-Hispanic White men of this age group have similar case numbers.[2]

Cases of all stages of syphilis increased in 2020 and were reported at 133,945 (40.8 cases per 100,000).[2] Primary and secondary (P&S) syphilis, the most infectious stage of this disease, saw the highest reported cases since its historic low in the early 2000s with 41,655 (12.7 cases per 100,000 population) cases in 2020.[2] Approximately 7% of P&S syphilis cases in 2020 were among older persons. Notably, most of these cases were among men, with similar case numbers among those identifying as Black and non-Hispanic White. Gay, bisexual, and other men who have sex with men (MSM) comprised more than half (53%) of all cases of P&S syphilis in older adults.[2]

Although the annual number of new HIV diagnoses in the US went from approximately 44,000 in 2009 to a little more than 37,000 in 2018, representing a 16% decline over a decade, the numbers of new diagnoses in those older than 55 years have remained largely flat over this period.[7] In 2018, persons older than 50 years accounted for 17% of the new HIV diagnoses in the US, representing approximately 1 in 6 of those who received an HIV diagnosis.[3] Furthermore, largely due to the success of antiretroviral therapy (ART), persons older than 50 years now represent more than half of all people with HIV (PWH) in the US. Lastly, the many inequities that have perpetuated over the last 40 years of the HIV epidemic across all age groups remain relevant in older adults as well. Illustrating that point is this alarming statistic: Black men older than 55 years represent nearly 1 in 2 new HIV diagnosis in this age group.[2] In 2020 there were 30,635 new diagnoses of HIV in the US reported in adolescents and adults, showing a decrease in the number of cases from the prior reporting year; however, this should be interpreted with caution due to disruptions in services and surveillance activities in the setting of the COVID-19 pandemic.[8] Racial/ethnic disparities persisted, in that Black persons had an HIV diagnosis rate 8.1 times as high as White persons did.[8] MSM age 55 years and older were the only age group with increased (5%) diagnoses of HIV noted.

Other infections affecting aging persons include herpes simplex virus (HSV) and *Trichomonas vaginalis*, both of which serve as risk factors for HIV acquisition and transmission.[9] HSV-1 and HSV-2 are common viral infections that can be associated with genital herpes. Because HSV is a lifelong infection, prevalence increases with age; however, seroprevalence data are only available for people younger than 50 years with an estimated half a billion people worldwide reported to be infected with HSV-1 or HSV-2.[10] *T vaginalis* is the most prevalent non-viral STI worldwide. *T vaginalis* is not a reportable disease, and routine screening recommendations do not exist outside of those for women living with HIV.[9] As such, data on *T vaginalis* infections in older adults are not available.

Epidemiologic data for acute viral hepatitis B (HBV), hepatitis C (HCV), and hepatitis A (HAV) are available through 2019.[2] Although not the primary mode of transmission, HCV can be sexually transmitted.[11] There have been several HCV outbreaks reported among MSM and PWH sexual networks over the last few years, highlighting the role of sexual transmission.[12,13] Rates of acute HCV have been increasing over the past few years with more than 4000 cases reported in 2019; nearly 600 of those were in people older than 55 years. On the other hand, rates of acute HBV have been essentially stable in the general population over the last decade except for adults older than 55 years in whom cases have been steadily increasing since 2015, with this group making up greater than 20% of all reported cases of acute HBV in 2019 (700 out of 3192).[2] Acute HAV was in decline in the US until 2017 when a sharp increase occurred in 2018, a pattern that was mimicked in people older than 55 years, with about 15% (2854) of all cases reported in this age group.[2] Epidemiologic studies have demonstrated that this increase may be linked to sexual transmission of HAV, particularly in MSM networks.[14,15] Lastly, although HPV is the most prevalent STI in the US making nearly all sexually active individuals vulnerable to exposure, surveillance data are largely only available for individuals younger than 65 years.[16] In older adults, lower rates of oncogenic strains of HPV have been reported compared with their younger counterparts; however, the incidence of HPV-associated oropharyngeal squamous cell carcinoma is increasing among older adults.[17] It is not clear though whether this is related to HPV reactivation in older adults or improved prognosis.

In review, STI epidemiologic trends among older adults largely mirror those seen in younger individuals underscoring the need to address sexual health in this population.

SEXUALITY AND AGING: FACTS VERSUS FICTION

One of the most pervasive societal myths is that older adults are asexual beings. Sexuality is a basic human need, and although normal aging results in an overall waning in physiological sexual response, many older adults continue to enjoy sex as they age. In this section, the authors discuss changes in sexuality as people age and explore factors associated with aging that may affect sexuality.

Frequency of Sexual Activity

Although it is true that there is decline in frequency of sexual activity in later decades of life, the decrease is not as much as is generally believed. According to the National Social Life, Health, and Aging Project (NSHAP), a landmark cohort study of more than 3000 men and women in the US aged 57 years and older, greater than 75% of adults between the ages of 57 and 65 years reported being sexually active. Sexual activity was reported in about half in the 65 to 74 years age range and about a quarter of adults older than 75 years.[5] Older men were more likely to be sexually active than women. NSHAP has also reported on sexuality in older adults with neurocognitive decline. In a survey of more than 3000 community-dwelling adults between the ages of 62 and 91 years with cognitive impairment, 46% of men and 18% of women reported sexual activity at least once a month.[18] Whereas among partnered persons, rates of sexual activity were even higher with 59% of men and 51% of women reporting sexual activity, including 41% of those older than 80 years. Another prevailing myth is that older adults in long-term care facilities (LTCF) are not sexually active. Although it is true that LTCF residents are much less likely to be sexually active than their peers in the community, some remain sexually active. Qualitative studies examining sexual expression in LTCFs have identified several barriers to sexuality in these settings. These barriers include poor health, cognitive decline, sexual dysfunction, disinterest, lack of privacy, and LCTF staff attitudes and policies.[19–21] Lesbian, gay, bisexual, transgender, queer (LGBTQ) older adults who reside in LTCFs face yet additional roadblocks related to stigma and negative views of staff surrounding same sex intimacy.[22] A focus group of 16 gay and bisexual LTCF residents reported that sexual expression may result in rejection by HCPs, aids, and fellow residents.[23] These fears may not be unfounded with data showing that LTCF staff view same sex sexual expression much more negatively than heterosexual sex.[24]

Physiologic Changes and Sexual Disorders

Beyond societal barriers, there are physiologic changes that also contribute to decline in sexuality in aging. Increasing comorbidities, cognitive decline, and lack of desire all play a role in this drop.[25] In women, onset of menopause is the formative change affecting sexuality in later decades. With menopause there are many physiologic changes that result in reduced sexual desire and activity: vaginal atrophy and dryness, decline in sensitivity of sex organs, decrease in libido, and pain during intercourse.[26] Men, on the other hand, experience gradual physiological changes, primarily related to decline in testosterone levels.[27] Although sexual desire remains largely stable in men as they age, sexual function such as erection and ejaculation are negatively affected. As testosterone levels decline, men can experience other adverse effects such as decrease in libido, loss of energy, and muscle and bone loss that can all contribute to decrease in sexual activity.[28]

Besides normal physiologic changes that occur with aging, older adults are also likely to experience sexual dysfunction. Several factors such as comorbid medical, or mental health conditions, medication adverse effects, and psychosocial issues may play a synergistic role in either triggering or exacerbating sexual dysfunction in older adults.[29–31] A myriad of sexual disorders such as sexual arousal disorder and genitopelvic pain can affect older women, with prevalence ranging from 68% to 87% in older women.[32] In men erectile dysfunction is the most frequent sexual disorder, affecting up to 40% of men in their 60s and between 50% and 70% of men older than 70 years.[33]

ADDRESSING SEXUAL HEALTH IN OLDER ADULTS: BARRIERS AND FACILITATORS

As illustrated in the previous section, sexuality remains a key component of overall health as people age. However, sexual health discussions within the health care space remain suboptimal.[34,35] Several themes emerge from studies exploring factors that hamper both older adults from seeking care related to sexuality and HCPs from addressing these health concerns in the clinic (**Fig. 1**).

First theme that emerges from these data is that frequently both patients and their HCPs avoid discussions of sex altogether, with cultural notions surrounding sexuality and aging having a profound negative impact. In a cross-sectional study examining comfort with sexual health discussions with HCPs among 474 older married adults, the investigators found that negative cultural views of sexuality had significant impact on women participants from raising these issues.[36] Low perceived risk for sexual problems may serve as a barrier to addressing sexual health as well. In a qualitative study of unmarried women aged 40 to 75 years, Politi and colleagues[37] reported that some participants felt that HCPs should ask about sexual health only if there was a specific health concern, and in turn HCPs were similarly hesitant to discuss sexual health with unmarried patients. Similarly, in a study of adults older than 55 years, most reported never discussing sexual health with their HCPs due to shame or embarrassment, and an overwhelming majority of participants reported that HCPs did not obtain a sexual history.[38] When sexual concerns were discussed with HCPs, negative experiences were common, ranging from encounters described as uncomfortable to dismissive.[38] Gender discordance between patients and HCPs was also reported as a barrier to discussions about sexuality, in particular women reporting that they are much more likely to discuss sexual concerns with a female HCPs.[38] Even when sexual health is discussed during health care visits, the content may be insufficient to fully assess risk for STIs in older adults. Ports and colleagues[39] found that among a cohort of persons aged 50 to 80 years while approximately half the participants had discussions about sexual performance with their HCPs, only 10% were asked if they were sexually active, and history of STIs was discussed in only 17% of the visits, whereas patients were never asked about anal or oral sex.

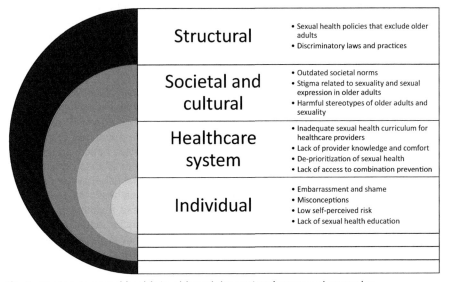

Fig. 1. Barriers to sexual health in older adults: major themes and examples.

Second theme, stigma and discrimination can be potent obstacles to sexual health seeking in older persons. When it comes to sexual expression, older adults are not a monolith, but instead a diverse group that includes persons who are gender diverse and identify as gay, bisexual, or heterosexual. LGBTQ older adults are likely to have grown up during an era when laws criminalizing homosexuality were ubiquitous and the practice was designated as a mental health disorder in the Diagnostic and Statistical Manual of Mental Disorders.[40] They are also likely to have lived through further marginalization of LGBTQ persons amid the rise of the HIV epidemic in the 1980s and resulting discriminatory state laws on criminalization of HIV transmission, many of which still exist on the books today. Within the shadows of these experiences, older LGBTQ persons are much less likely to seek sexual health care than their younger peers. In one study, within a cohort of unmarried women older than 40 years, women who self-identified as lesbians expressed more reluctance in sharing sexual history with HCPs than their heterosexual counterparts due to prior negative experiences related to perceived negative beliefs of HCPs surrounding sexual minorities.[37] In one survey study, older LGBTQ participants reported experiences where they were assumed to be heterosexual or entirely asexual by HCPs reflecting heterocentric practices.[41] Ageism more widely can also result in discrimination in other ways such as exclusion of older adults from policies on sexual health and research related to STIs, prevention, and treatment.[42]

Older adults also face provider or systems specific barriers when seeking sexual health care. Sexual health curriculums are inconsistent and inadequate during medical training and consequently; HCPs frequently lack the comfort or knowledge to address sexual health needs of their patients.[43,44] This problem is further compounded by the fact that sexual health is deprioritized in favor of other health concerns in older adults requiring HCPs attention during time-limited clinic visits.[45] The challenge is particularly acute when it comes to care of LGBTQ older adults as noted earlier. Despite increasing awareness of unique health care needs of LGBTQ individuals, when it comes to medical education, gaps remain. In a survey of 176 medical schools in Canada and the US, the median reported time dedicated to teaching LGBTQ specific content was 5 hours over the course of the entire medical education, with up to one-third reporting no content during clinical years.[46] One tangible impact of this lack of training shows up in provider knowledge and comfort with HIV testing. In a survey of primary care providers of individuals older than 50 years who received a late diagnosis of HIV, Youssef and colleagues[47] demonstrated that providers frequently lacked current HIV-related testing information and felt discomfort discussing details about sexuality with older adults.

Where there are obstacles, there are also several potential solutions. Normalizing sex as a vital component of healthy aging is the critical first step in maintaining sexual health of older individuals. Based on a survey of adults over the age of 60 years, Fileborn and colleagues[38] found that incorporating discussions about sex into general health care helped facilitate these conversations and minimized patient and clinician embarrassment. Use of electronic medical record–based data tools to obtain sexual orientation and gender identity information and assess sexual risk may not only help the HCPs develop a standardized approach but also address health care disparities experienced by LGBTQ persons.[48,49] By expanding access, health care policies such as the Affordable Care Act not only reduce stigmatization and discrimination of older LGBTQ and aging adults in general but can also serve as important solutions to tackling sexual health in this population.[50] Research that is inclusive of older adults and recognizes diverse expression of sexuality as part of healthy aging is another piece of the puzzle. A systematic review of clinical trials evaluating STI risk reduction published between 1994 and 2005 found that more than two-thirds of these trials excluded persons older than 50 years and approximately only 10% included persons older than 65 years.[51] Inclusion of older adults in these studies can help clinicians take a more evidence-based approach in reducing STI rates in this population. And lastly, expanding sexual health education early in medical training and maintaining training for practicing clinicians that incorporates a nonjudgmental, LGBTQ inclusive approach is critical in expanding both HCPs' comfort and skill, addressing sexual health needs of their diverse older patient populations.[52,53]

PREVENTING SEXUALLY TRANSMITTED INFECTIONS IN OLDER ADULTS: USING ALL THE TOOLS IN THE TOOLBOX

Combination STI prevention entails an array of biomedical, structural, and behavioral interventions tailored to the specific preferences and needs of the patient (**Fig. 2**). Biomedical interventions include testing and treatment, preexposure and postexposure prophylaxis (PrEP and PEP), condoms, and lubricants andvaccination for HAV and HBV. Behavioral interventions include education and counseling aimed at risk awareness and harm reduction. Structural strategies are aimed at affecting political and cultural change to protect marginalized individuals affected by HIV and other STIs. Despite proven efficacy of this combination approach in STI prevention, uptake in older population remains low.[54] Although these strategies are not unique to older adults, HCPs must be aware of how to tailor STI prevention strategies to serve the needs of older individuals.

Sexual History Taking

Accurate risk assessment through effective sexual history taking is the cornerstone of delivering quality preventative STI care. US Preventative Task Force (USPSTF) recommends that sexual history be obtained as part of comprehensive well visits along with

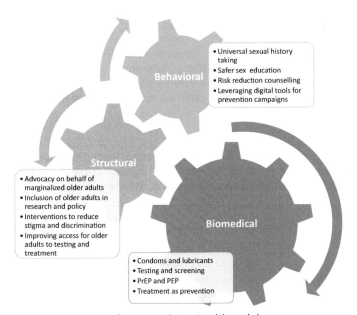

Fig. 2. Combination prevention for HIV and STIs in older adults.

acute visits related to sexual concerns.[55] CDC recommends framing sexual history around the 5 Ps (**Table 1**).[56] One approach that has been proposed to sexual history taking in older individuals is the Permission, Limited Information, Specific Suggestions, and Intensive Therapy model (PLISSIT) method.[57] This model begins with setting the stage by normalizing sex in aging, then stressing the importance of examining sexual history, followed by requesting permission to continue sexual history interview, followed by screening and open-ended questions to assess overall sexual health in older adults. The PLISSIT method is summarized in **Box 1** along with suggested examples of questions for HCPs. Although this model has not been exclusively studied in older adults, it has been shown to be a useful framework for addressing sexual health in other groups where sexual history taking may be challenging such as women with multiple sclerosis and gynecological cancer survivors.[58,59]

Education and Safer Sex Counseling

Safer sex counseling combines strategies on contraception alongside STI prevention. Because unintended pregnancies are of lower concern in older individuals, STI prevention counseling may get abandoned altogether by HCP and patient alike. Several studies have suggested that older adults do not consistently practice safe sex and many lack condom use skills.[60,61] Postmenopausal women and their partners are particularly vulnerable to decreased condom use due to lack of concern for unintended pregnancy.[62,63] Older men who suffer from erectile dysfunction may have difficulty navigating proper condom techniques or may deprioritize condoms in favor of sexual pleasure.[64] One study of adults older than 60 years concluded that although there was great variability in safer sex practices and STI knowledge, a range of misconceptions and issues related to physical limitations and embarrassment continue to serve as impediments to safer sex in this group.[65] A questionnaire study evaluating STI knowledge among a cohort of individuals aged 65 years and older demonstrated consistently low knowledge, with average score of 11 out of 27 questions assessed.[66] Consequently, safer sex counseling remains an important pillar of prevention in older adults. Various behavioral interventions such as online counseling, clinic-based education, and peer counseling have been found to be effective in reducing HIV and STI rates in youth and younger adults.[67–69] However, data on effective safer counseling strategies are limited in older adults. Gedin and colleagues[70] found a group-based sex educational intervention to be feasible in older adults living in a senior living center. Whether such an approach is efficacious remains unknown and as such there remains a knowledge gap when it comes to safer sex counseling strategies tailored toward older adults.

Screening and Testing

STIs are often part of a complex symbiotic relationship that predisposes hosts to other infections with similar mode of transmission, making coinfections common. STI screening is intended for asymptomatic persons, whereas testing is intended for those

Table 1	
The five Ps: a guide to major aspects of a sexual history	
Partners	Inquire about number and gender of your patient's sex partners
Practices	Ask about sex practices
Protection from STIs	Determine the level of risk-reduction counseling needed
Past history of STIs	Question regarding history of prior STIs
Pregnancy intention	Establish patient or the patient's partner's chances of pregnancy

Box 1
Permission, limited information, specific suggestions, and intensive therapy model method with suggested questions for sexual history taking

Sexual Health Assessment for Older Adults
1. Permission:
    "Sexual health is an important component of your physical and emotional well-being. May we further discuss your sexual health?"
2. Limited Information:
    "Our sexual function may change as we age. In what ways has your sexual function changed?"
    "Do you have any concerns or questions related to sex or your overall sexual health?"
    "Have you been sexually active in the past year? If so, how many sexual partners have you had?"
    "Do you have sex with men, women, or both?"
3. Specific Suggestions:
    "I think it is important that you openly discuss your sexual health with your partners."
    "We should discuss how your chronic medications might be affecting your sexual health."
4. Intensive Therapy:
    "What information or referrals can I provide to help you fulfill your goals regarding your sexual health?"

exhibiting symptoms or have had a potential exposure to an STI. CDC recommends screening for the 3 most prevalent bacterial STIs (chlamydia, gonorrhea, and syphilis) every 3 to 6 months in persons at increased risk of infection including sexually active MSM, transgender women (TGW), and PWH, regardless of age[9]; this includes screening in persons who report risk of exposure at extragenital anatomic sites. Trichomonas screening is recommended in women in high prevalence settings or sexually active women with HIV at least annually. Risk-based screening is recommended for HBV and HCV regardless of age. HSV serotype–specific serologic testing may be conducted in persons presenting for an STI evaluation. HPV cytology and cervical cancer screening is recommended in women 21 to 29 years of age every 3 years and women between 30 and 65 years of age every 3 years or every 5 years with a combination of cytology and HPV testing. Per the CDC, there are currently insufficient data for specific HPV cytology and anal cancer screening recommendations among men with increased risk.

Lastly, at least once in a lifetime HIV screening is recommend for persons aged 13 to 64 years, with more frequent screening based on risk and risk-based screening in persons older than 64 years. Some have advocated for eliminating the upper age limit for HIV screening in favor of screening for all adults, arguing that broadening the screening guidelines will not only enable us to capture this important, largely unscreened age demographic but also open opportunities for discussions about HIV, its predisposing factors, and modes of prevention between providers and their older patients.[71] There is also evidence to suggest that although risk-based testing may be a more efficient and cost-effective approach in persons 65 years and older, Black men remain at or greater than 0.1% prevalence threshold for population-based screening to remain efficient in this group.[72] Although discussions regarding upper age limit for HIV testing may be nuanced, what is quite clear is that delay in diagnosis and treatment of HIV in older adults has led to poorer outcomes, including lower baseline CD4 counts, decreased time to onset of AIDS, and increased mortality from AIDS-related illness.[73] Yet, uptake of HIV testing in older adults remains suboptimal with less than 15% of sexually active older adults ever tested for HIV.[74] Evidence suggests that interpersonal influences and sociodemographic characteristics are associated with

HIV testing among older adults.[6] Several surveys have indicated older adults were less likely than younger adults to be tested simply to find out their HIV status.[75] Interventions aimed at improving policies and practices that will increase HIV screening within the older adult population must be encouraged.

Preexposure and Postexposure Prophylaxis

According to the CDC, PrEP for HIV prevention should be considered in any adult and their partners with a history of anal or vaginal sex with a substantial risk of acquiring HIV such as bacterial STI in the last 6 months, history of inconsistent condom use with partners, HIV positive partner not on ART, or person who injects drugs.[76] Despite several clinical trials proving the effectiveness and safety of PrEP, no studies have focused specifically on individuals older than 50 years.[77] Renal toxicity and reduction in bone mineral density, attributed to the use of tenofovir disoproxil fumarate/emtricitabine (FTC), have raised concerns about safety of PrEP in older patients.[78] However, tenofovir alafenamide/FTC and possibly cabotegravir long-acting for PrEP are seemingly safer and equally effective alternatives for PrEP in older patients.[79,80] Studies have shown higher adherence to PrEP in older adults aged 50 to 64 years compared with adults younger than 35 years.[81] As such, there are no plausible reasons why PrEP for HIV would not be as effective in older adults as it is in younger individuals, and both strategies should be offered to older adults at risk for HIV acquisition. In an observational cohort of US Veterans that skewed older than those studied in clinical trials (mean age 41 years, range 21–77 years), PrEP remained highly effective.[82] Admittedly, longitudinal studies in the elderly are needed to substantiate the potential uptake, safety, and efficacy of PrEP in this population.

The success of HIV prevention using PrEP and PEP has paved the way for the use of other antimicrobial agents for prevention of other STIs. Currently under review by CDC is doxycycline PEP taken within 72 hours of condomless sex was demonstrated to reduce gonorrhea, chlamydia, and syphilis incidence in MSM and TGW.[83] PrEP and PEP for STI prevention are proving to be well tolerated and effective tools that should be considered for all at-risk adults regardless of age. Lastly, vaccines provide another safe and effective tool in STI prevention. The Advisory Committee on Immunization Practices (ACIP) recommends universal HBV vaccination among all adults aged 19 to 59 years and adults aged 60 years or older with risk factors for hepatitis B such as sexual exposure.[84] HAV vaccination is recommended among others to those with increased risk of HAV through sexual contact and all MSM regardless of age.[85] HPV vaccine is approved by Food and Drug Administration for up to age 45 years, as its role in older adults is undefined. Other strategies combining PEP and vaccines for STI prevention are currently in the pipeline and will provide additional tools for HIV prevention.

TREATMENT OF SEXUALLY TRANSMITTED INFECTIONS IN OLDER ADULTS: SPECIAL CONSIDERATIONS

Treatment of STIs is a critical piece of breaking the cycle of transmission and ultimately controlling the STI epidemics. One of the best pieces of evidence for "treatment as prevention" comes from the HIV literature where treatment of HIV has shown to be a potent tool for curbing transmission.[86] A comprehensive review of treatment recommendations is beyond the scope of this review; however, the CDC STI treatment guideline update from 2021 can serve as comprehensive guide for the diagnosis and management of STIs in all adults.[9] The aim of this section is to focus on issues to consider when treating older individuals for STIs. Special considerations during treatment of HIV infection in older adults is covered elsewhere in this issue.

Adverse Effects

Overall, the antimicrobial regimens used to treat STIs are generally short in duration, well tolerated with minimal to no clinically significant drug interactions to consider, even among older individuals. Doxycycline is now considered the drug of choice for chlamydia and remains alternative therapy in management of P&S syphilis. The most frequently reported side effect of doxycycline is dermatologic photosensitivity and is exacerbated in older adults with other potentiating agents. Drug-induced photosensitivity, however, can often be mitigated by limiting prolonged sun exposure, sun protective clothing, and broad-spectrum protective sunscreen.[87] Penicillin remains the drug of choice for all stages of syphilis. Treatment of early syphilis can result in Jarisch-Herxheimer reaction, an acute febrile reaction frequently accompanied by headache, myalgia, and fever that can occur within the first 24 hours after the initiation of any syphilis therapy. It occurs most frequently among persons who have early syphilis, presumably because bacterial loads are higher during these stages. There is no association between this paradoxical reaction and age. Ceftriaxone is primarily used for gonococcal infections and is generally well tolerated with no renal or hepatic dosage adjustments provided in the manufacturer's labeling. However, in patients with concurrent hepatic dysfunction and severe kidney impairment, use of more than 2 g/d should be done with caution and close monitoring for toxicity.[88] Similar to other beta lactams, ceftriaxone is one of the most common causes for *Clostridium difficile* colitis particularly in older adults who themselves are predisposed to higher rates of *C diff*.[89] These concerns may be of relevance in individuals with anaphylaxis to penicillin in whom ceftriaxone is used as alternate therapy for neurosyphilis.

Polypharmacy

Polypharmacy is common in older adults. Photosensitivity to oral therapeutic drugs such as doxycycline is relatively common in older individuals, probably because of the comparatively large use of therapeutic drugs by this age group.[90] Similarly, macrolides if prescribed for treating chlamydial STIs, must be used cautiously in patients with other drugs that potentiate QT prolongation.[91] As with other cephalosporins, ceftriaxone may enhance the anticoagulant effect of vitamin K Antagonists for patients on warfarin, a drug commonly used in older adults.[92]

SUMMARY

In summary, older adults are not immune to increasing STI rates in the US and are currently experiencing concerning increase in many STIs. Individual, provider, and systems barriers, can all lead to decreased access to safe sex counseling, prevention technologies, testing, and treatments of STIs in this age group. These barriers can be countered by normalizing sex as routine part of health care and aging. Deployment of combination prevention strategies and treatment of STIs tailored to older adults are the keys to stemming the tide of increasing STIs in people who are aging.

CLINICS CARE POINTS

- Despite prevailing beliefs regarding sexuality and aging, many older adults remain sexually active well into later decades of life.
- Incorporate sexual health into routine healthcare of older adults.
- Comprehensive STI prevention approach remains applicable in older adults.

DISCLOSURE

The authors have no disclosures.

REFERENCES

1. Prevention CfDCa. Sexually Transmitted Disease Surveillance. 2020. https://www.cdc.gov/std/statistics/2020. [Accessed 10 August 2022].
2. Prevention CfDCa. Atlas Plus: HIV, Hepatitis, STD, TB, social determines of health data. Available at:. https://www.cdc.gov/nchhstp/atlas/index.htm. Accessed August 10, 2022.
3. Centers for Disease Control and Prevention: HIV Surveillance Report, 2018 (Updated). Available at: https://www.cdc.gov/hiv/pdf/library/reports/surveillance/cdc-hiv-surveillance-report-2020-updated-vol-33.pdf. Accessed August 10, 2022.
4. Loeb DF, Lee RS, Binswanger IA, et al. Patient, resident physician, and visit factors associated with documentation of sexual history in the outpatient setting. J Gen Intern Med 2011;26(8):887–93.
5. Lindau ST, Schumm LP, Laumann EO, et al. A study of sexuality and health among older adults in the United States. N Engl J Med 2007;357(8):762–74.
6. Tillman JL, Mark HD. HIV and STI testing in older adults: an integrative review. J Clin Nurs 2015;24(15-16):2074–95.
7. Sullivan PS, Satcher Johnson A, Pembleton ES, et al. Epidemiology of HIV in the USA: epidemic burden, inequities, contexts, and responses. Lancet 2021;397(10279):1095–106.
8. Centers for Disease Control and Prevention. HIV Surveillance Report, 2022. hwcghlrh-shPM. Available at: https://www.cdc.gov/hiv/pdf/library/reports/surveillance/cdc-hiv-surveillance-report-2020-updated-vol-33.pdf. Accecced August 15, 2022.
9. Workowski KA, Bachmann LH, Chan PA, et al. Sexually transmitted infections treatment guidelines, 2021. MMWR Recomm Rep 2021;70(4):1–187.
10. James C, Harfouche M, Welton NJ, et al. Herpes simplex virus: global infection prevalence and incidence estimates, 2016. Bull World Health Organ 2020;98(5):315–29.
11. Tohme RA, Holmberg SD. Is sexual contact a major mode of hepatitis C virus transmission? Hepatology 2010;52(4):1497–505.
12. Charre C, Cotte L, Kramer R, et al. Hepatitis C virus spread from HIV-positive to HIV-negative men who have sex with men. PloS one 2018;13(1):e0190340.
13. Bradshaw D, Vasylyeva TI, Davis C, et al. Transmission of hepatitis C virus in HIV-positive and PrEP-using MSM in England. J Viral Hepat 2020;27(7):721–30.
14. Marciano S, Arufe D, Haddad L, et al. Outbreak of hepatitis A in a post-vaccination era: high rate of co-infection with sexually transmitted diseases. Ann Hepatol 2020;19(6):641–4.
15. Saito R, Imamura A, Nishiura H. Assessing countermeasures during a hepatitis A virus outbreak among men who have sex with men. Theor Biol Med Model 2021;18(1):19.
16. Dickson EL, Vogel RI, Luo X, et al. Recent trends in type-specific HPV infection rates in the United States. Epidemiol Infect 2015;143(5):1042–7.
17. Windon MJ, D'Souza G, Rettig EM, et al. Increasing prevalence of human papillomavirus-positive oropharyngeal cancers among older adults. Cancer 2018;124(14):2993–9.

18. Lindau ST, Dale W, Feldmeth G, et al. Sexuality and cognitive status: a U.S. Nationally Representative Study of home-dwelling older adults. J Am Geriatr Soc 2018;66(10):1902–10.
19. Villar F, Celdran M, Faba J, et al. Barriers to sexual expression in residential aged care facilities (RACFs): comparison of staff and residents' views. J Adv Nurs 2014;70(11):2518–27.
20. Roelofs TS, Luijkx KG, Embregts PJ. Intimacy and sexuality of nursing home residents with dementia: a systematic review. Int Psychogeriatr 2015;27(3):367–84.
21. Lester PE, Kohen I, Stefanacci RG, et al. Sex in nursing homes: a survey of nursing home policies governing resident sexual activity. J Am Med Dir Assoc 2016;17(1):71–4.
22. Mahieu L, Gastmans C. Older residents' perspectives on aged sexuality in institutionalized elderly care: a systematic literature review. Int J Nurs Stud 2015; 52(12):1891–905.
23. Stein GL, Beckerman NL, Sherman PA. Lesbian and gay elders and long-term care: identifying the unique psychosocial perspectives and challenges. J Gerontol Soc Work 2010;53(5):421–35.
24. Hinrichs KL, Vacha-Haase T. Staff perceptions of same-gender sexual contacts in long-term care facilities. J Homosex 2010;57(6):776–89.
25. Schick V, Herbenick D, Reece M, et al. Sexual behaviors, condom use, and sexual health of Americans over 50: implications for sexual health promotion for older adults. J Sex Med 2010;7(Suppl 5):315–29.
26. Thomas HN, Hamm M, Hess R, et al. Changes in sexual function among midlife women: "I'm older... and I'm wiser". Menopause 2018;25(3):286–92.
27. Saad F, Rohrig G, von Haehling S, et al. Testosterone deficiency and testosterone treatment in older men. Gerontology 2017;63(2):144–56.
28. Jia H, Sullivan CT, McCoy SC, et al. Review of health risks of low testosterone and testosterone administration. World J Clin Cases 2015;3(4):338–44.
29. Raheem OA, Su JJ, Wilson JR, et al. The association of erectile dysfunction and cardiovascular disease: a systematic critical review. Am J Mens Health 2017; 11(3):552–63.
30. Thomas DR. Medications and sexual function. Clin Geriatr Med 2003;19(3): 553–62.
31. Basson R, Gilks T. Women's sexual dysfunction associated with psychiatric disorders and their treatment. Womens Health (Lond). 2018;14. 1745506518762664.
32. Ambler DR, Bieber EJ, Diamond MP. Sexual function in elderly women: a review of current literature. Rev Obstet Gynecol 2012;5(1):16–27.
33. Laumann EO, Waite LJ. Sexual dysfunction among older adults: prevalence and risk factors from a nationally representative U.S. probability sample of men and women 57-85 years of age. J Sex Med 2008;5(10):2300–11.
34. Lanier Y, Castellanos T, Barrow RY, et al. Brief sexual histories and routine HIV/STD testing by medical providers. AIDS Patient Care and STDs 2014;28(3): 113–20.
35. Loeb DF, Aagaard EM, Cali SR, et al. Modest impact of a brief curricular intervention on poor documentation of sexual history in university-based resident internal medicine clinics. J Sex Med 2010;7(10):3315–21.
36. Adams SA. Marital quality and older men's and women's comfort discussing sexual issues with a doctor. J Sex Marital Ther 2014;40(2):123–38.
37. Politi MC, Clark MA, Armstrong G, et al. Patient-provider communication about sexual health among unmarried middle-aged and older women. J Gen Intern Med 2009;24(4):511–6.

38. Fileborn B, Lyons A, Heywood W, et al. Talking to healthcare providers about sex in later life: Findings from a qualitative study with older Australian men and women. Aust J Ageing 2017;36(4):E50–6.

39. Ports KA, Barnack-Tavlaris JL, Syme ML, et al. Sexual health discussions with older adult patients during periodic health exams. J Sex Med 2014;11(4):901–8.

40. Drescher J. Queer diagnoses: parallels and contrasts in the history of homosexuality, gender variance, and the diagnostic and statistical manual. Arch Sex Behav 2010;39(2):427–60.

41. Boggs JM, Dickman Portz J, King DK, et al. Perspectives of LGBTQ older adults on aging in place: a qualitative investigation. J Homosex 2017;64(11):1539–60.

42. Ezhova I, Savidge L, Bonnett C, et al. Barriers to older adults seeking sexual health advice and treatment: a scoping review. Int J Nurs Stud 2020;107:103566.

43. Palaiodimos L, Herman HS, Wood E, et al. Practices and barriers in sexual history taking: a cross-sectional study in a public adult primary care clinic. J Sex Med 2020;17(8):1509–19.

44. Shindel AW, Baazeem A, Eardley I, et al. Sexual health in undergraduate medical education: existing and future needs and platforms. J Sex Med 2016;13(7): 1013–26.

45. Gott M, Hinchliff S, Galena E. General practitioner attitudes to discussing sexual health issues with older people. Soc Sci Med 2004;58(11):2093–103.

46. Obedin-Maliver J, Goldsmith ES, Stewart L, et al. Lesbian, gay, bisexual, and transgender-related content in undergraduate medical education. JAMA 2011; 306(9):971–7.

47. Youssef E, Wright J, Kevin AD, et al. Factors associated with offering HIV testing to people aged $\geq$ 50 years: a qualitative study. Int J STD AIDS 2022;33(3): 289–95.

48. Cahill S, Makadon H. Sexual orientation and gender identity data collection in clinical settings and in electronic health records: a key to ending lgbt health disparities. LGBT Health 2014;1(1):34–41.

49. Pappas Y, Anandan C, Liu J, et al. Computer-assisted history-taking systems (CAHTS) in health care: benefits, risks and potential for further development. Inform Prim Care 2011;19(3):155–60.

50. Gonzales G, Henning-Smith C. The affordable care act and health insurance coverage for lesbian, gay, and bisexual adults: analysis of the behavioral risk factor surveillance system. LGBT Health 2017;4(1):62–7.

51. Levy BR, Ding L, Lakra D, et al. Older persons' exclusion from sexually transmitted disease risk-reduction clinical trials. Sex Transm Dis 2007;34(8):541–4.

52. Sekoni AO, Gale NK, Manga-Atangana B, et al. The effects of educational curricula and training on LGBT-specific health issues for healthcare students and professionals: a mixed-method systematic review. J Int AIDS Soc 2017; 20(1):21624.

53. Rubin ES, Rullo J, Tsai P, et al. Best practices in North American pre-clinical medical education in sexual history taking: consensus from the summits in medical education in sexual health. J Sex Med 2018;15(10):1414–25.

54. Roberson DW. Meeting the HIV prevention needs of older adults. J Assoc Nurses AIDS Care 2018;29(1):126–9.

55. US preventative services taskforce: sexually transmitted infections: behavioral counseling. Available at: https://www.uspreventiveservicestaskforce.org/uspstf/recommendation/sexually-transmitted-infections-behavioral-counseling. Accessed September 12, 2022.

56. Center for Disease Control and Prevention. A guide to taking a sexual history. Available at: https://www.cdc.gov/std/treatment/sexualhistory.pdf. Accessed August 3, 2022.

57. Rutte A, van Oppen P, Nijpels G, et al. Effectiveness of a PLISSIT model intervention in patients with type 2 diabetes mellitus in primary care: design of a cluster-randomised controlled trial. BMC Fam Pract 2015;16:69.

58. Khakbazan Z, Daneshfar F, Behboodi-Moghadam Z, et al. The effectiveness of the permission, limited information, specific suggestions, intensive therapy (PLISSIT) model based sexual counseling on the sexual function of women with multiple sclerosis who are sexually active. Mult Scler Relat Disord 2016;8:113–9.

59. Almeida NG, Britto DF, Figueiredo JV, et al. PLISSIT model: sexual counseling for breast cancer survivors. Rev Bras Enferm 2019;72(4):1109–13.

60. Cheng Y, McGeechan K, Bateson D, et al. Age differences in attitudes toward safer sex practices in heterosexual men using an Australian Internet dating service. Sexual health 2018;15(3):223–31.

61. Lyons A, Heywood W, Fileborn B, et al. Sexually active older Australian's knowledge of sexually transmitted infections and safer sexual practices. Aust N Z J Public Health 2017;41(3):259–61.

62. Bateson DJ, Weisberg E, McCaffery KJ, et al. When online becomes offline: attitudes to safer sex practices in older and younger women using an Australian internet dating service. Sex Health 2012;9(2):152–9.

63. Paranjape A, Bernstein L, St George DM, et al. Effect of relationship factors on safer sex decisions in older inner-city women. J women's Health 2006;15(1):90–7.

64. Jones SG, Fenkl EA, Patsdaughter CA, et al. Condom attitudes of heterosexual men ages 50 and older using prescribed drugs (viagra, cialis, levitra) to treat erectile dysfunction. Am J Mens Health 2013;7(6):504–15.

65. Fileborn B, Brown G, Lyons A, et al. Safer sex in later life: qualitative interviews with older Australians on their understandings and practices of safer sex. J Sex Res 2018;55(2):164–77.

66. Smith ML, Bergeron CD, Goltz HH, et al. Sexually transmitted infection knowledge among older adults: psychometrics and test-retest reliability. Int J Environ Res Public Health 2020;17(7). https://doi.org/10.3390/ijerph17072462.

67. Mustanski B, Greene GJ, Ryan D, et al. Feasibility, acceptability, and initial efficacy of an online sexual health promotion program for LGBT youth: the queer sex ed intervention. J Sex Res 2015;52(2):220–30.

68. Crosby RA, Mena L, Salazar LF, et al. Efficacy of a clinic-based safer sex program for human immunodeficiency virus-uninfected and human immunodeficiency virus-infected young black men who have sex with men: a randomized controlled trial. Sex Transm Dis 2018;45(3):169–76.

69. Darbes L, Crepaz N, Lyles C, et al. The efficacy of behavioral interventions in reducing HIV risk behaviors and incident sexually transmitted diseases in heterosexual African Americans. Aids 2008;22(10):1177–94.

70. Gedin TC, Resnick B. Increasing risk awareness and facilitating safe sexual activity among older adults in senior housing. J Community Health Nurs 2014;31(4): 187–97.

71. Chowdhury PP, Mawokomatanda T, Xu F, et al. Surveillance for certain health behaviors, chronic diseases, and conditions, access to health care, and use of preventive health services among states and selected local areas- behavioral risk factor surveillance system, United States, 2012. MMWR Surveill Summ 2016; 65(4):1–142.

72. Goetz MB, Hoang T, Kan VL, et al. Rates and predictors of newly diagnosed hiv infection among veterans receiving routine once-per-lifetime hiv testing in the veterans health administration. J Acquir Immune Defic Syndr 2015;69(5):544–50.

73. Cuzin L, Delpierre C, Gerard S, et al. Immunologic and clinical responses to highly active antiretroviral therapy in patients with HIV infection aged >50 years. Clin Infect Dis 2007;45(5):654–7.

74. Oraka E, Mason S, Xia M. Too old to test? Prevalence and correlates of HIV testing among sexually active older adults. J Gerontol Soc Work 2018;61(4):460–70.

75. Adekeye OA, Heiman HJ, Onyeabor OS, et al. The new invincibles: HIV screening among older adults in the U.S. PloS one 2012;7(8):e43618.

76. Centers for Disease Control and Prevention: Pre exposure prophylaxis for the prevention of HIV infection in the United States: 2021 an update. Available at: https://www.cdc.gov/hiv/pdf/risk/prep/cdc-hiv-prep-guidelines-2021.pdf. Accessed October 23, 2022.

77. Franconi I, Guaraldi G. Pre-exposure prophylaxis for HIV infection in the older patient: what can be recommended? Drugs Aging 2018;35(6):485–91.

78. Fioroti CEA, Distenhreft JIQ, Paulino BB, et al. Tenofovir-induced renal and bone toxicity: report of two cases and literature review. Rev Inst Med Trop Sao Paulo 2022;64:e10.

79. Mayer KH, Molina JM, Thompson MA, et al. Emtricitabine and tenofovir alafenamide vs emtricitabine and tenofovir disoproxil fumarate for HIV pre-exposure prophylaxis (DISCOVER): primary results from a randomised, double-blind, multicentre, active-controlled, phase 3, non-inferiority trial. Lancet 2020;396(10246):239–54.

80. Fernandez C, van Halsema CL. Evaluating cabotegravir/rilpivirine long-acting, injectable in the treatment of HIV infection: emerging data and therapeutic potential. HIV AIDS (Auckl) 2019;11:179–92.

81. van Epps P, Maier M, Lund B, et al. Medication adherence in a nationwide cohort of veterans initiating pre-exposure prophylaxis (prep) to prevent HIV infection. J Acquir Immune Defic Syndr 2018;77(3):272–8.

82. Van Epps P, Wilson BM, Garner W, et al. Brief report: incidence of HIV in a Nationwide cohort receiving pre-exposure prophylaxis for HIV prevention. J Acquir Immune Defic Syndr 2019;82(5):427–30.

83. Stewart J, Bukusi E, Sesay FA, et al. Doxycycline post-exposure prophylaxis for prevention of sexually transmitted infections among Kenyan women using HIV pre-exposure prophylaxis: study protocol for an open-label randomized trial. Trials 2022;23(1):495.

84. Weng MK, Doshani M, Khan MA, et al. Universal hepatitis B vaccination in adults aged 19-59 years: updated recommendations of the advisory committee on immunization practices - United States, 2022. MMWR Morb Mortal Wkly Rep 2022;71(13):477–83.

85. Nelson NP, Weng MK, Hofmeister MG, et al. Prevention of hepatitis a virus infection in the United States: recommendations of the advisory committee on immunization practices, 2020. MMWR Recomm Rep 2020;69(5):1–38.

86. Cohen MS, Chen YQ, McCauley M, et al. Antiretroviral therapy for the prevention of HIV-1 transmission. N Engl J Med 2016;375(9):830–9.

87. Goetze S, Hiernickel C, Elsner P. Phototoxicity of doxycycline: a systematic review on clinical manifestations, frequency, cofactors, and prevention. Skin Pharmacol Physiol 2017;30(2):76–80.

88. Stoeckel K, Koup JR. Pharmacokinetics of ceftriaxone in patients with renal and liver insufficiency and correlations with a physiologic nonlinear protein binding model. Am J Med 1984;77(4C):26–32.
89. McDonald LC, Gerding DN, Johnson S, et al. Clinical practice guidelines for clostridium difficile infection in adults and children: 2017 update by the infectious diseases society of America (IDSA) and society for healthcare epidemiology of America (SHEA). Clin Infect Dis 2018;66(7):e1–48.
90. Morin L, Johnell K, Laroche ML, et al. The epidemiology of polypharmacy in older adults: register-based prospective cohort study. Clin Epidemiol 2018;10:289–98.
91. Fung KW, Baye F, Kapusnik-Uner J, et al. Using medicare data to assess the proarrhythmic risk of non-cardiac treatment drugs that prolong the qt interval in older adults: an observational cohort study. Drugs Real World Outcomes 2021; 8(2):173–85.
92. Baillargeon J, Holmes HM, Lin YL, et al. Concurrent use of warfarin and antibiotics and the risk of bleeding in older adults. Am J Med 2012;125(2):183–9.

Health Care-Associated Infections in Older Adults
Epidemiology and Prevention

Brenda L. Tesini, MD*, Ghinwa Dumyati, MD

KEYWORDS

- Health care-associated infection (HAI) • Nosocomial infection • Long-term care
- Infection prevention • Older adults • Health care-associated pneumonia
- Urinary tract infection

KEY POINTS

- Older adults are at an increased risk of acquiring health care-associated infections.
- Host-specific and environmental factors contribute to the heightened risk of infection in older adults.
- The long-term care setting presents unique infection prevention challenges.
- Preventing health care-associated infections in older adults requires coordination between acute care and long-term care.

INTRODUCTION

Age-associated physiologic changes, unique geriatric syndromes, and frequent, prolonged health care interactions make older adults uniquely vulnerable to infections. The accumulation of health issues makes older adults more likely to be hospitalized or reside in long-term care facilities (LTCFs) and more susceptible to infection than younger individuals. These healthcare interactions present opportunities to acquire infections connected to health care environment, personnel, or procedures.

Healthcare-associated infections (HAIs) are infections that occur while receiving care at a facility for another condition. They represent a global public health issue and estimated attributable mortality place HAIs as a top 10 cause of death in the United States.[1–4] Many of these deaths occur in patients with underlying medical conditions but whose death was not anticipated; one-third of unexpected in-hospital mortality is attributed to HAIs.[5] These infections threaten patient safety, leading to prolonged hospital length of stay, additional procedures, and antibiotic use. HAIs

Division of Infectious Diseases, Department of Medicine, University of Rochester School of Medicine and Dentistry, 601 Elmwood Avenue, Rochester, NY 14642, USA
* Corresponding author.
E-mail address: brenda_tesini@urmc.rochester.edu

Infect Dis Clin N Am 37 (2023) 65–86
https://doi.org/10.1016/j.idc.2022.11.004
0891-5520/23/© 2022 Elsevier Inc. All rights reserved.

also place a substantial financial and emotional toll on society and health care. More than half of HAIs are preventable; the large burden coupled with the preventable nature of these infections makes their reduction a national priority.[6]

The risk of acquiring an HAI increases with age, and the exponential rise in the older population presents an infection prevention challenge. Older adults are projected to represent nearly a quarter of the US population by 2060 with a doubling of the population aged 65 years and older and tripling of those aged 85 years and older when compared with 2016.[7] Individuals need more health care services as they age and this is increasingly being delivered outside of the hospital, including ambulatory surgery centers, home health care, and post-acute and long-term care. The acuity and medical complexity of patients receiving care in these nonhospital locations continues to increase as economic pressure mounts to decrease hospital length of stay.[8,9] Understanding the diversity of older adults within the health care system is necessary to develop effective HAI prevention strategies. Roughly 1.16 million Americans reside in nursing homes (NHs), and residents have a median length of stay of greater than 1 year.[10] Most residents are admitted to NHs from the hospital and approximately 25% are transferred back to the hospital[11]; the proportion is even higher for those with chronic conditions such as dementia.[12] This highlights the interrelatedness of acute and post-acute care, as the risks from medical interventions such as device use, antibiotic use, and lapses in infection control span both settings.

This review summarizes the epidemiology and prevention of HAIs in older adults in acute and long-term care settings. It will focus on risk factors and prevention strategies unique to the older individual. The important related topics of multidrug-resistant organisms (MRDOs), *Clostridioides difficile* infection (CDI), COVID-19, and antibiotic stewardship will be covered elsewhere in this issue.

Epidemiology

Health care-associated infection burden in acute care hospitals

Centers for Disease Prevention and Control (CDC) estimates that one in 31 hospitalized patients has an HAI on any given day, leading to approximately 687,000 infections annually.[2] Older age is an independent risk factor for HAI along with longer hospital stay, presence of a central venous catheter (CVC), receipt of mechanical ventilation, critical care unit location, and large hospital size.[2] HAIs are associated with increased mortality; approximately 72,000 hospitalized patients with HAIs died in 2015.[2] The financial burden of HAIs on the hospital system is substantial, estimated at over $28 billion in excess costs annually.[13]

The current hospital-associated HAI surveillance system in the United States is robust and evolved over several decades. Early efforts to estimate the HAI burden in the United States were generally single-site or small multisite studies using various methodologies. By the 1970s, a national multisite HAI surveillance system (National Nosocomial Infections Surveillance (NNIS)) was formed and found through the Study of the Efficacy of Nosocomial Infection Control that 5.25% of patients experienced an HAI during their hospitalization.[14–17] NNIS was eventually replaced by the current National Healthcare Safety Network (NHSN) to expand surveillance to all hospitals for a limited number of high-risk infectious conditions.

Using NHSN HAI definitions, CDC has conducted multisite point prevalence studies to obtain standardized HAI prevalence rates. The first of these studies in 2011 found that 4% of hospitalized patients had an HAI on any given day with an estimated 648,000 patients experiencing 721,800 HAIs annually.[3] The most recently published CDC data from 199 hospitals in 2015 found that the overall HAI prevalence has declined to 3.2%.[2] Pneumonia represented over a quarter of all HAIs, and most of the cases were not ventilator-associated. The next most common HAIs included gastro-intestinal infections (21%), surgical site infections (SSIs) (16%), bloodstream infections (12%), and urinary tract infections (UTIs) (9%). Two-thirds of UTIs were catheter-associated. Most gastrointestinal infections were due to *C difficile*.[2]

The most common organism identified was *C difficile*, representing 15% of all HAI organisms in the survey. *Staphylococcus aureus* and *Escherichia coli* were the next most prevalent pathogens, representing 11% and 10% of infections, respectively. Overlap between HAI and MDRO burden was also noted. Nearly half of all *S aureus* isolated with antibiotic susceptibility results available were methicillin resistant (MRSA) and 5% of *E coli* isolates demonstrated resistance to at least one carbape-nem.[2] These two organisms, *S aureus* and *E coli*, are also prevalent in HAI surveys from other countries.[18,19]

Hospital-submitted NHSN data have indicated a steady decline in most reported infections from 2010 until the COVID-19 pandemic.[20] In 2020 and 2021, dramatic increases were seen in central line-associated bloodstream infections, catheter-associated urinary tract infections (CAUTIs), ventilator-associated events, and MRSA bloodstream infection rates.[21,22] Infection peaks corresponded to periods of high-COVID-19 hospitalizations. Inability to adhere to basic infection prevention prac-tices in the context of personal protective equipment (PPE) supply limitations, shifting patient populations, and staffing challenges are hypothesized as main drivers of the increased HAI burden. These troublesome findings underscore the need for ongoing HAI surveillance and prevention efforts.

The prevalence studies of HAI from outside of the United States estimate that 3.5% to 12% of patients hospitalized in high-income countries experience an HAI on any given day.[23] A recent European Centre for Disease Prevention and Control (ECDC) study conducted in 29 European countries found an HAI point prevalence of 5.9% (country range 2.9% to 10%) in 2016 to 2017.[19] The burden of HAIs is even higher in low- and middle-income countries with estimates ranging from 5.7% to 19.1%, although studies are limited and often of low quality.[24]

Health care-associated infection burden in hospitalized older adults

Despite the increased HAI risk in older hospitalized adults, our understanding of the epidemiology in this population is limited. Based on the latest CDC data, over a third of hospital-associated HAIs occur in patients aged over 65 years.[2] A study conducted in the United States between 1986 and 1990 using NNIS data found that over half of all HAIs were in older adults aged above 65 years.[17] UTI was the most common HAI in this age group, representing 44% of infections, followed by pneumonia (18%) and SSI (11%). An HAI point prevalence study of hospitalized older adults from all 45 hos-pitals in Scotland in 2005 to 2006 showed similar results.[25] Both studies identified age as an independent risk factor for developing an HAI, and the study from Scotland showed a linear relationship between prevalence of HAI and increasing age (*P* < .0001).[25] The study found that UTI and gastrointestinal infections (50% due to *C difficile* diarrhea) represented the largest burden of HAI in the 75 to 84 year and over 85-year age groups, whereas SSIs represented the largest burden in inpatients less than 75 years of age.[25]

These studies are older, and it is unknown whether these remain the most common types of infection in older hospitalized adults. Similarly, the attributable cost of HAIs in older adults is unknown. However, Nelson and colleagues estimate that the five most prevalent MDROs (MRSA, vancomycin-resistant *Enterococci*, extended-spectrum beta-lactamase-producing and carbapenem-resistant Enterobacterales (CRE), carbapenem-resistant *Acinetobacter*, and multidrug-resistant *Pseudomonas*) caused nearly 8000 invasive infections in hospitalized older adults in the United States in 2017. These infections contributed to over 1000 deaths and up to $300 million in associated health care costs.[26]

Health care-associated infection burden in long-term care facilities

Infections are nearly as common in LTCF setting as they are in acute care hospitals. The CDC estimates that one in 43 US NH residents has an HAI on any given day.[27] Approximately 1.13 to 2.68 million infections occurred in US NHs in 2013 based on NH-reported data available through the Minimum Data Set, which is a mandated process for periodic clinical assessment of residents in Medicare and Medicaid certified NHs.[28] A 2017 US HAI point prevalence survey led by the CDC across 161 NHs found that the most common sites for infection were skin (32%), respiratory tract (29%), and urinary tract (20%). The most prevalent syndromes within each of these categories were cellulitis, soft tissue, or wound infection; cold or pharyngitis; and symptomatic UTI (without presence of a catheter).[27] Although UTI was not the most common infection, it is the most common reason for antibiotic use in the NH.[29] The ECDC 2016 HAI point prevalence data show a roughly similar distribution of HAI types with respiratory tract (33%), urinary tract (32%), and skin (24%) as the most common sites of infection.[30] Although respiratory infections are common in both acute and LTCF settings, viral upper respiratory infections predominate in LTCFs, whereas bacterial pneumonia is more prevalent in the hospital.

Outbreaks of gastrointestinal, respiratory, and MDRO infections are also common in LTCFs due to the communal environment and dependence on care (**Table 1**). The recent public health crisis of COVID-19 underscores the devastating impact of outbreaks in the LTCF setting.[31] The rapid spread of multidrug-resistant *Candida auris* among LTCFs also highlights infection prevention challenges in this environment. *C auris* can be resistant to all three classes of antifungal agents, and infection is associated with 30% mortality.[32] LTCF-associated infections also represent a substantial financial burden to the health care system. The cost of LTCF-associated infections must consider the cost of resultant hospitalizations which is estimated to be $673 million to $2 billion in the United States annually as well as medication expenses for antimicrobials which cost LTCFs an additional $38 million to $137 million per year.[33]

Table 1
Outbreaks in long-term care facilities

Bacterial	Viral
Group A *Streptococcus*	Influenza
Multidrug-resistant organisms (eg, CRE, CRAB)	SARS-CoV-2
Mycoplasma pneumoniae	Human metapneumovirus
S pneumoniae	Rhinovirus
Mycobacterium tuberculosis	Hepatitis B
Legionella species	Norovirus
Fungal	Rotavirus
C auris	**Parasitic**
	Scabies

Abbreviations: CRAB, carbapenem-resistant *Acinetobacter baumannii*; CRE, carbapenem-resistant Enterobacterales.
(*Data from Refs*[31,104,121–125])

The 2017 CDC HAI point prevalence study estimated that 2.3% of residents in US NHs had an HAI on any given day using the 2012 revised McGeer surveillance definition.[27] Prior US estimates, using different methodologies, were higher and ranged from 4.4% to 12%.[34–37] Comparing trends of infections over time and by location is difficult due to changing in infection surveillance definitions. Variations in types of facilities, patient populations, and data analyses also impact comparisons and applicability of studies on the epidemiology of LTCF-associated infections.

Point prevalence studies in other high-income countries show similar HAI rates to that in the United States. For instance, the HAI prevalence was 2.9% in Australian LTCFs in 2014 using the revised McGeer criteria.[38] The ECDC demonstrated HAI rates of 2.6%, 3.4%, and 3.6% in European LTCF in 2010, 2013, and 2016, respectively, using similar methodology with some modification.[18,19,30] This corresponds to an estimated 130,000 residents experiencing at least one HAI on any given day, resulting in 4.4 million infections per year in Europe. An up to date total HAI burden estimate for US NHs is not yet available.

In summary, HAIs affect older adults in both acute and post-acute care settings, leading to substantial morbidity, mortality, and health care and societal cost. Understanding the predisposing factors and their interactions that lead to the development of HAI in the older adult is important to guide prevention. These factors are related to the host, the procedures, and devices that patients receive and the setting in which care is delivered.

Risk Factors for Health Care-Associated Infection in Older Adults

Older adults are at increased risk for infection due to interrelated host and environmental factors (**Fig. 1**). Host factors include decline in organ-specific and immune system function due to the natural aging process, specific geriatric syndromes, and accumulation of medical comorbidities. As a result, older adults have more health care exposure including medical devices and procedures, polypharmacy and antibiotics, and prolonged stays in acute and LTCFs with need for assistance with activities

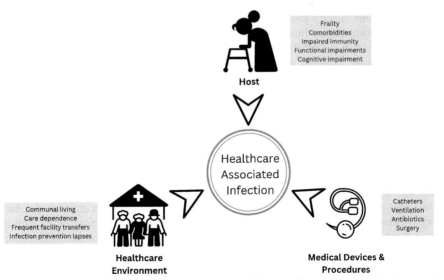

Fig. 1. Medical treatments, host and environmental factors all contribute to the increased susceptibility of health care-associated infections in the older adult.

of daily living (ADLs). Understanding which of these risk factors are modifiable allows for broad and targeted prevention strategies.

The aging process is accompanied by physiologic changes in multiple organ systems such as reduced cough reflex, decreased urinary flow, thinning of the skin, and alterations in the gut microbiome predisposing older adults to the most common HAIs: pneumonia, skin and soft tissue infections, and UTIs (**Table 2**). Alterations also occur in the innate and adaptive immune system characterized by a shift from naive to memory T and B cells and a more pro-inflammatory state.[39] This dysfunction, termed immunosenescence, contributes to blunted responses to both vaccinations and infections, thereby increasing susceptibility to and severity of infection. The presence of chronic medical conditions rather than chronologic age correlates more strongly with markers of impaired immunity, presumably mediated through chronic inflammation that accompanies many chronic illnesses.[40] Older adults residing in LTCFs have a mean of six comorbidities;[41] 77% of LTCF residents have hypertension; other common comorbidities include depression (49%), diabetes (35%), and cardiac disease (20%).[42] Multimorbidity also increases HAI risk through other means such as increased health care contact and medical procedures such as joint replacements, cardiac devices, hemodialysis, and urinary catheters.

In addition to these age-associated changes, LTCF residents have high rates of cognitive impairments, malnutrition and are generally more frail than community dwelling older adults. Roughly half of all LTCF residents have Alzheimer's disease or another form of dementia; this proportion is higher among long-stay residents.[42] Infection and sepsis contribute to further cognitive decline.[43] Cognitive dysfunction decreases the ability to care for oneself, increasing contact with health care personnel and the opportunity for pathogen transmission. In addition, residents with cognitive dysfunction are frequently unable to express symptoms of infection, leading to diagnostic uncertainty. This results in increased inappropriate antibiotic use, contributing to antimicrobial resistance.

Cognitive impairment frequently overlaps with frailty, a distinct syndrome that includes physical and functional impairments as well. It impacts up to one-third of adults aged 80 years and older.[44,45] It is a state of low reserve and chronic inflammation that contributes to poor health outcomes. Frailty can predispose to pneumonia, sepsis, SSI, and viral respiratory illness.[46] Studies regarding the impact of frailty on HAI development are complicated by the heterogeneity of frailty and HAI definitions.

Another HAI risk is malnutrition, which is common among older adults. Over half of older hospitalized patients are undernourished on admission.[47] Up to two-thirds of LTCF residents meet criteria for protein calorie malnutrition and 40% to 50% have specific micronutrient deficiencies.[48,49] A combination of factors related to physical conditions, psychosocial, and cultural concerns, and system barriers can all contribute to malnutrition in LTCF residents. For example, the inability to feed oneself coupled with low staffing levels is linked to the increased risk of malnutrition highlighting the complex interplay between intrinsic and environmental factors.[50]

Institutionalized older adults have increased dependence on others for many aspects of daily care. This increased health care staff contact predisposes them to colonization with MDROs and aids in the transmission of communicable diseases.[51,52] Over 85% of LTCF residents require support to complete ADLs such as bathing, toileting, walking, and transfers out of bed with the majority requiring assistance with at least three ADLs. In addition, urinary and stool incontinence is common in this population.[42] This both increases the risk of UTI and skin and soft tissue infections as well as need for care.[53,54] One-third of hospitalized patients aged 70 years or older lose independence with at least one ADL during an acute hospitalization.[55] This stepwise decline can mark a transition from community dwelling to LTCF residence.

Table 2
Predisposing factors and prevention measures for common health care-associated infections in older adults

Infection Sites	Common Infection Syndromes	Predisposing Factors		Prevention Measures
		Intrinsic Factors	Health Care Environmental Factors	
Respiratory Infections	Ventilator-associated pneumonia Hospital and long-term care associated bacterial pneumonia Viral respiratory infection (upper and lower respiratory tract)	General Decreased mobility Malnutrition Frailty Immunosenescence Smoking Organ Specific Decreased cough and other protective reflexes Decreased elastic tissue, mucociliary clearance and chest compliance Dysphagia Colonization of oral mucosa with bacteria due to poor oral care Underlying lung disease	Medical Interventions Mechanical ventilation Tracheostomy Feeding tubes Environment Low staffing (less assistance with feeding and oral care) Communal living	Vaccination for pneumococcus, influenza, COVID-19 Oral care Early diagnosis of dysphagia Early mobilization during hospitalization Prompt response to outbreaks
Urinary tract Infections (UTIs)	Symptomatic UTIs Catheter-related UTIs	General Diabetes mellitus Estrogen changes in postmenopausal women Organ Specific Decreased urine flow, reduction in bladder capacity, uninhibited contractions Increased bacterial adherence to uroepithelial cells Prostate enlargement	Medical Interventions Bladder catheterization Antibiotic exposures and multidrug-resistant organism (MDRO) colonization	Avoid unnecessary catheterization Appropriate maintenance of urinary catheters Avoid treatment of asymptomatic bacteriuria Vaginal estrogen Managing comorbid conditions

(continued on next page)

Table 2
(continued)

Infection Sites	Common Infection Syndromes	Predisposing Factors		Prevention Measures
		Intrinsic Factors	Health Care Environmental Factors	
Skin and soft tissue infections	Decubitus ulcer-related infection Cellulitis	General Malnutrition Peripheral vascular disease Diabetes mellitus Urinary incontinence Decreased mobility and bedridden status Organ Specific Epidermal thinning and decreased skin elasticity Flattening of dermal epidermal junction Decreased subcutaneous tissues Decreased blood vessels in dermis	Medical Interventions Percutaneous feeding tube Environment Low staffing (less assistance with patient positioning and mobilization) Poor infection control practices	Repositioning Mobilization Optimizing nutritional status Good compliance with hand hygiene Managing comorbid conditions
Gastrointestinal infections	Viral gastroenteritis C difficile infection	General Immunosenescence Organ Specific Decreased gastric acidity Decreased intestinal mobility Change in intestinal microbiome	Medical Interventions Antibiotic exposures Environment Communal living	Good compliance with hand hygiene Adequate environmental cleaning Prompt response to outbreaks Optimize antibiotic use
Surgical Site Infections	Superficial and deep surgical site infections	General Frailty Immobility Malnutrition Diabetes mellitus Peripheral Vascular diseases Obesity Cancer Smoking S aureus colonization	Environment Residence in long-term care facility before surgery MDRO exposure	Enhanced recovery after surgery protocols and prehabilitation Managing comorbid conditions S aureus decolonization

Bacteremia and sepsis	Central line associated bloodstream infection UTI	General Compromised skin integrity Immunosenescence Malnutrition Cancer Cognitive dysfunction with difficulty in communicating symptoms Atypical presentation of infection	Medical Interventions Device use (central venous catheter, urinary catheter) Environment Residing in a long-term care facility	Early diagnosis of sepsis

(*Data from* Refs[44,45,97–99,101,126,127])

Functional impairment is frequently compounded by medical device use in LTCF residents. Over 12% of residents had a device based on a CDC survey of 161 NHs in 2017.[27] Urinary catheters and percutaneous gastrostomy (PEG) tubes were the most common, present in approximately 5% of residents each, followed by CVC and tracheostomy tubes in almost 2% of patients. The presence of these devices further increases the risk of infection and MRDO acquisition through the breakdown of skin integrity, the formation of catheter-associated biofilm, and even greater dependence on others for care.[52,56]

Health Care-Associated Infection Prevention in Older Adults

HAI prevention requires developing infection risk reduction strategies at the individual patient level as well as institutional and regional levels. Infection prevention programs are well established in acute care hospitals with extensive national guidelines and detailed bundled care approaches to HAI prevention. These are often adapted to LTCFs but outcomes data are limited. Specific prevention strategies in older adults should target modifiable risk factors. Detailed below are risks and prevention approaches related to the two most common HAIs in older adults.

Respiratory Infections in Acute and Long-Term Care Settings

Pneumonia is the most common HAI in hospitalized adults. Presently, most infections are not ventilator related due to successful ventilator-associated pneumonia prevention campaigns.[2] Non-ventilator hospital-acquired pneumonia (HAP) affects roughly one in 100 hospitalized patients and is associated with significant morbidity and mortality.[57] There is a national call to action to better understand HAP risk factors to inform prevention strategies. The fundamental pathophysiology of HAP involves the introduction of endogenous oropharyngeal contents into the lower respiratory tract through aspiration and impaired airway clearance. Host, microbial, and environmental factors combined drive the progression to infection. Age-associated physiologic changes increase the frequency and severity of aspiration in older adults, particularly older frail adults. These include changes that impede the clearance of secretions such as decreased respiratory muscle strength and chest wall compliance and the increased prevalence of chronic obstructive pulmonary disease.[58] Neurologic conditions that impair swallowing such as Alzheimer's disease, Parkinson's disease, and posterior cerebrovascular disease are also common in older adults.[59] Hospitalization further increases the risk of HAP through the administration of medications such as narcotics, gabapentin, and benzodiazepines that lead to lower levels of alertness that in turn impair one's ability to protect the airway.[60,61] Additional predisposing factors for HAP that are prevalent in older adults include poor dentition and immobility.[57,62] Poor dentition is associated with increased oropharyngeal colonization with pathogenic bacteria; immobility is a risk factor for aspiration, delirium, and pneumonia.[63] Inability to maintain independence and/or inconsistent assistance with ADLs such as walking, oral care, and eating upright during hospitalization and LTCF stays further exacerbates these risks.

Several HAP prevention strategies are particularly relevant to older adults and predominantly focus on primary prevention of aspiration. This starts with assessing the patient's aspiration risk including evaluation of the patient's cognitive, frailty, and nutrition status. Identified needs can alert providers to screen for dysphagia, modify diets, and reduce sedating medications. Oral care is the most well-studied HAP prevention modality. Robust data link oral flora to bacteria present in aspiration pneumonia and demonstrate that oral care can restore a healthier oral microbiome.[64,65] However, data are less conclusive as to whether hospital- or LTCF-based oral hygiene programs reduce HAP rates. The role of chlorhexidine in oral care is particularly controversial as a meta-analysis of its use in critical care units raised the possibility of increased harm.[66] A meta-analysis of five RTCs evaluating various oral care regimens in either hospitals or NHs through 2014 found evidence of HAP prevention benefit.[67] However, two subsequent large cluster randomized trials in LTCFs failed to show sustained reductions in pneumonia.[68,69] Zimmerman and colleagues implemented an oral health care program which focuses on staff education in NHs with high pneumonia rehospitalization rates with no pneumonia reduction seen after 2 years. Post hoc analysis, however, showed a significant reduction in pneumonia in the first year of the program, suggesting that ongoing education and/or dedicated oral care staff are needed to sustain benefit.[69] In the other study, Juthani-Mehta and colleagues found no reduction in pneumonia with twice daily tooth brushing and chlorhexidine rinses in residents with impaired oral hygiene and/or swallowing difficulties.[68] This study notably excluded residents at high risk of aspiration due to nasogastric or PEG tubes. Based on the limited available evidence from heterogeneous studies, current national acute care guidelines for HAP recommend oral care with daily tooth brushing but not chlorhexidine rinses.[61] Programs that encourage patient independence and mobility are associated with less delirium, a reduction in sedating medication use, and fewer aspiration events; these lower pneumonia risk as well.[62,70,71] This is best accomplished in specific geriatric units, but the principles can be applied to general inpatient settings as well. Despite the limited evidence in LTCF, many of principles also apply to older LTCF residents.

Other Respiratory Infections in Older Adults

In addition to bacterial pneumonia, older adults are at risk of viral respiratory illnesses. These infections are associated with significant morbidity, hospitalization, and death especially for infections due to influenza, respiratory syncytial virus (RSV), and SARS-CoV-2. Other respiratory viruses such as rhinovirus, seasonal coronaviruses, human metapneumovirus, parainfluenza, and adenovirus are all prevalent in the LTCF setting.[72,73] These often cause LTCF outbreaks due to the increased susceptibility of the older population, the communal living environment, and their frequent contact with staff. Secondary bacterial pneumonia, most commonly due to *Streptococcus pneumoniae*, can occur concomitantly or after the viral illness and is an additional source of morbidity and mortality.[74]

Vaccination is the most effective primary preventive measure. It is currently available for influenza, SARS-CoV-2, and pneumococcus, and RSV vaccines are in late-stage clinical trials.[75] Outbreak prevention focuses on early identification, pathogen-specific transmission-based precautions, and hand hygiene as well as chemoprophylaxis (primarily for influenza).[76] Vaccination of staff and sick leave policies that do not incentivize presenteeism are also critical for outbreak management.[77,78]

Urinary Tract Infections in Acute and Long-Term Care Settings

Common comorbidities and geriatric syndromes are associated with the development of UTIs. Many of the same neurologic impairments that contribute to the increased risk of respiratory infections such as dementia and stroke also increase the chance of UTIs by promoting incomplete bladder emptying and urinary and/or fecal incontinence. Diabetes is also associated with UTI in all ages, including in older adults. The pathogenesis is multifactorial, including autonomic neuropathy leading to incomplete bladder emptying.[79] Poor functional status and cognitive impairment with ADL dependence correlate with UTI in LTCF residents. Women are at higher risk of UTI than men in any age group, and a history of UTIs when younger correlates strongly with recurrent

UTI in postmenopausal women.[80,81] The postmenopausal low estrogen state may further contribute to both urinary symptoms and infection through alteration in the vaginal mucosa and pH causing dysuria and changes to genitourinary flora. The UTI risk increases with age in men due to prostatic enlargement which contributes to bladder outflow obstruction and prostatitis.[54]

Older adults have high rates of asymptomatic bacteriuria with up to 50% in women and 40% in men residing in LTCFs experiencing it.[54] This complicates the diagnosis of UTI, particularly when compounded by chronic symptoms from other genitourinary issues and communication difficulties common in LTCF residents and hospitalized older adults. The high prevalence of urinary voiding issues in older adults also leads to high utilization of indwelling urinary catheters in this population. Bacteriuria is present in virtually all chronically catheterized individuals due to biofilm formation.[82] The risk of symptomatic UTI in this population is over twice that of non-catheterized LTCF residents, and the risk of infection increases 3% to 7% per day of catheterization.[83] The use of suprapubic catheters in the LTCF setting is associated with a reduction in CAUTI but an increase in colonization with MDRO.[84] Although external catheter devices for men are associated with a lower risk of infection than indwelling, they still increase the risk compared with no catheterization.[54,85,86] There are limited data on the risk of infection with external catheter devices for women.[87,88]

Much of the prevention of UTI targets urinary catheter removal as catheter related UTIs is associated with higher morbidity. This is particularly relevant in the acute care and post-acute care settings; indwelling urinary catheters are present in around 12% of patients transferred from the hospital to LTCF.[89] A marked reduction in catheter use in LTCFs was achieved along with the institution of surveillance programs and public reporting of catheter utilization. Catheter removal, however, may not be possible for many LTCF residents. Gurwitz and colleagues found that most urinary catheters present in Connecticut NH residents over a 1-year period were necessary.[90] Furthermore, nearly half of residents admitted with catheters in place for less than 3 months had them removed during the study period. Therefore, prevention of catheter-related UTI in LTCF should be shifted to proper catheter maintenance. The urinary drainage bag represents a reservoir for bacteria and should be cleaned, dried, and handled appropriately. Urinary reflux through the catheter can be reduced by avoiding dependent loops of catheter, maintaining a downward flow of urine and not irrigating the catheter. A multimodal study by Mody and colleagues in 12 NHs evaluated the impact of intensive staff education and preemptive barrier precautions (gown and gloves) during high-risk activities of residents with indwelling devices; such activities included morning and evening care and device care.[91] Active surveillance for device-associated infections and MDRO colonization showed a reduction in CAUTI incidence and the acquisition of MRSA. Similarly, a national multimodal study in 404 NHs across the United States investigated the effectiveness of an intervention that included diagnostic stewardship for UTI and education on indwelling urinary catheter maintenance along with active CAUTI surveillance. The intervention led to a 54% decrease in CAUTI over 1 year along with a reduction in urine cultures.[89] These studies demonstrate the effectiveness of comprehensive approaches to HAI prevention in LTCFs that include active surveillance and feedback in addition to periodic education.

The prevention of non-catheter-related UTI in older adults is more challenging. Topical (vaginal) estrogen therapy may reduce the frequency of symptomatic UTI in postmenopausal women, but systemic replacement therapy is not recommended.[92] A randomized clinical study using cranberry capsules in women residing in NH showed no reduction in the frequency of bacteriuria, pyuria, or symptomatic UTI.[93]

Treatment of asymptomatic bacteriuria does not prevent the occurrence of symptomatic UTI, other complications, or death and is not recommended[94]; moreover, treatment predisposes to future symptomatic infection with more resistant organisms. Vaccines for the most common UTI pathogen, *E coli*, have been in development for decades with several new promising candidates.[95] This would be an ideal prevention strategy given the large burden of disease and difficulty in modifying the predisposing factors in older adults.

Additional Health Care-Associated Infections in Older Adults

Older adults are at the increased risk of additional HAIs both in acute and long-term care settings through combinations of the risk factors that are outlined above. Older individuals are at high risk for CDI as a result of age-related microbiome disruptions, overuse of antibiotics, and increased health care contact. Fortunately, healthcare-associated CDI rates are declining in the US hospitals and NHs due to several drivers, notably improved diagnostic and antibiotic stewardship and the decrease prevalence of the epidemic strain, NAP1/BI/027.[96] *C difficile* in older adults will be covered elsewhere in this issue. Additional infections include skin and soft tissues infections, CVC-related bloodstream infections, and SSIs. Salient predisposing factors for skin infections secondary to pressure ulcers include malnutrition, diabetes, vascular disease, and immobility.[97] The increasing medical complexity of patients outside of acute care setting, particularly with indwelling devices such as peripherally inserted central catheters, raises the likelihood of bloodstream infections and sepsis.[98–100] The geriatric syndromes of frailty and malnutrition contribute to SSI risk.[101,102] Awareness and identification of these predisposing factors in older patients and LTCF residents will enable providers to develop tailored prevention plans and early intervention to combat HAIs in older adults. Risk assessment and prevention tools are available for many of these conditions (see **Table 2**, for details on risk factors and prevention strategies).

Outbreaks in Long-Term Care Facilities

The presence of a susceptible population with high care needs in the communal setting of long-term care, coupled with infection control challenges, creates the perfect conditions for disease outbreaks such as COVID-19 (see **Table 1**, for commonly identified outbreak pathogens). Transmission of organisms among residents and between staff and residents in LTCFs is facilitated by lapses in infection prevention and control practices. Before COVID-19, roughly half of reported outbreaks were spread via direct person-to-person contact. A recent systematic review found common themes of poor adherence to hand hygiene as well as inadequate equipment and environmental cleaning as further propagating outbreaks.[103] Staff presenteeism with the absence of work restrictions is another important contributor to outbreak transmission.[104]

Outbreak mitigation measures focus on addressing these lapses in infection control. Active monitoring of hand hygiene and other infection prevention practices, with feedback and education, as well as policies that make it feasible for staff to stay home when sick can help limit spread.[76–78,105] Additional measures to control outbreaks in LTCFs include screening of asymptomatic individuals. This approach was successful to control COVID-19 outbreaks in LFTCs by identifying asymptomatic and presymptomatic residents and staff.[106,107] Similarly, screening strategies are used at times for other pathogens such as Group A *Streptococcus*, *C auris*, and CRE to detect colonization and facilitate isolation, decolonization, or preemptive treatment.[108,109]

Details of these approaches are beyond the scope of this review, but several tools are available for LTCFs.[110,111]

The Interrelatedness of Health Care-Associated Infection in Hospitals and Long-Term Care Facilities

Acute care hospitals are impacted by HAIs that occur in the LTCF setting and vice versa. A quarter to half of hospital transfers from LTCFs are due to infection.[112] Similarly, experiencing an HAI during hospitalization increases the chance of discharge to an LTCF, and half of all older adults who acquire an HAI during a hospital admission get discharged to an LTCF.[113] For example, one study of 21 US hospitals found that although only 25% of patients who developed a non-ventilator HAP had come from an LTCF, nearly half of them required discharge to one.[114]

Patients who enter LTCFs from hospitals rather than the community are also at higher risk of developing an HAI while in the facility, and the risk is highest immediately following the transfer.[27,36,115] Dwyer and colleagues found increased prevalence of infection in NH residents who had a hospital admission (20% vs 11%) or even an emergency department visit (17% vs 11%) in the previous 90 days.[36] This association is even more pronounced for specific HAIs. For instance, three-quarters of all CDI cases occurring in the NH were patients hospitalized in the preceding month, and most of them received antibiotics during that admission.[116] In addition to in-hospital antibiotic exposure, hospital discharge with a chronic wound, CVC, or other invasive device all increase the risk of having an HAI and receiving antibiotics in the post-acute care setting, particularly in association with an MDRO infection such as MRSA or C difficile.[29,115,117]

The interconnectedness of acute and LTCFs with frequent transfer of older adults between the settings also promotes the regional transmission of pathogens. This is particularly true for patients discharged to ventilator-capable skilled nursing facilities and long-term acute care hospitals. Owing to their underlying severe diseases, these patients experience frequent hospitalization with prolonged stays and antibiotic exposures. As an example, Lapp and colleagues identified dissemination of a carbapenemase-producing CRE *Klebsiella pneumonia* among a variety of post-acute care facilities across the Chicago area.[118] *C auris* transmission was similarly detected among a large network of acute and long-term health care facilities in New York City.[119]

The introduction and spread of MDROs across new geographic areas and populations highlights the necessity of a regional rather than facility-specific approach to combatting HAIs. Communication between facilities is paramount to interrupt the dissemination of these organisms. Other measures include screening for colonization, decolonization, environmental cleaning, appropriate use of PPE, and antibiotic stewardship.

The topics of MRDO infections in older adults as well as the importance of antibiotic stewardship to combat these threats are covered elsewhere in this issue.

SUMMARY

Along with an aging population comes an increased risk of infection associated with multiple health care environments. Many of the aging-related factors, such as dementia and frailty, that predispose older adults to infections, are not readily reversible. Unfortunately, primary prevention through immunization is only currently available for a few HAI pathogens (influenza, SARS-CoV-2, and S pneumoniae). However, promising vaccine candidates for additional organisms such as C difficile, MRSA, E coli, and RSV are in development, as are mechanisms to enhance vaccine responses in older adults.[75,95,120]

Multimodality prevention strategies are presently required to mitigate HAI risk in this vulnerable population. In addition to infection prevention efforts at the individual and institutional level, a coordinated approach between acute and long-term care teams is necessary to decrease the susceptibility of older individuals as they transfer among a network of interrelated facilities. Robust antibiotic stewardship infrastructure across the spectrum of health care is crucial to reduce older individuals' susceptibility to infection by minimizing microbiome disruptions and limiting the acquisition of MDROs.

Timely active HAI surveillance with reporting and feedback of process and outcomes measures in both acute and LTCFs is needed to drive ongoing improvement and risk reduction along the continuum of care. Infection prevention programs in LTCFs are currently not as developed and well-resourced as those in acute care facilities, and acute care facilities are not as well-equipped as LTCFs to meet the age-specific needs of the older population. The sharing of expertise between hospital-based infection prevention and infectious diseases specialists and LTCF-based geriatric specialists would improve outcomes in both health care environments.

CLINICS CARE POINTS

- Health care-associated infection (HAI) burden is high in older adults. HAI prevention should focus on identifying and addressing modifiable risk factors. This includes optimizing management of medical comorbidities and minimizing medical device use.

- Screening for geriatric syndromes that predispose older individuals to HAI can inform tailored prevention plans during hospitalizations and long-term care stays.

- A regional approach to infection prevention is required to address emerging HAI threats such as multidrug-resistant organisms. Enhanced communication between acute care and long-term care providers will facilitate HAI risk reduction along the continuum of care.

DISCLOSURE

Dr G Dumyati received grant funding from Pfizer, United States. The relationship ended December 2021. Dr B R. Tesini receives writing honoraria from Merck. The relationship is ongoing.

ACKNOWLEDGMENTS

The authors gratefully acknowledge Dr Paul Graman for assistance in manuscript review.

REFERENCES

1. Klevens RM, Edwards JR, Richards CL Jr, et al. Estimating health care-associated infections and deaths in U.S. hospitals, 2002. Public Health Rep 2007;122(2):160–6.
2. Magill SS, O'Leary E, Janelle SJ, et al. Changes in prevalence of health care-associated infections in U.S. hospitals. N Engl J Med 2018;379(18):1732–44.
3. Magill SS, Edwards JR, Bamberg W, et al. Multistate point-prevalence survey of health care-associated infections. N Engl J Med 2014;370(13):1198–208.

4. Murphy SLKK, Xu JQ, Arias E. Mortality in the United States, 2020. In: National center for health statistics, 427. Hyattsville, MD: Division of Vital S; 2021. p. 1–8.
5. Morgan DJ, Meddings J, Saint S, et al. Does nonpayment for hospital-acquired catheter-associated urinary tract infections lead to overtesting and increased antimicrobial prescribing? Clin Infect Dis 2012;55(7):923–9.
6. Umscheid CA, Mitchell MD, Doshi JA, et al. Estimating the proportion of healthcare-associated infections that are reasonably preventable and the related mortality and costs. Infect Control Hosp Epidemiol 2011;32(2):101–14.
7. Vespa J, Medina L, Armstrong DM. Demographic turning points for the United States. Washington, DC: Population Projections for 2020 to 2060; 2020. p. 25–1144.
8. Werner RM, Konetzka RT. Trends in post-acute care use among medicare beneficiaries: 2000 to 2015. Jama 2018;319(15):1616–7.
9. Werner RM, Bressman E. Trends in post-acute care utilization during the covid-19 pandemic. J Am Med Directors Assoc 2021;22(12):2496–9.
10. Jones AL, Dwyer LL, Bercovitz AR, et al. The National Nursing Home Survey: 2004 overview. Vital Health Stat 2009;13(167):1–155.
11. Ogata M, Takano K, Moriuchi Y, et al. Effects of Prophylactic Foscarnet on Human Herpesvirus-6 Reactivation and Encephalitis in Cord Blood Transplant Recipients: A Prospective Multicenter Trial with an Historical Control Group. Biol Blood Marrow Transplant : J Am Soc Blood Marrow Transplant 2018;24(6):1264 73.
12. McCarthy EP, Ogarek JA, Loomer L, et al. Hospital transfer rates among us nursing home residents with advanced illness before and after initiatives to reduce hospitalizations. JAMA Intern Med 2020;180(3):385–94.
13. Scott RD. The Direct medical costs of healthcare-associated infections in U.S. hospitals and the benefits of prevention. National Center for Preparedness, Detection, and Control of Infectious Diseases (U.S.). Division of Healthcare Quality Promotion. 2009.
14. Hughes JM. Study on the Efficacy of Nosocomial Infection Control (SENIC Project): Results and Implications for the Future. Chemotherapy 1988;34(6):553–61.
15. Haley RW, Culver DH, White JW, et al. The efficacy of infection surveillance and control programs in preventing nosocomial infections in US hospitals. Am J Epidemiol 1985;121(2):182–205.
16. Jarvis WR. Benchmarking for prevention: the Centers for Disease Control and Prevention's National Nosocomial Infections Surveillance (NNIS) system experience. Infection 2003;31(Suppl 2):44–8.
17. Emori TG, Banerjee SN, Culver DH, et al. Nosocomial infections in elderly patients in the United States, 1986-1990. National Nosocomial Infections Surveillance System. Am J Med 1991;91(3b):289s–93s.
18. ECDC. Point prevalence survey of healthcare-associated infections and antimicrobial use in European long-term care facilities. Stockholm: European Centre for Disease Prevention and Control (ECDC); 2014.
19. Suetens C, Latour K, Kärki T, et al. Prevalence of healthcare-associated infections, estimated incidence and composite antimicrobial resistance index in acute care hospitals and long-term care facilities: results from two European point prevalence surveys, 2016 to 2017. Euro Surveill 2018;23(46):1800516.
20. CDC. 2020 National and State Healthcare-Associated Infections Progress Report. 2021. Available at: https://www.cdc.gov/hai/data/portal/progress-report.html. Accessed September 2, 2022.

21. Weiner-Lastinger LM, Pattabiraman V, Konnor RY, et al. The impact of coronavirus disease 2019 (COVID-19) on healthcare-associated infections in 2020: A summary of data reported to the National Healthcare Safety Network. Infect Control Hosp Epidemiol 2022;43(1):12–25.
22. Lastinger LM, Alvarez CR, Kofman A, et al. Continued increases in the incidence of healthcare-associated infection (HAI) during the second year of the coronavirus disease 2019 (COVID-19) pandemic. Infect Control Hosp Epidemiol 2022;1–5.
23. Saleem Z, Godman B, Hassali MA, et al. Point prevalence surveys of healthcare-associated infections: a systematic review. Pathog Glob Health 2019; 113(4):191–205.
24. Allegranzi B, Bagheri Nejad S, Combescure C, et al. Burden of endemic healthcare-associated infection in developing countries: systematic review and meta-analysis. Lancet (London, England) 2011;377(9761):228–41.
25. Cairns S, Reilly J, Stewart S, et al. The prevalence of health care-associated infection in older people in acute care hospitals. Infect Control Hosp Epidemiol 2011;32(8):763–7.
26. Nelson RE, Hyun D, Jezek A, et al. Mortality, Length of Stay, and Healthcare Costs Associated With Multidrug-Resistant Bacterial Infections Among Elderly Hospitalized Patients in the United States. Clin Infect Dis 2022;74(6):1070–80.
27. Thompson N, Stone N, Brown C, et al. Prevalence and Epidemiology of Healthcare-Associated Infections (HAI) in US Nursing Homes (NH), 2017. Infect Control Hosp Epidemiol 2020;41(S1):s45–6.
28. Herzig CTA, Dick AW, Sorbero M, et al. Infection Trends in US Nursing Homes, 2006-2013. J Am Med Dir Assoc 2017;18(7):635–e639.
29. Thompson ND, Stone ND, Brown CJ, et al. Antimicrobial Use in a Cohort of US Nursing Homes, 2017. JAMA 2021;325(13):1286–95.
30. ECDC. Distribution of HAI types in long-term care facilities in the EU/EEA, selected LTCF types, HALT point prevalence survey, 2016-2017. 2022. Available at: https://www.ecdc.europa.eu/en/all-topics-z/healthcare-associated-infections-long-term-care-facilities/surveillance-and-disease-3. Accessed September 6, 2022.
31. Chen MK, Chevalier JA, Long EF. Nursing home staff networks and COVID-19. Proc Natl Acad Sci 2021;118(1). e2015455118.
32. Sanyaolu A, Okorie C, Marinkovic A, et al. Candida auris: An Overview of the Emerging Drug-Resistant Fungal Infection. Infect Chemother 2022;54(2): 236–46.
33. Richards C. Infections in residents of long-term care facilities: an agenda for research. Report of an expert panel. J Am Geriatr Soc 2002;50(3):570–6.
34. Tsan L, Langberg R, Davis C, et al. Nursing home-associated infections in Department of Veterans Affairs community living centers. Am J Infect Control 2010;38(6):461–6.
35. Tsan L, Davis C, Langberg R, et al. Prevalence of nursing home-associated infections in the Department of Veterans Affairs nursing home care units. Am J Infect Control 2008;36(3):173–9.
36. Dwyer LL, Harris-Kojetin LD, Valverde RH, et al. Infections in Long-Term Care Populations in the United States. J Am Geriatr Soc 2013;61(3):341–9.
37. Danko L, Roselle G, Tsan L, et al. Prevalence of Long Term Care Healthcare-Associated Infections in U.S. Nationwide: San Diego, CA: Department of Veterans Affairs Community Living Centers (CLCs); 2013.

38. Bennett NJ, Johnson SA, Richards MJ, et al. Infections in Australian Aged-Care Facilities: Evaluating the Impact of Revised McGeer Criteria for Surveillance of Urinary Tract Infections. Infect Control Hosp Epidemiol 2016;37(5):610–2.
39. Aiello A, Farzaneh F, Candore G, et al. Immunosenescence and Its Hallmarks: How to Oppose Aging Strategically? A Review of Potential Options for Therapeutic Intervention. Front Immunol 2019;10:2247.
40. Ferrucci L, Fabbri E. Inflammageing: chronic inflammation in ageing, cardiovascular disease, and frailty. Nat Rev Cardiol 2018;15(9):505–22.
41. Moore KL, Boscardin WJ, Steinman MA, et al. Patterns of chronic co-morbid medical conditions in older residents of U.S. nursing homes: differences between the sexes and across the agespan. J Nutr Health Aging 2014;18(4):429–36.
42. Sengupta ML, Caffrey C, Melekin A, et al. Post-acute and long-term care providers and services users in the United States, 2017–2018. Vital Health Stat 3 2022;47:1–93. In: National Center for Health S, ed. Vol 3. Hyattsville, MD.
43. Hernandez-Ruiz V, Letenneur L, Fülöp T, et al. Infectious diseases and cognition: do we have to worry? Neurol Sci 2022;43(11):6215–24.
44. El Chakhtoura NG, Bonomo RA, Jump RLP. Influence of aging and environment on presentation of infection in older adults. Infect Dis Clin North Am 2017;31(4):593–608.
45. Clegg A, Young J, Iliffe S, et al. Frailty in elderly people. Lancet 2013;381(9868):752–62.
46. Cosentino CB, Mitchell BG, Brewster DJ, et al. The utility of frailty indices in predicting the risk of health care associated infections: a systematic review. Am J Infect Control 2021;49(8):1078–84.
47. Milne AC, Avenell A, Potter J. Meta-analysis: protein and energy supplementation in older people. Ann Intern Med 2006;144(1):37–48.
48. Morley JE, Silver AJ. Nutritional issues in nursing home care. Ann Intern Med 1995;123(11):850–9.
49. Norman K, Haß U, Pirlich M. Malnutrition in older adults—recent advances and remaining challenges. Nutrients 2021;13(8):2764.
50. Woo J, Chi I, Hui E, et al. Low staffing level is associated with malnutrition in long-term residential care homes. Eur J Clin Nutr 2005;59(4):474–9.
51. Roghmann MC, Johnson JK, Sorkin JD, et al. Transmission of methicillin-resistant staphylococcus aureus (mrsa) to healthcare worker gowns and gloves during care of nursing home residents. Infect Control Hosp Epidemiol 2015;36(9):1050–7.
52. Mody L, Maheshwari S, Galecki A, et al. Indwelling device use and antibiotic resistance in nursing homes: identifying a high-risk group. J Am Geriatr Soc 2007;55(12):1921–6.
53. Gray M. Incontinence-related skin damage: essential knowledge. Ostomy/wound Manag 2007;53(12):28–32.
54. Nicolle LE. Urinary Tract Infections in the Older Adult. Clin Geriatr Med 2016;32(3):523–38.
55. Covinsky KE, Pierluissi E, Johnston CB. Hospitalization-associated disability: "She was probably able to ambulate, but I'm not sure". JAMA 2011;306(16):1782–93.
56. Schrank G, Branch-Elliman W. Breaking the chain of infection in older adults: a review of risk factors and strategies for preventing device-related infections. Infect Dis Clin North Am 2017;31(4):649–71.

57. Munro SC, Baker D, Giuliano KK, et al. Nonventilator hospital-acquired pneumonia: A call to action: Recommendations from the National Organization to Prevent Hospital-Acquired Pneumonia (NOHAP) among nonventilated patients. Infect Control Hosp Epidemiol 2021;42(8):991–6.

58. van der Maarel-Wierink CD, Vanobbergen JNO, Bronkhorst EM, et al. Risk Factors for Aspiration Pneumonia in Frail Older People: A Systematic Literature Review. J Am Med Directors Assoc 2011;12(5):344–54.

59. González-Fernández M, Daniels SK. Dysphagia in stroke and neurologic disease. Phys Med Rehabil Clin 2008;19(4):867–88.

60. Park CM, Inouye SK, Marcantonio ER, et al. Perioperative gabapentin use and in-hospital adverse clinical events among older adults after major surgery. JAMA Intern Med 2022;e223680.

61. Klompas M, Branson R, Cawcutt K, et al. Strategies to prevent ventilator-associated pneumonia, ventilator-associated events, and nonventilator hospital-acquired pneumonia in acute-care hospitals: 2022 Update. Infect Control Hosp Epidemiol 2022;43(6):687–713.

62. Surkan MJ, Gibson W. Interventions to Mobilize Elderly Patients and Reduce Length of Hospital Stay. Can J Cardiol 2018;34(7):881–8.

63. El-Solh AA. Association between pneumonia and oral care in nursing home residents. Lung 2011;189(3):173–80.

64. Sumi Y, Miura H, Michiwaki Y, et al. Colonization of dental plaque by respiratory pathogens in dependent elderly. Arch Gerontol Geriatr 2007;44(2):119–24.

65. Mammen MJ, Scannapieco FA, Sethi S. Oral-lung microbiome interactions in lung diseases. Periodontol 2000 2020;83(1):234–41.

66. Price R, MacLennan G, Glen J. Selective digestive or oropharyngeal decontamination and topical oropharyngeal chlorhexidine for prevention of death in general intensive care: systematic review and network meta-analysis. BMJ : Br Med J 2014;348:g2197.

67. Kaneoka A, Pisegna JM, Miloro KV, et al. Prevention of healthcare-associated pneumonia with oral care in individuals without mechanical ventilation: a systematic review and meta-analysis of randomized controlled trials. Infect Control Hosp Epidemiol 2015;36(8):899–906.

68. Juthani-Mehta M, Van Ness PH, McGloin J, et al. A cluster-randomized controlled trial of a multicomponent intervention protocol for pneumonia prevention among nursing home elders. Clin Infect Dis 2015;60(6):849–57.

69. Zimmerman S, Sloane PD, Ward K, et al. Effectiveness of a mouth care program provided by nursing home staff vs standard care on reducing pneumonia incidence: a cluster randomized trial. JAMA Netw Open 2020;3(6):e204321.

70. McAuley S, Price R, Phillips G, et al. Interventions to prevent non-critical care hospital acquired pneumonia–a systematic review. Eur Geriatr Med 2015;6(4):336–40.

71. Quinn B, Giuliano KK, Baker D. Non-ventilator health care-associated pneumonia (NV-HAP): Best practices for prevention of NV-HAP. Am J Infect Control 2020;48(5s):A23–7.

72. Falsey AR, Dallal GE, Formica MA, et al. Long-term care facilities: a cornucopia of viral pathogens. J Am Geriatr Soc 2008;56(7):1281–5.

73. Kodama F, Nace DA, Jump RLP. Respiratory syncytial virus and other noninfluenza respiratory viruses in older adults. Infect Dis Clin North Am 2017;31(4):767–90.

74. Falsey AR, Becker KL, Swinburne AJ, et al. Bacterial complications of respiratory tract viral illness: a comprehensive evaluation. J Infect Dis 2013;208(3): 432–41.
75. Shan J, Britton PN, King CL, et al. The immunogenicity and safety of respiratory syncytial virus vaccines in development: A systematic review. Influenza other Respir viruses 2021;15(4):539–51.
76. Uyeki TM, Bernstein HH, Bradley JS, et al. Clinical practice guidelines by the infectious diseases society of america: 2018 update on diagnosis, treatment, chemoprophylaxis, and institutional outbreak management of seasonal influenzaa. Clin Infect Dis 2018;68(6):e1–47.
77. O'Neil CA, Kim L, Prill MM, et al. Preventing respiratory viral transmission in long-term care: knowledge, attitudes, and practices of healthcare personnel. Infect Control Hosp Epidemiol 2017;38(12):1449–56.
78. O'Neil CA, Kim L, Prill MM, et al. Respiratory viral surveillance of healthcare personnel and patients at an adult long-term care facility. Infect Control Hosp Epidemiol 2019;40(11):1309–12.
79. Nitzan O, Elias M, Chazan B, et al. Urinary tract infections in patients with type 2 diabetes mellitus: review of prevalence, diagnosis, and management. Diabetes Metab Syndr Obes 2015;8:129–36.
80. Jackson SL, Boyko EJ, Scholes D, et al. Predictors of urinary tract infection after menopause: A prospective study. Am J Med 2004;117(12):903–11.
81. Raz R, Gennesin Y, Wasser J, et al. Recurrent urinary tract infections in postmenopausal women. Clin Infect Dis 2000;30(1):152–6.
82. Saint S, Chenoweth CE. Biofilms and catheter-associated urinary tract infections. Infect Dis Clin North Am 2003;17(2):411–32.
83. Garibaldi RA, Mooney BR, Epstein BJ, et al. An evaluation of daily bacteriologic monitoring to identify preventable episodes of catheter-associated urinary tract infection. Infect Control : IC. 1982;3(6):466–70.
84. Gibson KE, Neill S, Tuma E, et al. Indwelling urethral versus suprapubic catheters in nursing home residents: determining the safest option for long-term use. J Hosp Infect 2019;102(2):219–25.
85. Saint S, Kaufman SR, Rogers MAM, et al. Condom versus indwelling urinary catheters: a randomized trial. J Am Geriatr Soc 2006;54(7):1055–61.
86. Ouslander JG, Greengold B, Chen S. External catheter use and urinary tract infections among incontinent male nursing home patients. J Am Geriatr Soc 1987; 35(12):1063–70.
87. Rearigh L, Gillett G, Sy A, et al. Effect of an external urinary collection device for women on institutional catheter utilization and catheter-associated urinary tract infections. Infect Control Hosp Epidemiol 2021;42(5):619–21.
88. Lem M, Jasperse N, Grigorian A, et al. Effect of external urinary collection device implementation on female surgical patients. Infect Dis Health 2022;27(4): 227–34.
89. Mody L, Greene MT, Meddings J, et al. A national implem entation project to prevent catheter-associated urinary tract infection in nursing home residents. JAMA Intern Med 2017;177(8):1154–62.
90. Gurwitz JH, DuBeau C, Mazor K, et al. Use of indwelling urinary catheters in nursing homes: implications for quality improvement efforts. J Am Geriatr Soc 2016;64(11):2204–9.
91. Mody L, Krein SL, Saint S, et al. A targeted infection prevention intervention in nursing home residents with indwelling devices: a randomized clinical trial. JAMA Intern Med 2015;175(5):714–23.

92. Ashraf MS, Gaur S, Bushen OY, et al. Diagnosis, treatment, and prevention of urinary tract infections in post-acute and long-term care settings: a consensus statement from AMDA's infection advisory subcommittee. J Am Med Dir Assoc 2020;21(1):12–24, e12.

93. Juthani-Mehta M, Van Ness PH, Bianco L, et al. Effect of cranberry capsules on bacteriuria plus pyuria among older women in nursing homes: a randomized clinical trial. JAMA 2016;316(18):1879–87.

94. Zalmanovici Trestioreanu A, Lador A, Sauerbrun-Cutler MT, et al. Antibiotics for asymptomatic bacteriuria. Cochrane Database Syst Rev 2015;4(4):Cd009534.

95. Magistro G, Stief CG. Vaccine development for urinary tract infections: where do we stand? Eur Urol Focus 2019;5(1):39–41.

96. Guh AY, Mu Y, Winston LG, et al. Trends in U.S. burden of Clostridioides difficile infection and outcomes. N Engl J Med 2020;382(14):1320–30.

97. Boyko TV, Longaker MT, Yang GP. Review of the current management of pressure ulcers. Adv Wound Care 2018;7(2):57–67.

98. Rowe TA, McKoy JM. Sepsis in older adults. Infect Dis Clin North Am 2017; 31(4):731–42.

99. Esme M, Topeli A, Yavuz BB, et al. Infections in the Elderly Critically-Ill Patients. Front Med 2019;6:118.

100. Chopra V, Montoya A, Joshi D, et al. Peripherally inserted central catheter use in skilled nursing facilities: a pilot study. J Am Geriatr Soc 2015;63(9):1894–9.

101. Millan M. Enhanced recovery after surgery in elderly and high-risk patients. Ann Laparosc Endoscopic Surg 2020;5:39.

102. Tsantes AG, Papadopoulos DV, Lytras T, et al. Association of malnutrition with surgical site infection following spinal surgery: systematic review and meta-analysis. J Hosp Infect 2020;104(1):111–9.

103. Lee MH, Lee GA, Lee SH, et al. A systematic review on the causes of the transmission and control measures of outbreaks in long-term care facilities: Back to basics of infection control. PLoS One 2020;15(3):e0229911.

104. Kobayashi M, Lyman MM, Francois Watkins LK, et al. A Cluster of Group A Streptococcal Infections in a Skilled Nursing Facility-the Potential Role of Healthcare Worker Presenteeism. J Am Geriatr Soc 2016;64(12):e279–84.

105. Kovacs-Litman A, Muller MP, Powis JE, et al. Association Between Hospital Outbreaks and Hand Hygiene: Insights from Electronic Monitoring. Clin Infect Dis 2020;73(11):e3656–60.

106. Hatfield KM, Reddy SC, Forsberg K, et al. Facility-Wide Testing for SARS-CoV-2 in Nursing Homes - Seven U.S. Jurisdictions, March-June 2020. MMWR Morbidity mortality weekly Rep 2020;69(32):1095–9.

107. Vilches TN, Nourbakhsh S, Zhang K, et al. Multifaceted strategies for the control of COVID-19 outbreaks in long-term care facilities in Ontario, Canada. Prev Med 2021;148:106564.

108. Dooling KL, Crist MB, Nguyen DB, et al. Investigation of a prolonged Group A Streptococcal outbreak among residents of a skilled nursing facility, Georgia, 2009-2012. Clin Infect 2013;57(11):1562–7.

109. Magill SS, O'Leary E, Janelle SJ, et al. Changes in Prevalence of Health Care–Associated Infections in U.S. Hospitals. N Engl J Med 2018;379(18):1732–44.

110. CDC. Facility Guidance for control of carbapenemase-resistant Enterobacteriaceae. CRE); 2019. Available at: https://www.cdc.gov/hai/pdfs/cre/cre-guidance-508.pdf. Accessed October 7, 2022.

111. Jordan HT, Richards CL Jr, Burton DC, et al. Group a streptococcal disease in long-term care facilities: descriptive epidemiology and potential control measures. Clin Infect Dis : official Publ Infect Dis Soc America 2007;45(6):742–52.
112. Dick A, Sorbero M, Furuya EY, et al. The Burden of Infection in Transfers from Nursing Homes to Hospitals. Infect Control Hosp Epidemiol 2020;41(S1):s80–1.
113. Hoffman GJ, Min LC, Liu H, et al. Role of Post-Acute Care in Readmissions for Preexisting Healthcare-Associated Infections. J Am Geriatr Soc 2020;68(2):370–8.
114. Baker D, Quinn B. Hospital Acquired Pneumonia Prevention Initiative-2: Incidence of nonventilator hospital-acquired pneumonia in the United States. Am J Infect Control 2018;46(1):2–7.
115. Gontjes KJ, Gibson KE, Lansing BJ, et al. Association of Exposure to High-risk Antibiotics in Acute Care Hospitals With Multidrug-Resistant Organism Burden in Nursing Homes. JAMA Netw Open 2022;5(2):e2144959.
116. Hunter JC, Mu Y, Dumyati GK, et al. Burden of Nursing Home-Onset Clostridium difficile Infection in the United States: Estimates of Incidence and Patient Outcomes. Open Forum Infect Dis 2016;3(1):ofv196.
117. Epstein L, Mu Y, Belflower R, et al. Risk Factors for Invasive Methicillin-Resistant Staphylococcus aureus Infection After Recent Discharge From an Acute-Care Hospitalization, 2011-2013. Clin Infect Dis : official Publ Infect Dis Soc America 2016;62(1):45–52.
118. Lapp Z, Crawford R, Miles-Jay A, et al. Regional Spread of blaNDM-1-Containing Klebsiella pneumoniae ST147 in Post-Acute Care Facilities. Clin Infect Dis 2021;73(8):1431–9.
119. Adams E, Quinn M, Tsay S, et al. Candida auris in Healthcare Facilities, New York, USA, 2013-2017. Emerg Infect Dis 2018;24(10):1816–24.
120. Anderson AS, Scully IL, Pride MW, et al. Vaccination against Nosocomial Infections in Elderly Adults. Interdiscip Top Gerontol Geriatr 2020;43:193–217.
121. Strausbaugh LJ, Sukumar SR, Joseph CL, et al. Infectious Disease Outbreaks in Nursing Homes: An Unappreciated Hazard for Frail Elderly Persons. Clin Infect Dis 2003;36(7):870–6.
122. CDC. Serious Infections and outbreaks occurring in LTCFs. 2020. Available at: https://www.cdc.gov/longtermcare/staff/report-publications.html. Accessed September 5, 2022.
123. Rossow J, Ostrowsky B, Adams E, et al. Factors Associated With Candida auris Colonization and Transmission in Skilled Nursing Facilities With Ventilator Units, New York, 2016–2018. Clin Infect Dis 2020;72(11):e753–60.
124. Calderwood LE, Wikswo ME, Mattison CP, et al. Norovirus Outbreaks in Long-term Care Facilities in the United States, 2009–2018: A Decade of Surveillance. Clin Infect Dis 2021;74(1):113–9.
125. Cassell JA, Middleton J, Nalabanda A, et al. Scabies outbreaks in ten care homes for elderly people: a prospective study of clinical features, epidemiology, and treatment outcomes. Lancet Infect Dis 2018;18(8):894–902.
126. Buetti N, Marschall J, Drees M, et al. Strategies to prevent central line-associated bloodstream infections in acute-care hospitals: 2022 Update. Infect Control Hosp Epidemiol 2022;43(5):1–17.
127. AHRQ. Toolkit for Reducing CAUTI in Hospitals. 2018. Content last reviewed March 2018. Available at: https://www.ahrq.gov/hai/tools/cauti-hospitals/index.html. Accessed September 5, 2022.

Update on *Clostridioides difficile* Infection in Older Adults

Curtis J. Donskey, MD[a,b,*]

KEYWORDS

- Older adults • Long-term care facility • *Clostridioides difficile* infection
- Fecal microbiota transplant

KEY POINTS

- *Clostridioides difficile* infection (CDI) disproportionately affects older persons.
- Asymptomatic carriage of toxigenic *C difficile* is common, particularly in health care settings.
- The diagnosis of CDI requires a combination of clinical symptoms consistent with the diagnosis and laboratory tests confirming presence of a toxigenic strain or toxin in stool.
- Many cases of CDI have their onset in long-term care facilities (LTCFs), and many hospital-onset cases are transferred to LTCFs.
- CDI has substantial adverse effects on quality of life in older individuals, particularly in cases involving multiple recurrences.

INTRODUCTION

Clostridioides difficile is the most common infectious cause of health care-associated diarrhea in developed countries.[1] The incidence of *C difficile* infection (CDI) increased dramatically in North America and Northern Europe beginning in the early 2000s in association with emergence of an epidemic strain termed 027/BI/NAP1.[1] Control of outbreaks often required sequential implementation of multiple control measures, including antimicrobial stewardship.[2] Many health care facilities continue to struggle with high endemic rates of CDI. Current estimates from the Centers for Disease Control and Prevention suggest that CDI now causes more health care-associated infections than any other pathogen. In 2017, it was estimated that there were 462,100 total CDI cases in the United States that were associated with 20,500 deaths.[1]

Disclosure statement: This work was supported by the Department of Veterans Affairs. C.J. Donskey has received research grants from Pfizer, Clorox, and Ecolab.
[a] Geriatric Research Education and Clinical Center, Cleveland Veterans Affairs Medical Center, Cleveland, OH, USA; [b] Case Western Reserve University School of Medicine, Cleveland, OH, USA
* Infectious Diseases Section, Louis Stokes Cleveland Veterans Affairs Medical Center, 10701 East Boulevard, Cleveland, OH 44106.
E-mail address: Curtis.Donskey@va.gov

The increase in the incidence of CDI during the past 2 decades occurred in all age groups, but older adults were disproportionately affected, and long-term care facilities (LTCFs) have borne a substantial proportion of the burden of CDI.[3–9] Older individuals may be at increased risk for initial CDI cases and recurrences of infection due to intrinsic factors associated with aging such as waning immunity and altered intestinal microbiota. In addition, increased exposure to health care and antibiotics are major contributors to the risk for CDI in the older population. This review focuses on current concepts related to the pathogenesis, epidemiology, diagnosis, and management of CDI among older adults.

PATHOGENESIS

C difficile is acquired through ingestion of spores that are ubiquitous in the environment. In health care facilities, contaminated environmental surfaces, the skin and hands of colonized or infected patients, and the hands of health care workers are common sources.[10,11] After ingestion, spores pass through the stomach and germinate in the small intestine in response to germinants, including bile salts.[11] Gastric acid provides an important host defense by killing ingested pathogens; however, the role of gastric acid as a defense against *C difficile* is controversial. Gastric acid does not kill *C difficile* spores, and whereas some studies have demonstrated an association between medications that inhibit stomach acid and CDI, others have not.[11]

In the colon, vegetative *C difficile* establishes colonization with production of toxin if the indigenous microbiota that provide colonization resistance are disrupted. The primary cause of altered colonization resistance is antibiotic therapy.[12] After establishment of colonization with toxigenic *C difficile* strains, ~10% to 60% of hospitalized patients develop CDI, with the remainder developing asymptomatic colonization (**Fig. 1**).[11] The immune system plays a crucial role in determining whether symptomatic illness occurs. An anamnestic antibody response to toxins protects against initial and recurrent CDI.[13] Other host factors may play a role in determining if symptomatic illness occurs, including innate immune responses. For example, a common polymorphism in the interleukin 8 gene promoter has been associated with initial and recurrent CDI.[14]

Older individuals may be at increased risk for CDI in part due to waning of natural defenses with advanced age. Gastric acid production may be reduced in the older adults.[15] The intestinal microbiota of older individuals may be altered when compared

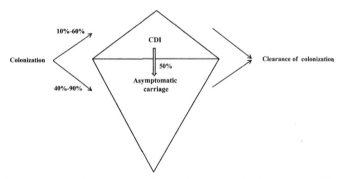

Fig. 1. Outcomes after establishment of colonization by toxigenic *Clostridium difficile*. (*From* Donskey CJ, Kundrapu S, Deshpande A. Colonization versus carriage of *Clostridium difficile*. Infect Dis Clin North Am 2015; 29:13-28; with permission.)

with that of younger individuals,[16,17] and may be less inhibitory to growth of *C diffi-cile*.[18] It is plausible that changes associated with aging may contribute to the increased frequency of CDI in this population. However, it is likely that loss of natural defense mechanisms among older persons is primarily iatrogenic because older adults are frequently prescribed proton pump inhibitors and antibiotics, often unnec-essarily.[19,20] Given alteration of defenses due to these therapies and increased risk for exposure to spores during hospital and long-term care admissions, it is not surprising that CDI predominantly affects older adults.

ASYMPTOMATIC CARRIAGE OF TOXIGENIC *C DIFFICILE*

Asymptomatic carriage of toxigenic *C difficile* is common, particularly in health care settings.[11] Rea and colleagues[17] reported *C difficile* carriage in 2% of subjects older than 65 years in the community versus 10% in the community with outpatient health care exposures and 21% in hospital or LTCF settings. Others have demonstrated that asymptomatic carriage of *C difficile* is common in LTCFs, including upon admis-sion.[3–6,11] In an outbreak setting, Riggs and colleagues[3] found that 51% of asymptom-atic patients in 2 LTCF wards were colonized with toxigenic *C difficile*. Residents with asymptomatic carriage outnumbered those with CDI by a factor of 7 to 1. Antibiotic exposure and recent CDI were risk factors for asymptomatic carriage.

The fact that toxigenic *C difficile* is often carried asymptomatically has important clinical and infection control implications. First, diarrhea due to non-CDI causes is very common in health care facilities.[21] Testing for CDI in an asymptomatic carrier who develops diarrhea due to a non-CDI cause can lead to a diagnosis of CDI and exposure to CDI therapy that is not needed.[22] Second, although current infection con-trol strategies for *C difficile* focus primarily on symptomatic CDI cases, several studies suggest that asymptomatic carriers of toxigenic *C difficile* may be an underappreci-ated source of transmission.[23–26] Based on molecular typing, incident CDI cases in a tertiary care hospital were as frequently linked to asymptomatic carriers of toxigenic *C difficile* as to CDI cases (29% vs 30%, respectively).[23] In another recent study, LTCF residents with asymptomatic carriage of *C difficile* contributed to transmission both in the LTCF and in the affiliated hospital during acute care admissions.[26]

EPIDEMIOLOGY

After the emergence of the NAP1/BI/027 strain in the early 2000s, the incidence of CDI increased dramatically in North America and Northern Europe and many facilities experienced large outbreaks.[1] The increase in CDI disproportionately involved older adults. In 2009, the incidence of CDI-related hospitals stays for adults aged 65 to 84 years and 85 years or older was 4- and 10-fold greater, respectively, than for adults aged 45 to 64 years.[27]

LTCFs have borne a significant proportion of the increasing burden of CDI. Hospi-talized patients with CDI are often discharged to LTCFs.[11] In a recent national surveil-lance study, it was estimated that 36% of health care-associated CDI cases in the United States had their onset in LTCFs versus 37% in hospitals.[28] Many LTCF-associated CDI cases occur within 1 month after hospital discharge.[6,11] For example, 85% of LTCF-onset CDI cases in a Department of Veterans Affairs' LTCF had their onset within 1 month after transfer from the hospital (**Fig. 2**).[6]

Studies demonstrating onset of CDI soon after transfer from the hospital suggest that many cases of LTCF-onset CDI may be acquired during hospital stays. How-ever, studies that include serial cultures and molecular typing are needed to defin-itively determine the source of acquisition. In such a study, we found that LTCF

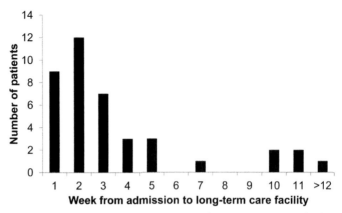

Fig. 2. Timing of onset of CDI in LTCF residents in relation to the time of admission to the LTCF from the hospital. (*From* Guerrero DM, Nerandzic MM, Jury LA, Chang S, Jump RL, Donskey CJ. Clostridium difficile infection in a Department of Veterans Affairs long-term care facility. Infect Control Hosp Epidemiol 2011;32:513-5.)

residents frequently acquired colonization with toxigenic *C difficile* after transfer from the hospital, and 3 of 4 initial CDI cases with onset within 1 month of transfer occurred in residents who acquired colonization in the LTCF.[29] These findings suggest that both the hospital and LTCF may be important sources of *C difficile* acquisition.

During the past few years, there have been some promising developments in the epidemiology of CDI. Between 2011 and 2017, the total burden of CDI in the United States decreased by 24%.[1] The reduction was driven by a 36% reduction in health care-associated CDI. There was no change in the burden of community-associated CDI during that period. Similar reductions in health care-associated CDI were observed in England.[30] Infections due to the fluoroquinolone-resistant NAP1/BI/027 epidemic strain decreased dramatically in the United States and England in conjunction with reduced use of fluoroquinolones.[30,31] Although rates of several health care-associated infections increased during the first year of the coronavirus disease 2019 pandemic, there was no increase in CDI rates in the United States based on data from the National Healthcare Safety Network.[32]

CLINICAL PRESENTATION

For patients who develop CDI, the typical clinical presentation is diarrhea, ranging in severity from mild to profuse.[11] In most cases, the diarrhea is antibiotic associated, occurring either during or after completion of antibiotic therapy. Although most cases occur during or within 1 to 2 weeks after completion of antibiotic therapy, increased risk for CDI may persist for up to 90 days after antibiotic exposure.[33] The diarrhea may include presence of mucus in stools and may be associated with abdominal cramping. Fever occurs in a minority of cases. Leukocytosis is a frequent laboratory finding in patients with CDI and may precede the onset of diarrhea. In patients with antibiotic exposure, a peripheral white blood cell count greater than 20,000/mm^3 with no alternative explanation should raise concern for CDI. A small percentage of patients with CDI never develop diarrhea due to the presence of an ileus. Patients with ileus are at risk for severe complications including hypotension or shock, toxic megacolon, and intestinal perforation. Factors that reduce bowel motility may increase the risk for ileus (eg, narcotic or antidiarrheal medication exposure, recent intra-abdominal surgery).

Some presentations are not typical of CDI and should lead to consideration of alternative diagnoses. For example, although presence of occult blood is common in stool of CDI cases, frank melena and hematochezia are rare. Vomiting is also uncommon in the absence of ileus. A syndrome with acute onset of vomiting and diarrhea would be more consistent with viral gastroenteritis (eg, *Norovirus*) or staphylococcal food poisoning than CDI, particularly if multiple patients or LTCF residents and staff members present with similar symptoms. In fact, several pseudo-outbreaks of CDI have been attributed to CDI testing during *Norovirus* outbreaks, with positive CDI results representing detection of asymptomatic carriers of toxigenic *C difficile*.[34] Similarly, a positive test for *C difficile* in a patient with diarrhea after receiving a laxative in the absence of prior antibiotic exposure would suggest asymptomatic carriage rather than CDI.[11]

Although effective treatments are available for CDI, 20% to 30% of patients who respond to initial courses of treatment develop recurrent CDI, usually within 1 to 4 weeks of completing treatment with either vancomycin or metronidazole.[11] The risk of recurrent CDI is even higher in patients who have already had one or more recurrences, and many patients develop repeated episodes that may continue to occur over a period of months or years. Recurrent CDI has a significant impact on health care systems due to need for multiple courses of treatment, increased average length of stay, and increased costs.[27,35] Recurrent episodes of CDI can also be associated with adverse outcomes. For example, in a study conducted in the setting of an outbreak associated with the BI/NAP1/027 strain, 11% of patients with a first recurrence of CDI had serious complications, including shock, toxic megacolon, colectomy, and death.[35]

The presentation of CDI is similar in older and younger adults, but older adults may suffer much greater adverse consequences due to comorbid conditions or debility. In a relatively healthy young adult, having to urgently use the bathroom 8 times per day may be an inconvenience. In an older person with decreased mobility, visual impairment, or dementia, having to urgently use the bathroom multiple times per day can be a nearly impossible situation to manage independently. Older individuals with multiple medical problems are often in a tenuous state, and CDI can lead to institutionalization. For older adults able to live at home, recurrent CDI often has a significant negative impact on quality of life of patients and their families.[36] Common complaints of patients include loss of independence and inability to travel or enjoy normal activities due to fear of uncontrolled episodes of fecal incontinence or diarrhea.

DIAGNOSIS

The diagnosis of CDI is based on a combination of clinical symptoms consistent with the diagnosis and laboratory tests confirming presence of a toxigenic strain or toxin in stool.[11,37] To avoid diagnosis of CDI in asymptomatic carriers, laboratories should only accept unformed stools (defined as stools taking the shape of the container) for testing unless ileus due to CDI is suspected.[37,38] In the absence of a positive laboratory test, histopathologic or endoscopic findings may be used to support the diagnosis.

Many laboratories in the United States currently use nucleic acid amplification tests (NAATs) for diagnosis of CDI. Although NAATs have excellent sensitivity, there is concern that they may identify asymptomatic carriers of toxigenic *C difficile* with unformed stool due to other causes (eg, laxatives), resulting in unnecessary treatment and inflation of CDI rates.[11,38,39] One strategy to address this concern has been to implement stewardship interventions to restrict testing to patients with 3 or more unformed stools within 24 hours with no alternative explanation for diarrhea.[37] Alternatively, multistep testing algorithms can be used in which results of stool toxin testing and clinical assessments are used to guide management for patients with positive initial screening assays for *C difficile*.[37–39] **Fig. 3** shows a 2-step test algorithm in which the first step is an NAAT that detects toxin B genes indicating the presence a toxin-producing *C difficile* strain that may either be asymptomatically colonizing or infecting a patient. If the NAAT test is positive, the stool specimen undergoes a second step test with an enzyme immunoassay that detects free toxin. A positive toxin assay indicates CDI, whereas a negative toxin assay suggests either asymptomatic carriage of toxigenic *C difficile* or relatively mild CDI that may resolve without treatment.[37–39] Patients with a positive NAAT but negative toxin assay may contribute to transmission and should be isolated even if treatment is not prescribed.[37–39]

The multistep algorithm approach is supported by some studies that have demonstrated that patients with evidence of toxigenic *C difficile* in stool (eg, positive NAAT) but with absence of free toxin based on negative enzyme immunoassay for toxin infrequently suffer adverse outcomes if they are not treated.[38,39] However, clinical assessment remains essential because some NAAT-positive-only patients do have severe, complicated infections.[40,41] Recently, ultrasensitive and quantitative toxin measurement has been shown to correlate with severe disease, severe CDI-attributable outcomes, and recurrence.[42] Although promising, ultrasensitive *C difficile* toxin assays are not commonly available.

Because all CDI testing methods have limitations, it is essential that clinicians and nursing staff understand the advantages and disadvantages of the approach used in their facility. For facilities using NAATs as standalone tests, ongoing education of providers and nursing staff regarding appropriate indications for CDI testing is needed

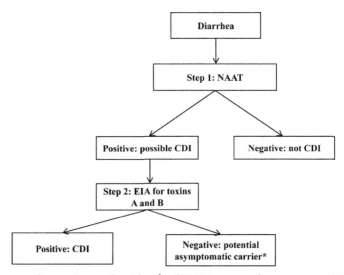

Fig. 3. Two-step diagnostic test algorithm for CDI. EIA, enzyme immunoassay; NAAT, nucleic acid amplification test. Asterisk indicates patients with positive NAAT but negative EIA for toxin may be asymptomatic carriers of toxigenic *C difficile* or may have relatively mild CDI that may resolve without treatment; however, clinical assessment is needed because some NAAT-positive-only patients do have severe, complicated infections.

to reduce the risk that asymptomatic carriers will be diagnosed with CDI and treated unnecessarily. In settings in which sensitive screening tests are followed by a relatively sensitive enzyme immunoassay for toxins A and B, it must be appreciated that even relatively sensitive toxin tests miss some patients with CDI. Planche and Wilcox[39] cautioned that the need for CDI treatment in toxin-negative patients is a clinical decision.

Performance of a test of cure after CDI treatment is not recommended.[37,39] It has been demonstrated that polymerase chain reaction (PCR) and glutamate dehydrogenase tests often remain positive after resolution of symptoms, and ~20% of patients may have positive tests at the end of treatment.[43] Moreover, after discontinuation of metronidazole or vancomycin treatment, as many as 56% of patients who remain asymptomatic have positive cultures 1 to 4 weeks after treatment cessation.[43] The efficacy of treatment should be determined based on resolution of diarrhea.

Repeat testing during the same episode of diarrhea is a common practice that is also discouraged in current guidelines.[37] Repeat testing increases the possibility of false-positive results and does not substantially increase the yield of true-positives. In practice, some laboratories prohibit repeat testing after an initial negative test for 5 or 7 days to avoid inappropriate repeat testing.

In severe CDI cases, computed tomography findings may include colonic mural thickening, pericolonic fat changes, trapping of contrast material between thickened folds (accordion sign), and ascites.[37] Sigmoidoscopy or colonoscopy may also be useful in these cases to evaluate for the presence of pseudomembranous colitis. Perirectal swab specimens could potentially be useful as a diagnostic approach in patients with suspected CDI and ileus. In a study of 139 patients tested for CDI by PCR (Xpert *C difficile*), perirectal swab testing was 96% sensitive when compared with stool specimens.[44]

Efforts to assess the timeliness of CDI diagnostic testing and to expedite the diagnosis of CDI may be beneficial. Efficient diagnostic testing for CDI will minimize delays in initiation of isolation and treatment of confirmed cases, while also allowing rapid discontinuation of empirical therapy and isolation when testing is negative. However, delays in diagnosis are common in practice. In the VA hospital and adjacent LTCF, the average time between placing an order and obtaining a test result from the on-site laboratory was 1.8 days, with the time required for collection of stool specimens contributing most to the delay.[45] An intervention focused on expediting stool sample collection and testing and reducing rejection of specimens was effective in significantly reducing the time from test order to diagnosis. Quinn and colleagues[46] found that most Iowa LTCFs did not have a protocol to identify residents with CDI and did not perform diagnostic testing unless a resident had severe diarrhea. Given that many LTCFs use off-site laboratories, improving the timeliness of diagnostic testing may be a particular challenge in this setting.

MANAGEMENT

General measures for all patients with CDI include replacing fluid and electrolyte losses, avoiding antiperistaltic agents and, whenever possible, stopping the inciting antibiotic. In debilitated older adults, it is necessary to consider the potential for complications such as dehydration if it is not possible to maintain adequate fluid intake or falls if there is difficulty making multiple trips to the bathroom.

The Infectious Diseases Society of America (IDSA) in collaboration with the Society for Healthcare Epidemiology of America (SHEA) and the American College of Gastroenterology (ACG) have published recent guidelines for management of CDI.[37,47,48] The recommendations are similar with some differences related to treatment choices and when fecal microbiota transplantation (FMT) should be recommended. **Table 1** provides a modified version of treatment regimens recommended by the IDSA/SHEA in a 2021 focused update,[47] including comments on how the IDSA/SHEA and ACG guidelines differ.

For initial episodes of CDI, the IDSA/SHEA guidelines recommend a 10-day course of fidaxomicin if resources are available, whereas the ACG guidelines recommend either fidaxomicin or a 10-day course of oral vancomycin.[47,48] The rationale for preferring fidaxomicin is that multiple studies have demonstrated a comparable treatment response for fidaxomicin and vancomycin but lower rates of recurrence.[47,49] The lower recurrence rate is microbiologically plausible because fidaxomicin causes less alteration of the indigenous intestinal microbiota that compete with *C difficile*.[49] The potential benefit of fidaxomicin may be particularly great in older individuals because they are at relatively high risk for recurrence of CDI.[50] Although there is a strong rationale for preferred use of fidaxomicin in older individuals with CDI, the relatively high cost of this medication has limited widespread adoption of this treatment.

CDI is deemed to be fulminant if hypotension or shock, ileus, or toxic megacolon is present.[37,48] These patients have a high risk for mortality and may require surgical intervention. Patients with fulminant CDI should ideally be managed in an intensive care unit and surgery should be consulted. The management of such cases is outside the scope of this review.

For patients who develop first recurrences of CDI, the IDSA/SHEA guidelines recommend fidaxomicin and the ACG guidelines recommend either fidaxomicin or a vancomycin taper and pulse regimen.[47,49] For fidaxomicin, an extended-pulsed regimen using the same total dose as the standard 10-day regimen resulted in a low rate of recurrence when compared with a 10-day course of vancomycin.[50] For the extended-pulsed regimen, fidaxomicin is prescribed at the standard dose of 200 mg twice daily for 5 days followed by once every other day for 20 days. The extended-pulsed regimen should only be used if there is evidence of substantial improvement in symptoms by day 5. For patients with a second recurrence of CDI, the IDSA/SHEA guidelines recommend a standard or extended-pulsed regimen of fidaxomicin or a vancomycin taper and pulse regimen.[47] The ACG guidelines recommend referral of patients with a second recurrence for FMT, whereas the IDSA/SHEA guidelines only recommend FMT after 3 or more recurrences.

Bezlotoxumab is a monoclonal antibody against *C difficile* toxin B approved for the prevention of recurrent CDI in high-risk adults in conjunction with antibiotic treatment.[47] Bezlotoxumab is given as a one-time infusion over 60 minutes and provides measurable antibody concentrations for up to 3 months. In phase 3 clinical studies, bezlotoxumab reduced rates of CDI recurrence compared with placebo. History of congestive heart failure is a relative contraindication for bezlotoxumab. The 2021 IDSA/SHEA guidelines for CDI recommends addition of bezlotoxumab to antibiotic treatment of patients with CDI with at least 1 risk factor for recurrence (recurrent CDI episode within the last 6 months, age ≥65 years, immunocompromised host, and severe CDI on presentation), particularly in patients with multiple risk factors for recurrence.[47] For primary care providers, it is recommended that bezlotoxumab be prescribed only in consultation with infectious diseases specialists.

Given the delays in diagnosis that often occur in outpatients or in LTCFs with off-site laboratories, it is often necessary to consider empirical treatment of CDI in older adults. Current practice guidelines recommend empirical treatment of only patients suspected to have severe CDI.[37] Empirical treatment of patients with suspected recurrence of infection is also reasonable given the high likelihood of infection in

Table 1
Recommendations for treatment of *Clostridium difficile* infection (CDI)

Clinical Definition	Preferred Treatment	Alternative Treatments	Other Considerations
Initial episode	Fidaxomicin 200 mg given twice daily for 10 d[a]	Vancomycin 125 mg 4 times daily for 10 d; for nonsevere CDI, metronidazole 500 mg 3 times daily for 10–14 d can be considered but is not recommended in elderly patients[b]	Nonsevere CDI: white blood cell count ≤15,000 cells/μL and serum creatinine <1.5 mg/dL
First CDI recurrence	Fidaxomicin 200 mg given twice daily for 10 d OR fidaxomicin extended-pulsed regimen (200 mg twice daily for 5 d followed by once every other day for 20 d)[c]	Vancomycin taper and pulse regimen[d], adjunctive bezlotoxumab 10 mg/kg given once intravenously[e]	Vancomycin 125 mg 4 times daily for 10 d can be given if metronidazole used for initial episode
Second or subsequent CDI recurrence	FMT OR fidaxomicin 200 mg given twice daily for 10 d OR fidaxomicin 200 mg twice daily for 5 d followed by once every other day for 20 d OR vancomycin taper and pulse regimen	Consider adjunctive bezlotoxumab 10 mg/kg given once intravenously	ACG guidelines recommend FMT for second or further recurrence; IDSA guidelines recommend antibiotic treatment of at least 2 recurrences before considering FMT
Fulminant CDI	Vancomycin, 500 mg 4 times daily by mouth or by nasogastric tube plus metronidazole 500 mg every 8 h intravenously	If complete ileus, consider adding rectal instillation of vancomycin	Surgical consultation recommended; FMT can be considered for fulminant CDI refractory to antibiotic therapy, particularly if poor surgical candidates

[a] IDSA guidelines recommend fidaxomicin but acknowledge that implementation depends on available resources because fidaxomicin is more expensive than vancomycin, whereas ACG guidelines recommend either fidaxomicin or vancomycin.

[b] Not recommended for elderly patients; ACG guidelines note that metronidazole can be considered in low-risk patients (younger outpatients with minimal comorbidities) and specifically cite evidence that metronidazole may be inferior in older patients.

[c] ACG guidelines recommend either fidaxomicin or vancomycin taper and pulse regimen; the extended-pulsed regimen should only be used if symptoms are improving after 5 d of twice-daily fidaxomicin.

[d] No standard protocol; vancomycin taper and pulse regimen example: 125 mg 4 times daily for 10 to 14 d, 2 times daily for 7 d, once daily for 7 d, and then every 2 to 3 d for 2 to 8 wk.

[e] Bezlotoxumab may be considered for patients with risk factors for recurrence (>65 y and immunocompromise) or severe CDI if resources and logistics for intravenous administration are available; history of congestive heart failure is a relative contraindication for bezlotoxumab and should be reserved for when the benefit outweighs the risk.

From Johnson S, Lavergne V, Skinner AM, Gonzales-Luna AJ, Garey KW, Kelly CP, Wilcox MH. Clinical practice guideline by the Infectious Diseases Society of America (IDSA) and Society for Healthcare Epidemiology of America (SHEA): 2021 focused update guidelines on management of Clostridioides difficile infection in adults. Clin Infect Dis 2021;73:755-757.

the setting of typical symptoms recurring after discontinuation of therapy. If significant delays in testing are anticipated, empirical treatment for frail older adults with high clinical suspicion for CDI but mild to moderate symptoms may be reasonable in some settings (eg, an LTCF with a high incidence of CDI). If empirical treatment is considered for suspected mild to moderate CDI, the risks of adverse effects of treatment (eg, adverse drug reactions, promotion of colonization by vancomycin-resistant enterococci) must be balanced against the risks of adverse outcomes due to delays in treatment. Clinicians should also be aware that empirical CDI therapy can convert CDI test results from positive to negative.[51] Thus, if empirical treatment is prescribed it is important to ensure that a stool sample is collected before the start of therapy.

FECAL MICROBIOTA TRANSPLANTATION

FMT is an effective therapy for patients with multiple recurrences of CDI.[48,52] During the past decade, use of FMT for CDI has increased dramatically. During that time, the method of administration has transitioned from colonoscopy, nasoduodenal infusion, and enema to use of frozen or freeze-dried oral capsules.[53–55] The ability to administer FMT via capsules is much more convenient for patients and health care facilities. In a systematic review and meta-analysis of oral FMT formulations, the estimated efficacy of oral FMT for recurrent CDI was 82%, which is similar to the efficacy of FMT via other routes of administration.[54] At MetroHealth Medical Center in Cleveland, the efficacy of FMT via freeze-dried capsules was 68% after a single transplant, but increased to greater than 90% after 1 to 3 additional FMT procedures.[55] Although adverse effects have been uncommon with FMT, safety remains an important consideration due to occasional reports of illness due to pathogens transmitted via transplant material.[56] In a recent report, an FMT product that is modified to contain only spore-forming bacteria rather than the complete fecal microbiota was effective in patients with recurrent CDI.[57] Such modified commercial preparations could potentially address safety concerns related to transplantation of feces. At present, it is recommended that patients being considered for FMT be referred to specialists with experience and expertise in providing this procedure.

If fecal transplantation is not available or if medical therapy is preferred, there are options for medical treatment of patients with multiple recurrences. One approach that was effective in a small observational trial was fidaxomicin prescribed as a tapering course over 14 to 33 days or as a "chaser" after completion of oral vancomycin therapy.[58] Only 2 of 11 (18%) patients with multiple recurrences of CDI developed recurrence after completion of the fidaxomicin taper or chaser. A second approach for management of patients with multiple recurrences is chronic suppressive therapy (eg, once daily oral vancomycin 125 mg). This approach may be appropriate for patients with relatively short life expectancy or for patients who are not good candidates for fecal transplantation due to frequent requirement for antibiotic therapy that would lead to a high risk for failure of the transplant. Preferably, patients such as these with multiple recurrences would be referred to infectious diseases for management.

EDUCATING AND EMPOWERING PATIENTS

In recent years there has been increasing interest in the empowerment of patients to serve as partners in efforts to prevent health care-associated infections.[59] CDI is an attractive target for patient empowerment initiatives because patients experience

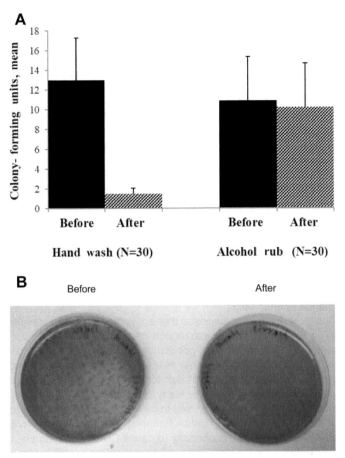

Fig. 4. Effect of soap and water hand wash versus alcohol hand sanitizer on the mean number of spores recovered from hands of patients with CDI or asymptomatic carriage (*A*) and pictures of *C difficile* colonies recovered from hands of a patient with CDI before versus after soap and water hand washing (*B*). Error bars show standard error. (*Adapted from* Soriano MM, Danziger LH, Gerding DN, Johnson S. Novel fidaxomicin treatment regimens for patients with multiple *Clostridium difficile* infection recurrences that are refractory to standard therapies. Open Forum Infect Dis 2014;1:ofu069; with permission.)

reduced quality of life and are motivated to avoid recurrence and to prevent transmission to family members. However, a recent study demonstrated that current education provided to patients with CDI is often suboptimal.[60] Although most facilities surveyed had educational materials or protocols for education of patients with CDI, approximately half of the patients with CDI did not recall receiving education during their admission, and knowledge deficits regarding CDI prevention were common.[60]

Older patients with CDI and family members should be aware of the risk for recurrence and measures that they may take to reduce their risk. These measures include frequent hand washing with soap and water, cleaning and disinfection of bathrooms and other high-touch areas with bleach or other sporicidal disinfectants, frequent laundering of clothing and bedding, and avoidance of unnecessary antibiotic prescriptions.[60] Hand washing with soap and water is effective in reducing the burden of spores on hands through mechanical removal, whereas alcohol hand sanitizer is ineffective (**Fig. 4**).[61] Thorough showering by patients with CDI is also recommended when spore contamination of skin is common.[10,43] It is important to reassure patients that the risk for transmission to family members is low unless those individuals are receiving antibiotic therapy. Moreover, the measures taken to reduce risk for recurrence will also reduce the risk for transmission of spores.

Prescription of antibiotics other than those used to treat CDI is a major risk factor for recurrence of CDI, including after initially successful FMT.[12] Given that a significant proportion of antibiotic therapy is unnecessary, it is important for FMT providers to make efforts to avoid overuse of antibiotics after FMT. At MetroHealth Medical Center and the Cleveland VA Medical Center, FMT recipients are encouraged to contact their FMT providers and/or have their physicians contact the FMT providers for consultation regarding antibiotic prescriptions after the transplant. We recently reported our experience with this stewardship intervention.[62] Of 73 FMT recipients, 25 (34%) consulted their FMT physicians, either directly or through their non-FMT providers, regarding a total of 43 antibiotic prescriptions. Of the 43 consultations, 26 (60%) antibiotic courses were deemed unnecessary, 7 (16%) were deemed necessary but an alternative regimen less frequently associated with CDI was recommended, and 10 (23%) were deemed necessary and the regimen was considered appropriate. The recommendations were accepted in 39 of 41 (95%) cases. There were no adverse effects attributable to avoidance of antibiotics.

The author's experience demonstrates that engaging patients in stewardship interventions can be an effective strategy to reduce inappropriate antibiotic use after FMT. Patients undergoing FMT are an ideal population for such interventions because they are motivated to avoid antibiotics as they fear failure of the transplant and are aware that antibiotics are the most important risk for recurrence. Other patients with CDI would also be excellent candidates for such interventions if they are educated that receipt of antibiotics other than those used to treat CDI is a major risk factor for recurrence of CDI.[63,64] In cases in which antibiotic therapy is indicated, it may be possible to select agents with a reduced propensity to cause CDI.[12] For example, clinical and animal model studies suggest that doxycycline presents a relatively low risk for promotion of CDI.[65]

SUMMARY

CDI disproportionately affects the older adults, particularly those requiring frequent hospital stays or LTCF admission. Recurrences of CDI are common in older adults and may have significant adverse effects on quality of life. Although intrinsic factors associated with aging contribute to the risk for CDI in this population, modifiable factors such as antibiotic therapy also play a major role. Ensuring appropriate diagnostic testing and management is challenging for older adults in the community and in LTCFs. FMT is a promising approach for older patients with multiple recurrences.

CLINICS CARE POINTS

- Antibiotic therapy is the most important risk factor for C. difficile infection
- A diagnosis of C. difficile infection should be based on a combination of clinical symptoms consistent with the diagnosis and a laboratory test confirming the presence of a toxigenic strain or toxin in stool

- A positive nucleic acid amplification test (NAAT) may indicate either asymptomatic carriage of toxigenic C. difficile or C. difficile infection
- Fidaxomicin or vancomycin are appropriate for treatment of initial cases of C. difficile infection
- Fecal microbiota transplantation is an effective therapy for patients with multiple recurrences of C. difficile infection

ACKNOWLEDGMENTS

This work was supported by the Veterans Integrated Service Network 10 Geriatric Research Education and Clinical Center (VISN 10 GRECC) and the Veterans Affairs Merit Review Program (C.J. Donskey.).

REFERENCES

1. Guh AY, Mu Y, Winston LG, et al. Trends in U.S. burden of *Clostridioides difficile* infection and outcomes. N Engl J Med 2020;382:1320–30.
2. Donskey CJ. Fluoroquinolone restriction to control fluoroquinolone-resistant *Clostridium difficile*. Lancet Infect Dis 2017;17:353–4.
3. Riggs MM, Sethi AK, Zabarsky TF, et al. Asymptomatic carriers are a potential source for transmission of epidemic and nonepidemic *Clostridium difficile* strains among long-term care facility residents. Clin Infect Dis 2007;45:992–8.
4. Simor AE, Bradley SF, Strausbaugh LJ, et al. *Clostridium difficile* in long-term-care facilities for the elderly. Infect Control Hosp Epidemiol 2002;23:696–703.
5. Marciniak C, Chen D, Stein AC, et al. Prevalence of *Clostridium difficile* colonization at admission to rehabilitation. Arch Phys Med Rehabil 2006;87:1086–90.
6. Guerrero DM, Nerandzic MM, Jury LA, et al. *Clostridium difficile* infection in a Department of Veterans Affairs long-term care facility. Infect Control Hosp Epidemiol 2011;32:513–5.
7. Pawar D, Tsay R, Nelson DS, et al. Burden of *Clostridium difficile* infection in long-term care facilities in Monroe County, New York. Infect Control Hosp Epidemiol 2012;33:1107–12.
8. Hunter JC, Mu Y, Dumyati GK, et al. Burden of nursing home-onset *Clostridium difficile* infection in the United States: Estimates of incidence and patient outcomes. Open Forum Infect Dis 2016;3:ofv196.
9. Jinno S, Kundrapu S, Guerrero DM, et al. Potential for transmission of *Clostridium difficile* by asymptomatic acute care patients and long-term care facility residents with prior *C. difficile* infection. Infect Control Hosp Epidemiol 2012;33:638–9.
10. Bobulsky GS, Al-Nassir WN, Riggs MM, et al. *Clostridium difficile* skin contamination in patients with *C. difficile*-associated disease. Clin Infect Dis 2008;46:447–50.
11. Donskey CJ, Kundrapu S, Deshpande A. Colonization versus carriage of *Clostridium difficile*. Infect Dis Clin North Am 2015;29:13–28.
12. Owens RC Jr, Donskey CJ, Gaynes RP, et al. Antimicrobial-associated risk factors for *Clostridium difficile* infection. Clin Infect Dis 2008;46(Suppl 1):S19–31.
13. Kyne L, Warny M, Qamar A, et al. Asymptomatic carriage of *Clostridium difficile* and serum levels of IgG antibody against toxin A. N Engl J Med 2000;342:390–7.
14. Jiang ZD, DuPont HL, Garey K, et al. A common polymorphism in the interleukin 8 gene promoter is associated with *Clostridium difficile* diarrhea. Am J Gastroenterol 2006;101:1112–6.

15. Bhutto A, Morley JE. The clinical significance of gastrointestinal changes with aging. Curr Opin Clin Nutr Metab Care 2008;11:651–60.
16. Hopkins MJ, Macfarlane GT. Changes in predominant bacterial populations in human faeces with age and with *Clostridium difficile* infection. J Med Microbiol 2002;51:448–54.
17. Rea MC, O'Sullivan O, Shanahan F, et al. *Clostridium difficile* carriage in elderly subjects and associated changes in the intestinal microbiota. J Clin Microbiol 2012;50:867–75.
18. Borriello SP, Barclay FE, Welch AR. Evaluation of the predictive capability of an in-vitro model of colonization resistance to *Clostridium difficile* infection. Microb Ecol Health Dis 1988;1:61–4.
19. Peron EP, Hirsch AA, Jury LA, et al. Another setting for stewardship: high rate of unnecessary antimicrobial use in a veterans affairs long-term care facility. J Am Geriatr Soc 2013;61:289–90.
20. Mafi JN, May FP, Kahn KL, et al. Low-value proton pump inhibitor prescriptions among older adults at a large academic health system. J Am Geriatr Soc 2019;67:2600–4.
21. Polage CR, Solnick JV, Cohen SH. Nosocomial diarrhea: Evaluation and treatment of causes other than *Clostridium difficile*. Clin Infect Dis 2012;55:982–9.
22. Kundrapu S, Sunkesula V, Tomas M, et al. Response to Prior and Fitzpatrick. Infect Control Hosp Epidemiol 2016;37:362–3.
23. Curry SR, Muto CA, Schlackman JL, et al. Use of multilocus variable number of tandem repeats analysis genotyping to determine the role of asymptomatic carriers in *Clostridium difficile* transmission. Clin Infect Dis 2013;57:1094–102.
24. Longtin Y, Paquet-Bolduc B, Gilca R, et al. Effect of detecting and isolating *C difficile* carriers at hospital admission on the incidence of *C difficile* infections: A quasi-experimental controlled study. JAMA Intern Med 2016;176:796–804.
25. Blixt T, Gradel KO, Homann C, et al. Asymptomatic carriers contribute to nosocomial *Clostridium difficile* infection: A cohort study of 4508 patients. Gastroenterol 2017;152:1031–41.
26. Donskey CJ, Sunkesula VCK, Stone ND, et al. Transmission of *Clostridium difficile* from asymptomatically colonized or infected long-term care facility residents. Infect Control Hosp Epidemiol 2018;39:909–16.
27. Lucado J, Gould C, Elixhauser A. Clostridium difficile Infections (CDI) in Hospital Stays, 2009 - Healthcare Cost and Utilization Project (HCUP) Statistical Briefs - NCBI Bookshelf.
28. Lessa FC, Mu Y, Bamberg WM, et al. Burden of *Clostridium difficile* infection in the United States. N Engl J Med 2015;372:825–34.
29. Ponnada S, Guerrero DM, Jury LA, et al. Acquisition of *Clostridium difficile* colonization and infection after transfer from a Veterans Affairs Hospital to an affiliated long-term care facility. Infect Control Hosp Epidemiol 2017;38:1070–6.
30. Dingle KE, Didelot X, Quan TP, et al. Effects of control interventions on *Clostridium difficile* infection in England: an observational study. Lancet Infect Dis 2017;17:411–21.
31. Silva SY, Wilson BM, Redmond SN, et al. Inpatient fluoroquinolone use in Veterans' Affairs hospitals is a predictor of *Clostridioides difficile* infection due to fluoroquinolone-resistant ribotype 027 strains. Infect Control Hosp Epidemiol 2021;42:57–62.
32. Weiner-Lastinger LM, Pattabiraman V, Konnor RY, et al. The impact of coronavirus disease 2019 (COVID-19) on healthcare-associated infections in 2020: A

summary of data reported to the National Healthcare Safety Network. Infect Control Hosp Epidemiol 2022;43:12–25.

33. Hensgens MP, Goorhuis A, Dekkers OM, et al. Time interval of increased risk for *Clostridium difficile* infection after exposure to antibiotics. J Antimicrob Chemother 2012;67:742–8.

34. Koo HL, Ajami NJ, Jiang ZD, et al. A nosocomial outbreak of Norovirus infection masquerading as CDI. Clin Infect Dis 2009;48:e75–7.

35. Pepin J, Routhier S, Gagnon S, et al. Management and outcomes of a first recurrence of *Clostridium difficile*-associated disease in Quebec, Canada. Clin Infect Dis 2006;42:758–64.

36. Garey KW, Aitken SL, Gschwind L, et al. Development and validation of a *Clostridium difficile* health-related quality-of-life questionnaire. J Clin Gastroenterol 2016;50:631–7.

37. McDonald LC, Gerding DN, Johnson S, et al. Clinical practice guidelines for *Clostridium difficile* infection in adults and children: 2017 update by the Infectious Diseases Society of America (IDSA) and Society for Healthcare Epidemiology of America (SHEA). Clin Infect Dis 2018;66:987–94.

38. Polage CR, Gyorke CE, Kennedy MA, et al. Overdiagnosis of *Clostridium difficile* infection in the molecular test era. JAMA Intern Med 2015;175:1792–801.

39. Planche T, Wilcox MH. Diagnostic pitfalls in *Clostridium difficile* infection. Infect Dis Clin North Am 2015;29:63–82.

40. Guerrero DM, Chou C, Jury LA, et al. Clinical and infection control implications of *Clostridium difficile* infection with negative enzyme immunoassay for toxin. Clin Infect Dis 2011;53:287–90.

41. Miller R, Morillas JA, Brizendine KD, et al. Predictors of *Clostridioides difficile* infection-related complications and treatment patterns among nucleic acid amplification test-positive/toxin enzyme immunoassay-negative patients. J Clin Microbiol 2020;58. e01764-19.

42. Alonso CD, Kelly CP, Garey KW, et al. Ultrasensitive and quantitative toxin measurement correlates with baseline severity, severe outcomes, and recurrence among hospitalized patients with *Clostridioides difficile* infection. Clin Infect Dis 2022;74:2142–9.

43. Sethi AK, Al-Nassir WN, Nerandzic MM, et al. Persistence of skin contamination and environmental shedding of *Clostridium difficile* during and after treatment of *C. difficile* infection. Infect Control Hosp Epidemiol 2010;31:21–7.

44. Kundrapu S, Sunkesula VC, Jury LA, et al. Utility of perirectal swab specimens for diagnosis of *Clostridium difficile* infection. Clin Infect Dis 2012;55:1527–30.

45. Kundrapu S, Jury LA, Sitzlar B, et al. Easily modified factors contribute to delays in diagnosis of *Clostridium difficile* infection: a cohort study and intervention. J Clin Microbiol 2013;51:2365–70.

46. Quinn LK, Chen Y, Herwaldt LA. Infection control policies and practices for Iowa long-term care facility residents with *Clostridium difficile* infection. Infect Control Hosp Epidemiol 2007;28:1228–32.

47. Johnson S, Lavergne V, Skinner AM, et al. Clinical practice guideline by the Infectious Diseases Society of America (IDSA) and Society for Healthcare Epidemiology of America (SHEA): 2021 focused update guidelines on management of *Clostridioides difficile* infection in adults. Clin Infect Dis 2021;73:755–7.

48. Kelly CR, Fischer M, Allegretti JR, et al. ACG clinical guidelines: Prevention, diagnosis, and treatment of *Clostridioides difficile* infections. Am J Gastroenterol 2021;116:1124–47.

49. Louie TJ, Miller MA, Mullane KM, et al. Fidaxomicin versus vancomycin for *Clostridium difficile* infection. N Engl J Med 2011;364:422–31.
50. Guery B, Menichetti F, Anttila VJ, et al. Extended-pulsed fidaxomicin versus vancomycin for *Clostridium difficile* infection in patients 60 years and older (EXTEND): a randomised, controlled, open-label, phase 3b/4 trial. Lancet Infect Dis 2018;18:296–307.
51. Sunkesula VC, Kundrapu S, Muganda C, et al. Does empirical *Clostridium difficile* infection (CDI) therapy result in false-negative CDI diagnostic test results? Clin Infect Dis 2013;57:494–500.
52. Van Nood E, Vrieze A, Nieuwdorp M, et al. Duodenal infusion of donor feces for recurrent *Clostridium difficile*. N Engl J Med 2013;368:407–15.
53. Hecker MT, Obrenovich ME, Cadnum JL, et al. Fecal Microbiota Transplantation by Freeze-Dried Oral Capsules for Recurrent *Clostridium difficile* Infection. Open Forum Infect Dis 2016;3:ofw091.
54. Du C, Luo Y, Walsh S, et al. Oral fecal microbiota transplant capsules are safe and effective for recurrent *Clostridioides difficile* infection: a systematic review and meta-analysis. J Clin Gastroenterol 2021;55:300–8.
55. Rosero C, Donskey CJ, Hecker MT. Long-term follow-up after fecal microbiota transplantation via colonoscopy or freeze-dried capsules for recurrent *Clostridioides difficile* infection. Open Forum Infect Dis 2021;8(Supplement 1):S599.
56. Wilcox MH, McGovern BH, Hecht GA. The efficacy and safety of fecal microbiota transplant for recurrent *Clostridium difficile* infection: current understanding and gap analysis. Open Forum Infect Dis 2020;7:ofaa114.
57. Feuerstadt P, Louie TJ, Lashner B, et al. SER-109, an Oral Microbiome Therapy for Recurrent *Clostridioides difficile* Infection. N Engl J Med 2022;386:220–9.
58. Soriano MM, Danziger LH, Gerding DN, et al. Novel fidaxomicin treatment regimens for patients with multiple *Clostridium difficile* infection recurrences that are refractory to standard therapies. Open Forum Infect Dis 2014;1:ofu069.
59. Sharp D, Palmore T, Grady C. The ethics of empowering patients as partners in healthcare-associated infection prevention. Infect Control Hosp Epidemiol 2014;35:307–9.
60. DeBenedictus CM, Hecker MT, Zuccaro PD, et al. What is the current state of patient education after *Clostridioides difficile* infection? Infect Control Hosp Epidemiol 2020;41:1338–40.
61. Kundrapu S, Sunkesula V, Jury I, et al. A randomized trial of soap and water hand wash versus alcohol hand rub for removal of *Clostridium difficile* spores from hands of patients. Infect Control Hosp Epidemiol 2014;35:204–6.
62. Hecker MT, Ho E, Donskey CJ. Fear of failure: Engaging patients in antimicrobial stewardship after fecal transplantation for recurrent *Clostridium difficile* infection. Infect Control Hosp Epidemiol 2017;38:127–9.
63. Hecker MT, Aron DC, Patel NP, et al. Unnecessary use of antimicrobials in hospitalized patients: current patterns of misuse with an emphasis on the antianaerobic spectrum of activity. Arch Intern Med 2003;163:972–8.
64. Hecker MT, Son AH, Alhmidi H, et al. Efficacy of a stewardship intervention focused on reducing unnecessary use of non-*Clostridioides difficile* antibiotics in patients with *Clostridioides difficile* infection. Infect Control Hosp Epidemiol 2020;41:216–8.
65. Xu D, Mana TSC, Cadnum JL, et al. Why Does Doxycycline Pose a Relatively Low Risk for Promotion of *Clostridioides difficile* Infection? Pathog Immun 2022;7:81–94.

Vaccine-Preventable Diseases in Older Adults

Maha Al-Jabri, MD[a,b,1], Christian Rosero, MD[a,b,1], Elie A. Saade, MD, MPH[a,*]

KEYWORDS

- Influenza • *Streptococcus pneumoniae* • Herpes zoster • Immunization schedule
- Older adults

KEY POINTS

- The accumulation of comorbidities with age, changes in organ systems, and immunosenescence contribute to the increased incidence, severity, and fatality of infections in older adults.
- Immunosenescence, the complex and interrelated changes that occur in the innate and adaptive system related to aging, contributes to the increased incidence and severity of infections in older adults and to the decreased effectiveness and waning of the effect of vaccines.
- On the basis of the immunologic and clinical evidence, the Centers for Disease Control and Prevention (CDC) recommend enhanced influenza vaccines (namely, the high-dose inactivated, the MF-59 adjuvanted inactivated, and the recombinant vaccines) for adults 65 years of age and older.
- The CDC recommends that most adults 65 years or older receive either a PCV15 or PCV20 pneumococcal vaccine; for those who receive the lower valence vaccine, a dose of PPSV23 is recommended after 1 year.
- The CDC recommends that most adults 50 years of age or older receive a series of two doses of the recombinant zoster vaccine separated by 2 to 6 months.
- Older adults with certain demographic or social risk factors or comorbidities might need to receive additional vaccines, such as vaccines against diphtheria, tetanus, pertussis, hepatitis A and/or B, meningococcus, and *Haemophilus influenzae* type B.

INTRODUCTION

With older age, humans are at a progressively higher risk of infection and increased morbidity and mortality related to vaccine-preventable infections, such as influenza, coronavirus disease-2019 (COVID-19), pneumococcal pneumonia, herpes zoster,

[a] Division of Infectious Diseases and HIV Medicine, University Hospitals Cleveland Medical Center, 11100 Euclid Avenue – Mailstop Fol. 5083, Cleveland, OH 44106, USA; [b] Case Western Reserve University, Cleveland, OH, USA
[1] Maha Al-Jabri and Christian Rosero contributed equally to the manuscript.
* Corresponding author.
E-mail address: elie.saade@uhhospitals.org

Infect Dis Clin N Am 37 (2023) 103–121
https://doi.org/10.1016/j.idc.2022.11.005

id.theclinics.com

pertussis, and others. Physiologic changes related to the immune system and other organ systems contribute to this increased vulnerability. Respiratory system changes, such as decreased respiratory muscle strength, reduced lung compliance, and impaired mucociliary function, lead to decreased clearance of infectious organisms. Neurocognitive changes and increased vulnerability to metabolic encephalopathy contribute to a delayed recognition of infectious syndromes; this is further complicated by the atypical presentation of infections commonly seen in older adults with frailty syndrome, which are commonly unrecognized until severe worsening related to the disease or another inciting event.[1] In addition, immunosenescence, the complex and interrelated changes that occur in the innate and adaptive immune system as part of the aging process, is thought to play a major role in this increased predisposition to infections and reduced response to vaccines occurring with advancing age.[2,3] For example, the efficacy of inactivated influenza vaccines decreases with age, from approximately 70% to 90% in children and younger adults, to 30% to 50% in older adults.[4] The duration of long-term protection is equally reduced.[4,5]

In this review, we address the following diseases, as well as the vaccines used to prevent them: influenza, pneumococcal disease, herpes zoster, tetanus, diphtheria, pertussis, hepatitis A, hepatitis B, meningococcal disease, and *H influenzae type B* infections. COVID-19 and the vaccines for severe acute respiratory syndrome coronavirus 2 (SARS-COV-2) will not be discussed in this review, as they will be covered in detail elsewhere in this issue.

AGING AND THE IMMUNE SYSTEM

The innate immune system includes physical barriers like epithelium from the skin, gastrointestinal and respiratory tracts, and immune cells that respond nonspecifically to pathogens, such as monocytes, neutrophils, natural killer (NK) cells, and dendritic cells (DC). Studies have shown extensive changes in the innate immune system related to age, including a decline in the function of the innate cells, such as impaired phagocytosis by monocytes and neutrophils, decreased bacterial killing by macrophages, and diminished cytotoxicity and cytokine production by NK cells.[4] Defects in pattern recognition receptors in DCs and decreased production of proinflammatory cytokines when stimulated contribute to a diminished activation of the adaptive immune system, which has been shown to be associated with response to influenza vaccination with older age.[4,6] In summary, the dysfunction of the different components of the innate immune system with alteration of antigen sensing, presentation, and cytokine response of innate cells affects the appropriate stimulation of the adaptive system and its response to immunization.[2,4]

The adaptive immune system provides a specialized response to infections and includes cell-mediated and humoral responses. It has the advantage of creating memory cells that can mount a defensive response to subsequent infections. Immunization needs a well-functioning adaptive immune system to provide the maximum benefit. Changes in the adaptive immune system related to aging are thought to play an important role in the altered response to vaccinations observed in older adults.[4,7] Overall T cell count seems to be unchanged during life, but the number of naïve Tcells decreases progressively after puberty due to thymic involution.[4,8] In addition, Tcells experience changes in the expression of T cell receptors and costimulatory molecules. The changes in the naïve T-cell subpopulation and the persistence of previously differentiated memory Tcells in older adults limit the ability to generate a protective immune response to a new antigen compared with young adults.[4] Humoral immunity plays a major role in protecting the host after vaccination and studies have shown a decreased production of antibodies in older adults after immunization against different pathogens including influenza and pneumococcus.[9,10] Like T cells, memory Bcell (class-switched) counts seem to be preserved in older adults, but naïve B cells experience a decrease in number resulting in a lower number of cells that can be stimulated by novel antigens from vaccination or thus leading to a limited repertoire of B cell receptors (BCR), immunoglobulin class switching, and plasma cell differentiation.[11,12] This alteration of the humoral immune response is associated with failure to elicit protective antibody titers (seroconversion) and lower functional activities of antibodies in response to vaccination.[4] In addition, structural changes,including fibrosis and decreased size of lymph nodes and lymphoid structures, have shown a negative impact on the appropriate immune response to vaccination in older adults.[13,14]

Although some components of the innate immune system suffer alterations that prevent them from functioning appropriately, aging is also characterized by a basal pro-inflammatory state with continuous low-grade activation of the innate immune system (inflammaging) that can amplify any damage caused by infections in older adults.[15,16] Inflammaging by itself seems to play an important role in abnormal vaccine responses in the elderly and thus,reducing this background inflammation might boost vaccine efficacy.[17]

Possible approaches to overcome the decreased response to immunizations associated with older age include:

- Higher antigen doses, which would generate greater levels of vaccine antigen presentation by DCs and, subsequently, an increase in B cell stimulation.[4]
- Adjuvants to increase the immunogenicity of vaccine antigens; these seem to induce a local pro-inflammatory environment with an increase in innate immune cell recruitment and amplification of the adaptive immune cell response.[4]
- Frequent boosters exposing the innate and adaptive immune system repeatedly to the same antigens.[4]
- Other novel strategies to generate a better immune response to vaccines in older adults are being studied and include: stimulating the innate immune system (eg, toll-like receptors and NK cells), targeting specifically T cells, and using inhibitors to block specific pathways in T or B cells (mTOR) to improve cell function.[17,18]

INFLUENZA
Epidemiology

Influenza is an acute respiratory infection caused by influenza virus, an RNA virus from the Orthomyxoviridae family.[19] Influenza spreads through aerosolized droplets, especially in crowded places, and by contaminated hands and fomites. It causes seasonal epidemics during the winter months in the southern and northern hemispheres and all year round in tropical climates, and occasional pandemics, such as the 2009 H1N1 Influenza pandemic.[20–22] Influenza has a high annual mortality, affecting mostly populations at high risk, including people at extremes of age (children and elderly), patients who are immunocompromised, and those with chronic medical problems.[23] In the United States, the Centers for Disease Control and Prevention (CDC) estimate that, between 2010 and 2020, influenza resulted in 9 to 41 million illnesses, 140 to 170 thousand hospitalizations, and 12 to 52 thousand deaths annually.[24] Furthermore, it is estimated that 50% to 70% of hospitalizations and 70% to 85% of deaths occurred in adults 65 years and older.[25] A startling decrease in influenza and other respiratory viral infections incidence was noted during the COVID-19 pandemic, thought to be related to non-pharmaceutical interventions to control the spread of SARS-CoV-2.[26]

Clinical Presentation and Complications

Influenza commonly presents as an acute illness with systemic symptoms (fever, myalgias, arthralgia, headaches) and respiratory symptoms (sore throat, rhinorrhea, nonproductive cough) that may last one to two weeks. The prevalence of fever and other typical symptoms decreases with advancing age, which is associated with delayed diagnosis, longer length of stay, and worse prognosis.[27–29] Based on data from prospective surveillance studies, Falsey and colleagues[30] found that a temperature of 37.3 C for older adults and 37.9 C in younger individuals, combined with an acute sore throat and/or cough, provided the optimal balance between sensitivity and specificity for the definition of influenza-like illness. The burden of influenza in older adults extends beyond classic respiratory symptoms and includes exacerbation of chronic underlying conditions, acute cardiovascular events, and functional decline.[31] For instance, influenza is associated with increased incidence of myocardial infarctions and strokes, particularly in people with underlying cardiovascular disease and older adults; these associations are thought to be related to the direct effect of the influenza virus on the cardiac tissues, but also to systemic inflammation induced by the acute illness.[31–33] Influenza illness is also associated with a functional decline and with a deterioration in the ability to perform basic activities of daily living, which might lead to loss of independence.[31,34] Influenza is associated with an increased risk of developing bacterial pneumonia as a co-infection or secondary infection, most commonly with *Streptococcus pneumoniae, H influenzae,* and *Staphylococcus aureus.*[35] A study looking into patients with influenza during the pandemic influenza A H1N1 of 2009 found that age >50 was predictive of bacterial co-infection.[36]

Most individuals recover from influenza without medical attention. However, influenza infection can progress to severe illness with respiratory failure due to pneumonia and multiorgan dysfunction, especially in medically vulnerable individuals, including older adults.[19,31] Given this population's vulnerability to infections, as well as its poor response to influenza vaccines, different strategies to enhance the effect of the vaccines on the elderly were developed, reviewed below.[37]

Immunization

There are four known types of influenza viruses (A, B, C, and D); types A and B are the most common to infect humans, but type C, though much less common, can cause severe illness.[38] Type A is further classified into subtypes based on hemagglutinin (HA) and neuraminidase (NA) combinations. HA and NA are key glycoproteins on the surface of the virus; there are 18 HA and 11 NA antigenic variants, with different combinations thereof.[39] The influenza A subtypes that are currently circulating in humans are H1N1 and H3N2.[40] Knowledge of currently circulating subtypes is essential for the development of annual influenza vaccines. HA and NA glycoproteins are prone to change, and they do so constantly. Small seasonal changes in circulating influenza viruses, called antigenic drift, are caused by accumulation of point mutations in HA and NA genes that occur due to lack of proofreading mechanism in the viral RNA polymerase.[19] Because of the antigenic drift, influenza vaccines composition is updated annually based on anticipated circulating subtypes, as antibodies from previous influenza infections or vaccinations may not provide sufficient immunity for newly mutated virus.[19] Influenza B has two lineages, Victoria and Yamagata, circulating in humans and contributing to seasonal influenza.[22,23] In the recent past, influenza vaccines were available in two formulations: trivalent or quadrivalent, which refers to the number of strains present in the virus. Trivalent vaccines contain two influenza A strains, H1N1 and H3N2, which are the currently circulating human influenza type A subtypes, as well as the dominant influenza B strain predicted to be circulating at the upcoming influenza season. Quadrivalent vaccines, on the other hand, contain the aforementioned influenza A subtypes, as well as the two influenza B strains.[41] All vaccines available for the 2021 to 2022 and 2022 to 2023 influenza seasons are quadrivalent, making trivalent vaccines more of an outdated concept[42] Trivalent vaccines are still important to discuss, however, given that recent literature still included them, including studies mentioned below.

Currently, three different types of influenza vaccines are available commercially in the United States: live attenuated, inactivated, and recombinant hemagglutinin vaccines. The live attenuated vaccine (LAIV), administered intranasally, is used for healthy individuals ages 2 to 49 years, and is contraindicated in older adults, and thus will not be discussed further in this review.[41] Inactivated influenza vaccines (IIV) can be divided into adjuvanted and non-adjuvanted, with the latter further divided into standard-dose (SD-IIV) and high-dose (HD-IIV) (Fig. 1). HD-IIV contains 60 μg of HA per strain, versus SD-IIV, which contains 15 μg of HA per strain.[19] HD-IIV has been shown to improve immunogenicity in older adults compared SD-IIV in a randomized controlled trial.[43] A meta-analysis by Ng and colleagues[44] also found that HD-IIV is associated with higher post-vaccination titers and a higher proportion of elevated titers compared with SD-IIV. Another meta-analysis showed a decrease in laboratory-confirmed influenza illness with HD-IIV compared with SD-IIV in adults 65 years or older.[45] In a cluster-randomized trial of nursing home (NH) residents, those randomized to the HD-IIV arm had significantly lower rates of respiratory-related hospital admissions compared with residents randomized to the SD-IIV arm.[46] Moreover, a double-blind, randomized controlled trial showed improved efficacy (against laboratory-confirmed influenza) of HD-IIV compared with SD-IIV; the study showed that about quarter of all breakthrough influenza infections could have been prevented if HD-IIV was used instead of SD-IIV.[47]

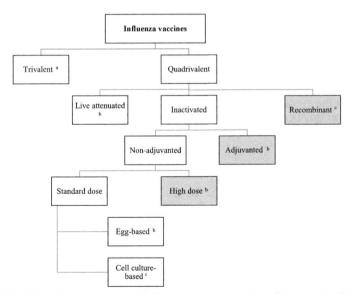

Fig. 1. 2022–2023 ACIP recommended influenza vaccines. ACIP, Advisory Committee on Immunization Practices.[a]Outdated.[b]Egg-based.[c]Egg-free.Grey-colored blocks: preferentially recommended in older adults ≥ 65 years.

The adjuvanted IIV (aIIV) vaccine components include MF-59, an oil-in-water emulsion (which essentially means a mixture with an aqueous solution as the predominant component with oil mixed in), with the oil component, in this case, being squalene.[48] Trivalent aIIV was first approved in Italy in 1997, and later approved in the United States in 2015. The quadrivalent version of the vaccine was recently approved in 2020 in the United States for use in adults aged 65 and above.[49] A meta-analysis of studies comparing MF59-aIIV against non-adjuvanted IIV found that the adjuvanted vaccine elicited significantly higher immunogenicity in older patients.[43] In addition, a meta-analysis of four identified case-control studies showed significant protection against hospitalization due to pneumonia and influenza (VE 51%, 95% CI 39%–61%).[50] Another meta-analysis found a decrease in medical encounters related to lab-confirmed influenza, non-emergency outpatient visits, and hospitalizations for aIIV compared with non-adjuvanted SD-IIV.[51] Further, a cluster-randomized trial of NH residents showed better outcomes (lower all-cause-, pneumonia-, and influenza-related hospitalizations) of residents randomized to aIIV arm compared with residents randomized to non-adjuvanted IIV.[52]

Recombinant influenza vaccine (RIV) has been approved in the United States since 2013.[53] The recombinant technology involves combining the genetic material coding for HA with the genome of a baculovirus, creating a recombinant virus. The recombinant baculovirus then acts as a viral vector to transport the HA genetic material into a host cell line, which in turns begins producing the HA proteins. The HA proteins are then purified and used as antigens for the RIV.[54] Of note, RIV contains 45 μg of HA, 3 times what is contained in SD-IIV. A randomized controlled multicenter trial in those age 50 and older comparing RIV with SD-IIV showed 30% lower probability of influenza-like illnesses in the RIV arm, satisfying both the non-inferiority and the exploratory superiority criteria.[55]

All current influenza vaccines are made using egg-based manufacturing process, with the notable exception of RIV and cell culture-based SD-IIV. Cell culture-based vaccine is produced using virus grown and replicated in cultured cells of mammalian origin, instead of hen eggs.[22] Multiple advantages to egg-free influenza vaccines have been proposed. First, they have the potential to accelerate vaccine production as they are not dependent on egg supply. Second, egg-based vaccines are thought to propagate egg-adaptive mutations that are mostly located in the genes encoding HA, thus affecting antigenicity of the vaccine.[56] Egg-free methods aim to avoid these mutations, therefore maintaining intended antigenicity.

Based on the available evidence, in June 2022, the CDC's Advisory Committee on Immunization Practices (ACIP) preferentially recommended HD-IIV, aIIV, and RIV for adults aged 65 years and older.[57]

PNEUMOCOCCAL INFECTIONS
Epidemiology

Streptococcus pneumoniae, alternatively known as pneumococcus, is a gram-positive, cocci-shaped bacterium that causes myriad of diseases, including otitis media, pneumonia, meningitis, and bacteremia.[58] According to the CDC, there were 30,000 cases of Invasive Pneumococcal Disease (IPD) and 3000 IPD-related deaths in adults in 2019%, 43% of which were in adults 65 years or older.[59] In 2017, 100,000 hospitalizations related to pneumococcal pneumonia occurred in the United States. The incidence of pneumococcal infections in the United States in adults ranges from 18 to 45.4 cases per 100,000 for people 65 and above, compared with 9.14 per 100,000 in the general population.[60] Similarly, mortality is higher in older adults, ranging from 2.17 to 11.4 per 100,000, compared with 1.01 per 100,000 in the general population.[60]

Clinical Presentation and Complications

S pneumoniae can cause non-invasive (otitis media, sinusitis, pneumonia) and invasive (bacteremia, meningitis) infections. Pneumococcal pneumonia is the most common clinical presentation of pneumococcal disease in adults. Epidemiologic studies indicate that *S pneumoniae* is the most common etiology of community-acquired pneumonia (CAP) in older adults, ranging from 20% to 80% depending on the setting and methodology of the specific study.[61] In a prospective study of adults (median age 67 years) hospitalized with CAP in the UK where comprehensive multibacterial and multiviral testing was performed on sputum or endotracheal samples, *S pneumoniae* was identified in 36% of cases, second only to *Haemophilus influenzae*.[62] 15% to 25% of pneumococcal pneumonia cases are associated with pneumococcal bacteremia; furthermore, pneumococcal bacteremia with or without pneumonia is associated with a case-fatality rate as high as 60% among older adults. Pneumococcal meningitis is the most common cause of bacterial meningitis in adults and has a high case-fatality rate and risk of severe neurologic sequelae in survivors.[63,64]

Older adults with pneumonia, including pneumococcal pneumonia, can present somewhat differently than their younger counterparts. They are less likely to complain of headaches, myalgias, and pleuritic chest pain.[65] They are also more likely to develop altered mental status and present without fevers, although this is thought to be associated with dementia and not with older age by itself.[65,66] In addition, older adults are at a high risk of in-hospital complications and death related to acute respiratory failure, shock and multiorgan failure.[65]

Immunization

Encapsulated strains of *S pneumoniae* have a polysaccharide capsule that forms the outer layer of the cell wall.[67] This polysaccharide capsule is considered among the most important virulence factors of *S pneumoniae* and acts by preventing opsonization of the bacteria, and thus phagocytosis.[67,68] The capsular polysaccharide is also the target of neutralizing antibodies produced by the host.[69] There are more than 100 serotypes of *S pneumoniae*; each serotype has its own distinct polysaccharide capsule, thus inducing unique antibodies in the host upon exposure, though cross-reactivity is possible.[70] Given high morbidity and mortality from infections caused by *S pneumoniae*, preventative efforts were underway soon after pneumococcal capsular polysaccharide structure was elucidated.[71] The first pneumococcal vaccine was a purified tetravalent polysaccharide vaccine in 1945, but that was unsuccessful due to lack of efficacy and due to introduction of penicillin, which shifted the aim from preventative to therapeutic for some time.[71] In 1977, a 14-valent purified polysaccharide vaccine was approved, followed by the 23-valent polysaccharide vaccine (PPSV23) in 1983. Pneumococcal polysaccharide vaccines (PPSV) containing the purified bacterial capsule polysaccharides have been recommended and used for decades in adults. However, PPSVs induce a T-cell-independent immune response that does not elicit formation of memory B cells, making the immunogenicity of PPSVs transient and short lived.[72] To address this, pneumococcal conjugated vaccines (PCV) were introduced, produced by covalently binding capsular polysaccharide to a carrier protein conjugate such as tetanus toxoid, for the purpose of increasing immunogenicity.[73] Conjugate vaccines induce a more durable T cell-dependent immune response, and their introduction played a clear role in the reduction of disease burden. PCV7 was included into childhood immunization in 2000. This did not only affect the rate of pneumococcal disease in children, but also affected the rates of pneumococcal infections in adults aged 65 and older, as the rate decreased by 45%.[60] PCV13 was then introduced in 2010 into the child and adolescent immunization schedule, and that decreased the rates of infection in older adults even further.[60] This effect is thought to be stemming from herd immunity which decreased transmission of S pneumoniae from children to older adults. In 2014, vaccination with PCV13 was implemented for older adults. A randomized double-blind clinical trial comparing the immunogenicity of older adults a month after receiving PCV13 versus PPSV23 found that PCV13 elicited greater immunogenicity for 8 out of 12 serotypes contained in both vaccines, and non-inferior immunogenicity for the rest of the serotypes.[74] Because PCV13 and PPSV23 together offer potentially additive advantages, the CDC recommended a schedule using both vaccines for older adults, where PCV13 was administered initially, followed by PPSV23 a year later (or shorter in some cases). Most recently, in June 2021, the FDA approved PCV15 and PCV20.[75](p20) PCV15 and PCV20 were approved based on meeting non-inferiority criteria relative to PCV13 in terms of immunogenicity, the incremental benefit of targeting additional serotypes, as well as meeting safety criteria.[76,77] No head-to-head comparison was done between PCV15 and PCV20. Effectiveness studies results are expected in the future.

Currently, the CDC recommends routine administration of PCV (PCV15 or PCV20) for all adults aged 65 or older who have not received a prior pneumococcal vaccine (**Fig. 2**). If PCV15 is used, a dose of PPSV23 is indicated 1 year later, but the interval may be shortened to 8 weeks in the presence of high-risk factors (immunocompromising condition, cochlear implant, or cerebrospinal fluid leak).[78] For individuals who previously received a dose of PPSV23 a dose of PCV15 or PCV20 is indicated at age 65 or older, at least a year after the latest PPSV23 dose. For individuals who received a dose of PCV13 previously, but have not received PPSV23, a dose of PPSV23 is recommended at age 65, at least 1 year after PCV13. They may instead receive a dose of PCV20, if PPSV23 is not available[78]

HERPES ZOSTER
Epidemiology

Varicella zoster virus (VZV) is responsible for two different infections in humans, varicella (chickenpox) and herpes zoster (HZ, shingles); the latter occurs as a reactivation of dormant VZV in nerve roots of the dorsal root ganglions. Before the introduction of the Zoster vaccine live (ZVL) in the United States in 2006, HZ affected one million people annually.[79] A recent systematic review estimates the cumulative incidence of HZ at 2.9 to 19.5 cases per 1,000 population and from 5.23 to 10.9 cases per 1,000 person-years in the general population $\geq$50 years of age.[80] The risk of HZ increases with age, from an average of 3 to 5/1000 person-years before age 50 to approximately 6 to 8/1000 person-years around 60 years of age and about 8 to 12/1000 person-years in older adults aged 80 or more.[81] The risk of reactivation and severe disease is higher in older adults due to changes in cell-mediated immunity with decreasing response of VZV-specific T cells observed with aging.[82]

Clinical Presentation

HZ typically presents as a maculopapular rash limited to 1 or 2 adjacent unilateral dermatomes and progresses to vesicles and pustules. In older adults, it can present as a limited patch of lesions in a dermatome and may not form pustules or as maculopapular lesions that do not progress to vesicles.[83] It is typically associated with severe burning and/or lancinating (neuropathic) pain over the involved area. The rash usually

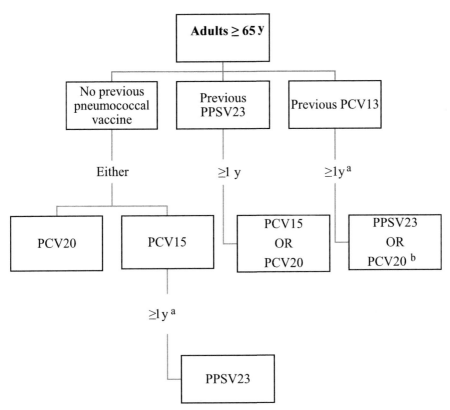

Fig. 2. ACIP recommended pneumococcal vaccines in adults ≥ 65 years. PPSV23, pneumo-coccal polysaccharide vaccine 23 valent; PCV13, pneumococcal conjugate vaccine 13 valent; PCV15, pneumococcal conjugate vaccine 15 valent; PCV20, pneumococcal conjugate vaccine 20 valent; yr, year; wk, week.[a]8 weeks can be considered in adults with immunocompromis-ing conditions, cochlear implants, or cerebrospinal fluid leak.[b]One dose of PCV20 can be given in place of PPSV23 if PPSV23 was not available.

resolves within 2 to 4 weeks. The mean duration of pain is around 45 days; however, in 5% to 30% of patients, the infection can be complicated by chronic pain (postherpetic neuralgia) that often requires chronic pain control and may disrupt the quality of life.[79,80] Other less common presentations include HZ ophthalmicus, acute retinal ne-crosis, herpes zoster oticus (Ramsay Hunt syndrome), aseptic meningitis, and en-cephalitis. These are often seen in immunocompromised patients and have significant associated morbidity.

Immunization

After the initial infection by VZV, the virus remains dormant in sensory neurons, where the cell-mediated immunity (CMI) plays a major role in maintaining latency.[84] However, CMI declines with age, which is associated with an increase in the incidence and severity of HZ.[84] Therefore, the goal of vaccination is to restore an adequate CMI. His-torically, the live attenuated zoster vaccine, ZVL, was available for adults 60 years and older but is no longer available for use in the United States as of November 2020. ZVL had an age-dependent effectiveness against HZ that ranged from 18% for those 80 years or older to 70% for those 50 to 59 years of age.[85,86] In addition, ZVL efficacy against HZ significantly decreased after 5 to 8 years of vaccination, albeit with a better persistence of efficacy against post-herpetic neuralgia.[87,88] Despite its limitations, ZVL was generally safe and well tolerated and is thought to have prevented more than 100,000 severe cases of HZ annually.[84] Currently, the only vaccine available for HZ is the recombinant zoster vaccine (RZV), which is based on VZV glycoprotein E combined with an adjuvant system AS01 B. Randomized placebo-controlled trials documented an efficacy of 97% for all participants (50 years or older), and 91% for those 70 years or older.[89,90] The ACIP recommends the use of RZV for people 50 years and older regardless of history of HZ, ZLV administration, or varicella vaccination, as well as adults 19 years and older with immunocompromising conditions.[91,92] RZV is a 2-dose vaccine, administered 2 to 6 months apart. One study examined the safety and immunogenicity of RZV administration after ZVL and found a robust immune response, with no safety concerns when vaccinated after 5 years.[93] For people with active HZ, vaccination should be delayed until the acute infection has resolved. In addition, RZV can be administered at the same time as other vaccines but at different sites.

TETANUS, DIPHTHERIA, AND PERTUSSIS
Epidemiology and Clinical Presentation

Tetanus
Caused by *Clostridium tetani*'s neurotoxin, it usually presents as generalized tetanus with trismus. The incidence of tetanus in the United States and other developed countries has decreased since the 1940s due to immunization. According to the CDC, 462 cases were reported from 2001 to 2016.[94] People 65 years and older are at increased risk of infection.[95]

Pertussis
Bordetella pertussis is a highly contagious infection, which presents with inspiratory whoop, paroxysmal cough, and post-tussive emesis. It is usually under-diagnosed in adults due to atypical presentation with only prolonged cough.[96] The incidence of pertussis decreased after universal vaccination.[16] However, more cases have been reported recently likely due to increased physician awareness and more sensitive diagnostic methods. Infected adults 65 years and older often require hospitalization.[97]

Diphtheria
A respiratory disease caused by *Corynebacterium diphtheriae* characterized by the formation of a white-gray pseudomembrane that can extend from the nasopharynx to the tracheobronchial tract. In severe cases it can involve the heart, nervous system, and kidneys.[98] Its incidence has decreased due to vaccination. According to the CDC, 13 cases of respiratory diphtheria were reported from 1996 to 2016.[94]

Immunization
The ACIP recommends tetanus, diphtheria, acellular pertussis (Tdap) vaccine or tetanus, diphtheria (Td) vaccine for adults 65 years or older as part of a booster every 10 years, as a catch-up vaccination if not previously vaccinated with Tdap, and for tetanus prophylaxis for wound management.[99]

HEPATITIS A
Epidemiology and Significance

Hepatitis A is usually a self-limited disease caused by the hepatitis A virus but rarely progresses to acute liver failure. It is transmitted via fecal-oral route after close contact with an infected person.[100] Hepatitis A incidence has increased during the last few years due to outbreaks in certain populations (people who inject drugs, people experiencing homelessness, men who have sex with men [MSM]) and related to contaminated food.[101]

Immunization

Two inactivated vaccines are available in the United States, Havrix and Vaqta, and one in combination with Hepatitis B vaccine, Twinrix. Older age is associated with lower vaccine response.[102] The ACIP recommends vaccination to individuals at risk of infection: MSM, people who use drugs (injected or noninjected), people at risk of occupational exposure, people experiencing homelessness, travelers to an endemic area, as well as people at increased risk for severe infection: people living with HIV or chronic liver disease.[100] No specific recommendations for older adults were issued.

HEPATITIS B
Epidemiology and Significance

Hepatitis B can present as icteric or anicteric hepatitis during the acute phase and progress to chronic asymptomatic carriage or cirrhosis with liver cancer.[102] Approximately 296 million people were living with chronic hepatitis B in 2019, and about 820 thousand deaths were associated with this infection.[103] Hepatitis B vaccines can be divided into three categories: mono-antigenic, tri-antigenic, and combination vaccines. Mono-antigenic vaccines include.

Recombivax HB, Engerix-B, and Heplisav-B, whereas the tri-antigenic vaccine is PreHevbrio. Combination vaccines include Twinrix, which is co-formulated with hepatitis A. Heplisav-B seems to be more effective in adults with comorbidities and older adults compared with Engerix-B.[104] The tri-antigenic vaccine, PreHevbrio, showed a better response in older adults compared with the mono-antigenic Engerix-B.[105]

Immunization

The ACIP recommends universal hepatitis B vaccination for adults aged 19 to 59 years and for adults 60 years or older at risk for infection, including people living with HIV, HCV infection, chronic liver disease, multiple sexual partners, MSM, people who inject drugs, hemodialysis, living with someone with chronic hepatitis B, travelers to endemic regions, and individuals at risk of blood exposure at work.[106]

MENINGOCOCCUS
Epidemiology and Significance

Neisseria meningitidis can cause severe meningitis and systemic infection. The overall incidence has decreased significantly during the last few years due to vaccination but the case fatality rate remains high in older adults.[107,108]

Immunization

Three quadrivalent (serogroups A, C, W, and Y; MenACWY) and two monovalent (serogroup B; MenB) vaccines are available in the United States. The MenACWY are all conjugate vaccines, whereas the MenB are recombinant vaccines. The ACIP recommends immunization for adults if they have anatomic or functional asplenia, HIV infection, complement component deficiency, using C5 inhibitors, traveling to regions where meningococcal disease is endemic or hyperendemic (Sub-Saharan Africa "meningitis belt") or microbiologists working with N meningitidis.[109] Any of the approved MenACYW and MenB vaccines can used, and a booster is recommended

Table 1
Vaccines recommended for older adults by the Centers for Disease Control and Prevention Advisory Committee on Immunization Practices

	Routine Schedule for Adults 65 y or Older
COVID-19	Indicated for all adults; variable schedule
Influenza	Yearly seasonal vaccination. High-dose inactivated, adjuvanted inactivated, and recombinant vaccines are preferred for adults 65 y or older.
Tetanus, diphtheria, and pertussis	1 dose Tdap, then Td or Tdap booster every 10 y
Measles, mumps, and rubella	Not indicated
Varicella	Not indicated for individuals born before 1980 with few exceptions[a]
Zoster recombinant vaccine (RZV)	Two doses starting at age 50
Human papillomavirus	Not indicated
Pneumococcal vaccines	PCV 15 followed by PPSV23, or PCV20
Hepatitis A	Indicated for nonimmune adults at high risk[b]
Hepatitis	Indicated for nonimmune adults at high risk[c]
Meningococcal	MenACWY[d] and/or MenB[e] for adults at high risk
Haemophilus influenzae type b	Indicated for nonimmune adults at high risk[f]

[a] Health care personnel born before 1980 without other evidence of immunity against varicella have an indication to receive a varicella vaccine.
[b] Chronic liver disease, HIV infection, men who have sex with men, injection or non-injection drug use, persons experiencing homelessness, household or equivalent contact with international adoptee, works with hepatitis A virus or in health care settings targeting services to high-risk individuals.
[c] Chronic liver disease, HIV infection, sexual risk exposure, injection drug use, percutaneous or mucosal risk for exposure to blood, incarcerated persons, travel in countries with high or intermediate endemic hepatitis B.
[d] Asplenia, travel in countries with hyperendemic or epidemic meningococcal disease, microbiologists routinely exposed to *N meningitidis*.
[e] Asplenia.
[f] Asplenia, Hematopoietic stem cell transplant.

for previously vaccinated individuals who become or remain at high risk. No special recommendations for older adults were issued.

HAEMOPHILUS INFLUENZAE TYPE B

The incidence of meningitis due to *H influenzae* has decreased due to universal vaccination.[107] Three monovalent and two combination vaccines against *H influenzae* are available in the United States. The ACIP recommends one dose of any of the approved vaccines for adults undergoing elective splenectomy if not immune. For recipients of hematopoietic stem cell transplant, three doses are recommended 6 to 12 months after the transplant.[110] No special recommendations for older adults were issued.

SUMMARY

In conclusion, older adults have weakened immune systems that provide a less robust response to vaccines than younger individuals. However, given the weaker immune system, they are at higher risk of severe disease and more pronounced complications of vaccine-preventable illnesses. Some of the vaccine strategies to increase immunogenicity in older adults were discussed in this review, including using higher antigenic doses, adjuvants, and conjugate proteins (**Table 1**). All these strategies have been shown in the literature to increase the immune response in older adults.

CLINICS CARE POINTS

- Except when there is a contraindication, adults 65 years of age and older should receive a yearly dose of enhanced inactivated influenza vaccine (high-dose IIV, adjuvanted IIV, or recombinant vaccine) before (preferably) or during the local influenza season.

- Most adults 65 years of age and older should receive a dose of 15-valent or 20-valent pneumococcal conjugate vaccine; those who receive the 15-valent formulation should also receive a dose of 23-valent pneumococcal polysaccharide vaccine a year later.

- Except when there is a contraindication, adults 50 years of age or older should receive a one-time dose of the recombinant zoster vaccine.

- Most adults of all ages should receive a booster dose of tetanus-diphtheria-acellular pertussis (Tdap) or tetanus-diphtheria (Td) every ten years.

- Adults of all ages with special indications may need to receive additional vaccines, including for the prevention of hepatitis A and B, *Neisseria meningitidis*, and *Haemophilus influenzae* type B infections.

DISCLOSURE

E. A. Saade reports the following relationships: Janssen Pharmaceuticals Inc that includes consulting or advisory and funding grants, Pfizer, United States that includes consulting or advisory and travel reimbursement, Sanofi Pasteur Inc that includes speaking and lecture fees and travel reimbursement, and Seqirus Inc. that includes funding grants. M. Al-Jabri and C. Rosero have nothing to disclose.

REFERENCES

1. Gavazzi G, Krause KH. Ageing and infection. Lancet Infect Dis 2002;2(11): 659–66.
2. Agrawal A, Weinberger B. Editorial: the impact of immunosenescence and senescence of immune cells on responses to infection and vaccination. Front Aging 2022;3:882494.
3. Gustafson CE, Kim C, Weyand CM, et al. Influence of immune aging on vaccine responses. J Allergy Clin Immunol 2020;145(5):1309–21.
4. Allen JC, Toapanta FR, Chen W, et al. Understanding immunosenescence and its impact on vaccination of older adults. Vaccine 2020;38(52):8264–72.
5. Shapiro ED, Berg AT, Austrian R, et al. The Protective Efficacy of Polyvalent Pneumococcal Polysaccharide Vaccine. N Engl J Med 1991;325(21):1453–60.
6. Panda A, Qian F, Mohanty S, et al. Age-Associated Decrease in TLR Function in Primary Human Dendritic Cells Predicts Influenza Vaccine Response. J Immunol 2010;184(5):2518–27.
7. Crooke SN, Ovsyannikova IG, Poland GA, et al. Immunosenescence: A systems-level overview of immune cell biology and strategies for improving vaccine responses. Exp Gerontol 2019;124:110632.
8. Haynes BF, Sempowski GD, Wells AF, et al. The human thymus during aging. Immunol Res 2000;22(2–3):253–61.

9. Sasaki S, Sullivan M, Narvaez CF, et al. Limited efficacy of inactivated influenza vaccine in elderly individuals is associated with decreased production of vaccine-specific antibodies. J Clin Invest 2011;121(8):3109–19.

10. Kolibab K, Smithson SL, Shriner AK, et al. Immune response to pneumococcal polysaccharides 4 and 14 in elderly and young adults. I. Antibody concentrations, avidity and functional activity. Immun Ageing A 2005;2:10.

11. Listì F, Candore G, Modica MA, et al. A study of serum immunoglobulin levels in elderly persons that provides new insights into B cell immunosenescence. Ann N Y Acad Sci 2006;1089:487–95.

12. Frasca D, Diaz A, Romero M, et al. B Cell Immunosenescence. Annu Rev Cell Dev Biol 2020;36:551–74.

13. Thompson HL, Smithey MJ, Surh CD, et al. Functional and Homeostatic Impact of Age-Related Changes in Lymph Node Stroma. Front Immunol 2017;8:706.

14. Kityo C, Makamdop KN, Rothenberger M, et al. Lymphoid tissue fibrosis is associated with impaired vaccine responses. J Clin Invest 2018;128(7):2763–73.

15. Shaw AC, Joshi S, Greenwood H, et al. Aging of the innate immune system. Curr Opin Immunol 2010;22(4):507–13.

16. Santoro A, Bientinesi E, Monti D. Immunosenescence and inflammaging in the aging process: age-related diseases or longevity? Ageing Res Rev 2021;71: 101422.

17. Pereira B, Xu XN, Akbar AN. Targeting Inflammation and Immunosenescence to Improve Vaccine Responses in the Elderly. Front Immunol 2020;11:583019.

18. Mannick JB, Del Giudice G, Lattanzi M, et al. mTOR inhibition improves immune function in the elderly. Sci Transl Med 2014;6(268):268ra179.

19. Paules C, Subbarao K. Influenza. Lancet 2017;390(10095):697–708.

20. Javanian M, Barary M, Ghebrehewet S, et al. A brief review of influenza virus infection. J Med Virol 2021;93(8):4638–46.

21. CDC. 2009 H1N1 Pandemic. Centers for Disease Control and Prevention. 2019. Available at: https://www.cdc.gov/flu/pandemic-resources/2009-h1n1-pandemic.html. Accessed July 23, 2022.

22. Bartoszko J, Loeb M. The burden of influenza in older adults: meeting the challenge. Aging Clin Exp Res 2021;33(3):711–7.

23. Influenza (Seasonal). Available at: https://www.who.int/news-room/fact-sheets/detail/influenza-(seasonal. Accessed July 23, 2022.

24. CDC. Burden of Influenza. Centers for Disease Control and Prevention. Available at: https://www.cdc.gov/flu/about/burden/index.html. Published January 7, 2022. Accessed August 20, 2022.

25. CDC. Flu & People 65 Years and Older. Centers for Disease Control and Prevention. Available at: https://www.cdc.gov/flu/highrisk/65over.htm. Published June 23, 2022. Accessed August 20, 2022.

26. Feng L, Zhang T, Wang Q, et al. Impact of COVID-19 outbreaks and interventions on influenza in China and the United States. Nat Commun 2021;12(1): 3249.

27. Pop-Vicas A, Gravenstein S. Influenza in the Elderly – A Mini-Review. Gerontology 2011;57(5):397–404.

28. Czaja CA, Miller L, Alden N, et al. Age-Related Differences in Hospitalization Rates, Clinical Presentation, and Outcomes Among Older Adults Hospitalized With Influenza-U.S. Influenza Hospitalization Surveillance Network (FluSurv-NET). Open Forum Infect Dis 2019;6(7):ofz225.

29. Smith BJ, Price DJ, Johnson D, et al. Influenza With and Without Fever: Clinical Predictors and Impact on Outcomes in Patients Requiring Hospitalization. Open Forum Infect Dis 2020;7(7):ofaa268.
30. Falsey AR, Baran A, Walsh EE. Should clinical case definitions of influenza in hospitalized older adults include fever? Influenza Other Respir Viruses 2015; 9(Suppl 1):23–9.
31. Macias AE, McElhaney JE, Chaves SS, et al. The disease burden of influenza beyond respiratory illness. Vaccine 2021;39(Suppl 1):A6–14.
32. FOSTER ED, CAVANAUGH JE, HAYNES WG, et al. Acute myocardial infarctions, strokes and influenza: seasonal and pandemic effects. Epidemiol Infect 2013; 141(4):735–44.
33. Warren-Gash C, Blackburn R, Whitaker H, et al. Laboratory-confirmed respiratory infections as triggers for acute myocardial infarction and stroke: a self-controlled case series analysis of national linked datasets from Scotland. Eur Respir J 2018;51(3):AR.
34. Gozalo PL, Pop-Vicas A, Feng Z, et al. The impact of influenza on functional decline. J Am Geriatr Soc 2012;60(7):1260–7.
35. Morris DE, Cleary DW, Clarke SC. Secondary Bacterial Infections Associated with Influenza Pandemics. Front Microbiol 2017;8:1041.
36. Dhanoa A, Fang NC, Hassan SS, et al. Epidemiology and clinical characteristics of hospitalized patients with pandemic influenza A (H1N1) 2009 infections: the effects of bacterial coinfection. Virol J 2011;8:501.
37. Haq K, McElhaney JE. Immunosenescence: influenza vaccination and the elderly. Curr Opin Immunol 2014;29:38–42.
38. CDC. Types of Influenza Viruses. Centers for Disease Control and Prevention. 2021. Available at: https://www.cdc.gov/flu/about/viruses/types.htm. Accessed August 16, 2022.
39. Kosik I, Yewdell JW. Influenza Hemagglutinin and Neuraminidase: Yin–Yang Proteins Coevolving to Thwart Immunity. Viruses 2019;11(4):346.
40. CDC. Types of Influenza Viruses. Centers for Disease Control and Prevention. 2021. Available at: https://www.cdc.gov/flu/about/viruses/types.htm. Accessed August 8, 2022.
41. Houser K, Subbarao K. Influenza Vaccines: Challenges and Solutions. Cell Host Microbe 2015;17(3):295–300.
42. TABLE. Influenza vaccines — United States, 2021–22 influenza season* | CDC. 2021. Available at: https://www.cdc.gov/flu/professionals/acip/2021-2022/acip-table.htm. Accessed July 26, 2022.
43. Falsey AR, Treanor JJ, Tornieporth N, et al. Randomized, Double-Blind Controlled Phase 3 Trial Comparing the Immunogenicity of High-Dose and Standard-Dose Influenza Vaccine in Adults 65 Years of Age and Older. J Infect Dis 2009;200(2):172–80.
44. Ng TWY, Cowling BJ, Gao HZ, et al. Comparative Immunogenicity of Enhanced Seasonal Influenza Vaccines in Older Adults: A Systematic Review and Meta-analysis. J Infect Dis 2019;219(10):1525–35.
45. Wilkinson K, Wei Y, Szwajcer A, et al. Efficacy and safety of high-dose influenza vaccine in elderly adults: A systematic review and meta-analysis. Vaccine 2017; 35(21):2775–80.
46. Gravenstein S, Davidson HE, Taljaard M, et al. Comparative effectiveness of high-dose versus standard-dose influenza vaccination on numbers of US nursing home residents admitted to hospital: a cluster-randomised trial. Lancet Respir Med 2017;5(9):738–46.

47. DiazGranados CA, Dunning AJ, Kimmel M, et al. Efficacy of High-Dose versus Standard-Dose Influenza Vaccine in Older Adults. N Engl J Med 2014;371(7): 635–45.
48. O'Hagan DT, Ott GS, De Gregorio E, et al. The mechanism of action of MF59 – An innately attractive adjuvant formulation. Vaccine 2012;30(29):4341–8.
49. Adjuvanted Flu Vaccine | CDC. 2021. Available at: https://www.cdc.gov/flu/prevent/adjuvant.htm. Accessed July 19, 2022.
50. Domnich A, Arata L, Amicizia D, et al. Effectiveness of MF59-adjuvanted seasonal influenza vaccine in the elderly: A systematic review and meta-analysis. Vaccine 2017;35(4):513–20.
51. Coleman BL, Sanderson R, Haag MDM, et al. Effectiveness of the MF59-adjuvanted trivalent or quadrivalent seasonal influenza vaccine among adults 65 years of age or older, a systematic review and meta-analysis. Influenza Other Respir Viruses 2021;15(6):813–23.
52. McConeghy KW, Davidson HE, Canaday DH, et al. Cluster-randomized trial of adjuvanted vs. non-adjuvanted trivalent influenza vaccine in 823 U.S. nursing homes. Clin Infect Dis 2020. https://doi.org/10.1093/cid/ciaa1233.
53. How Influenza (Flu) Vaccines Are Made | CDC. 2021. Available at: https://www.cdc.gov/flu/prevent/how-fluvaccine-made.htm. Accessed October 25, 2022.
54. Cox MMJ, Patriarca PA, Treanor J. FluBlok, a recombinant hemagglutinin influenza vaccine. Influenza Other Respir Viruses 2008;2(6):211–9.
55. Dunkle LM, Izikson R, Patriarca P, et al. Efficacy of Recombinant Influenza Vaccine in Adults 50 Years of Age or Older. N Engl J Med 2017;376(25):2427–36.
56. Zost SJ, Parkhouse K, Gumina ME, et al. Contemporary H3N2 influenza viruses have a glycosylation site that alters binding of antibodies elicited by egg-adapted vaccine strains. Proc Natl Acad Sci U S A 2017;114(47):12578–83.
57. Recombinant Influenza (Flu) Vaccine | CDC. 2022. Available at: https://www.cdc.gov/flu/prevent/qa_flublok-vaccine.htm. Accessed July 26, 2022.
58. Marquart ME. Pathogenicity and virulence of Streptococcus pneumoniae: Cutting to the chase on proteases. Virulence 2021;12(1):766–87.
59. Centers for Disease Control and Prevention. 2019. Active Bacterial Core Surveillance Report, Emerging Infections Program Network, Streptococcus pneumoniae, 2019.
60. Pneumococcal - Vaccine Preventable Diseases Surveillance Manual | CDC. 2022. Available at: https://www.cdc.gov/vaccines/pubs/surv-manual/chpt11-pneumo.html. Accessed July 29, 2022.
61. Henig O, Kaye KS. Bacterial Pneumonia in Older Adults. Infect Dis Clin North Am 2017;31(4):689–713.
62. Gadsby NJ, Russell CD, McHugh MP, et al. Comprehensive Molecular Testing for Respiratory Pathogens in Community-Acquired Pneumonia. Clin Infect Dis 2016;62(7):817–23.
63. Clinical Features of Pneumococcal Disease | CDC. 2022. Available at: https://www.cdc.gov/pneumococcal/clinicians/clinical-features.html. Accessed August 20, 2022.
64. Serrano Fernández L, Ruiz Iturriaga LA, España Yandiola PP, et al. Bacteraemic pneumococcal pneumonia and SARS-CoV-2 pneumonia: differences and similarities. Int J Infect Dis 2022;115:39–47.
65. Fernández-Sabé N, Carratalà J, Rosón B, et al. Community-Acquired Pneumonia in Very Elderly Patients: Causative Organisms, Clinical Characteristics, and Outcomes. Medicine (Baltimore) 2003;82(3):159–69.

66. Johnson JC, Jayadevappa R, Baccash PD, et al. Nonspecific Presentation of Pneumonia in Hospitalized Older People: Age Effect or Dementia? J Am Geriatr Soc 2000;48(10):1316–20.

67. Paton JC, Trappetti C. Streptococcus pneumoniae Capsular Polysaccharide. Microbiol Spectr 2019;7(2):33.

68. Mitchell AM, Mitchell TJ. Streptococcus pneumoniae: virulence factors and variation. Clin Microbiol Infect 2010;16(5):411–8.

69. Briles DE, Paton JC, Mukerji R, et al. Pneumococcal Vaccination. Microbiol Spectr 2019;7(6):2.

70. Geno KA, Gilbert GL, Song JY, et al. Pneumococcal Capsules and Their Types: Past, Present, and Future. Clin Microbiol Rev 2015;28(3):871–99.

71. Berical AC, Harris D, Dela Cruz CS, et al. Pneumococcal Vaccination Strategies. An Update and Perspective. Ann Am Thorac Soc 2016;13(6):933–44.

72. Vila-Corcoles A, Ochoa-Gondar O. Preventing Pneumococcal Disease in the Elderly. Drugs Aging 2013;30(5):263–76.

73. Rappuoli R, De Gregorio E, Costantino P. On the mechanisms of conjugate vaccines. Proc Natl Acad Sci U S A 2019;116(1):14–6.

74. Jackson LA, Gurtman A, van Cleeff M, et al. Immunogenicity and safety of a 13-valent pneumococcal conjugate vaccine compared with a 23-valent pneumococcal polysaccharide vaccine in pneumococcal vaccine-naive adults. Vaccine 2013;31(35):3577–84.

75. Research C for BE and. PREVNAR 20. FDA. 2021. Available at: https://www.fda.gov/vaccines-blood-biologics/vaccines/prevnar-20. Accessed August 1, 2022.

76. Food and Drug Administration. Summary basis for regulatory action— PREVNAR20. Silver Spring, MD: US Department of Health and Human Services, Food and Drug Administration, 2021. https://www.fda.gov/media/150388/download.

77. Food and Drug Administration. Summary basis for regulatory action—VAXNEUVANCE. Silver Spring, MD: US Department of Health and Human Services. Food and Drug Administration 2021;. https://www.fda.gov/media/151201/download.

78. Pneumococcal Vaccine Recommendations | CDC. 2022. Available at: https://www.cdc.gov/vaccines/vpd/pneumo/hcp/recommendations.html. Accessed August 20, 2022.

79. Tseng HF, Bruxvoort K, Ackerson B, et al. The Epidemiology of Herpes Zoster in Immunocompetent, Unvaccinated Adults ≥50 Years Old: Incidence, Complications, Hospitalization, Mortality, and Recurrence. J Infect Dis 2020;222(5):798–806.

80. van Oorschot D, Vroling H, Bunge E, et al. A systematic literature review of herpes zoster incidence worldwide. Hum Vaccin Immunother 2021;17(6):1714–32.

81. Kawai K, Gebremeskel BG, Acosta CJ. Systematic review of incidence and complications of herpes zoster: towards a global perspective. BMJ Open 2014;4(6):e004833.

82. Weinberg A, Lazar AA, Zerbe GO, et al. Influence of Age and Nature of Primary Infection on Varicella-Zoster Virus–Specific Cell-Mediated Immune Responses. J Infect Dis 2010;201(7):1024–30.

83. John AR, Canaday DH. Herpes Zoster in the Older Adult. Infect Dis Clin North Am 2017;31(4):811–26.

84. Levin MJ, Weinberg A. Immune responses to zoster vaccines. Hum Vaccin Immunother 2019;15(4):772–7.

85. Oxman MN, Levin MJ, Johnson GR, et al. A Vaccine to Prevent Herpes Zoster and Postherpetic Neuralgia in Older Adults. N Engl J Med 2005;352(22): 2271–84.

86. Tseng HF. Herpes Zoster Vaccine in Older Adults and the Risk of Subsequent Herpes Zoster Disease. JAMA 2011;305(2):160.

87. Morrison VA, Johnson GR, Schmader KE, et al. Long-term Persistence of Zoster Vaccine Efficacy. Clin Infect Dis 2015;60(6):900–9.

88. Baxter R, Bartlett J, Fireman B, et al. Long-Term Effectiveness of the Live Zoster Vaccine in Preventing Shingles: A Cohort Study. Am J Epidemiol 2018;187(1): 161–9.

89. Cunningham AL, Lal H, Kovac M, et al. Efficacy of the Herpes Zoster Subunit Vaccine in Adults 70 Years of Age or Older. N Engl J Med 2016;375(11): 1019–32.

90. Lal H, Cunningham AL, Godeaux O, et al. Efficacy of an Adjuvanted Herpes Zoster Subunit Vaccine in Older Adults. N Engl J Med 2015;372(22):2087–96.

91. Dooling KL, Guo A, Patel M, et al. Recommendations of the Advisory Committee on Immunization Practices for Use of Herpes Zoster Vaccines. MMWR Morb Mortal Wkly Rep 2018;67(3):103–8.

92. Anderson TC, Masters NB, Guo A, et al. Use of Recombinant Zoster Vaccine in Immunocompromised Adults Aged ≥19 Years: Recommendations of the Advisory Committee on Immunization Practices — United States, 2022. MMWR Morb Mortal Wkly Rep 2022;71(3):80–4.

93. Grupping K, Campora L, Douha M, et al. Immunogenicity and Safety of an Adjuvanted Herpes Zoster Subunit Vaccine in Older Adults Previously Vaccinated with a Live-Attenuated Herpes Zoster Vaccine: A Phase III, Group-Matched, Clinical Trial. Open Forum Infect Dis 2017;4(suppl_1):S414.

94. Liang JL, Tiwari T, Moro P, et al. Prevention of Pertussis, Tetanus, and Diphtheria with Vaccines in the United States: Recommendations of the Advisory Committee on Immunization Practices (ACIP). MMWR Recomm Rep 2018;67(2):1–44.

95. Centers for Disease Control and Prevention (CDC). Tetanus surveillance — United States, 2001-2008. MMWR Morb Mortal Wkly Rep 2011;60(12):365–9.

96. Choi JH, Correia de Sousa J, Fletcher M, et al. Improving vaccination rates in older adults and at-risk groups: focus on pertussis. Aging Clin Exp Res 2022; 34(1):1–8.

97. Skoff TH, Hadler S, Hariri S. The Epidemiology of Nationally Reported Pertussis in the United States, 2000–2016. Clin Infect Dis 2019;68(10):1634–40.

98. Truelove SA, Keegan LT, Moss WJ, et al. Clinical and Epidemiological Aspects of Diphtheria: A Systematic Review and Pooled Analysis. Clin Infect Dis 2020; 71(1):89–97.

99. Havers FP, Moro PL, Hunter P, et al. Use of Tetanus Toxoid, Reduced Diphtheria Toxoid, and Acellular Pertussis Vaccines: Updated Recommendations of the Advisory Committee on Immunization Practices — United States, 2019. MMWR Morb Mortal Wkly Rep 2020;69(3):77–83.

100. Nelson NP, Weng MK, Hofmeister MG, et al. Prevention of Hepatitis A Virus Infection in the United States: Recommendations of the Advisory Committee on Immunization Practices, 2020. MMWR Recomm Rep 2020;69(5):1–38.

101. Foster MA, Hofmeister MG, Kupronis BA, et al. Increase in Hepatitis A Virus Infections — United States, 2013–2018. MMWR Morb Mortal Wkly Rep 2019; 68(18):413–5.

102. Herzog C, Van Herck K, Van Damme P. Hepatitis A vaccination and its immunological and epidemiological long-term effects – a review of the evidence. Hum Vaccin Immunother 2021;17(5):1496–519.

103. Hepatitis B. Available at: https://www.who.int/news-room/fact-sheets/detail/hepatitis-b. Accessed July 29, 2022.

104. Jackson S, Lentino J, Kopp J, et al. Immunogenicity of a two-dose investigational hepatitis B vaccine, HBsAg-1018, using a toll-like receptor 9 agonist adjuvant compared with a licensed hepatitis B vaccine in adults. Vaccine 2018; 36(5):668–74.

105. Vesikari T, Langley JM, Segall N, et al. Immunogenicity and safety of a tri-antigenic versus a mono-antigenic hepatitis B vaccine in adults (PROTECT): a randomised, double-blind, phase 3 trial. Lancet Infect Dis 2021;21(9):1271–81.

106. Weng MK, Doshani M, Khan MA, et al. Universal Hepatitis B Vaccination in Adults Aged 19–59 Years: Updated Recommendations of the Advisory Committee on Immunization Practices — United States, 2022. MMWR Morb Mortal Wkly Rep 2022;71(13):477–83.

107. Castelblanco RL, Lee M, Hasbun R. Epidemiology of bacterial meningitis in the USA from 1997 to 2010: a population-based observational study. Lancet Infect Dis 2014;14(9):813–9.

108. MacNeil JR, Blain AE, Wang X, et al. Current Epidemiology and Trends in Meningococcal Disease—United States, 1996–2015. Clin Infect Dis 2018;66(8): 1276–81.

109. Mbaeyi SA, Bozio CH, Duffy J, et al. Meningococcal Vaccination: Recommendations of the Advisory Committee on Immunization Practices, United States, 2020. MMWR Recomm Rep 2020;69(9):1–41.

110. Briere EC, Rubin L, Moro PL, et al. Prevention and control of haemophilus influenzae type b disease: recommendations of the advisory committee on immunization practices (ACIP). MMWR Recomm Rep Morb Mortal Wkly Rep Recomm Rep 2014;63(RR-01):1–14.

Outpatient Parenteral Antibiotic Therapy in Older Adults

Nora T. Oliver, MD MPH[a],*, Marion J. Skalweit, MD PhD[b]

KEYWORDS

- Outpatient parenteral antibiotic therapy • Older adults • Intravenous antibiotics
- Adverse drug events

KEY POINTS

- Older age is not a contraindication to participating in outpatient parenteral antibiotic therapy (OPAT) when candidates are carefully vetted, and patient safety is a forefront consideration.
- OPAT in the home setting is preferred over OPAT given at skilled nursing facilities or infusion clinic because it optimizes patient comfort, satisfaction, and autonomy while minimizing health-care exposure amid the ongoing COVID-19 pandemic.
- Older persons have more comorbidities and are at risk for polypharmacy and drug–drug interactions that should be considered when selecting antibiotic and individualizing monitoring plans for the patient.
- Innovations in OPAT such as use of long-acting lipoglycopeptides and the use of telemedicine further increase patient-centered care and reduce health-care exposure.

INTRODUCTION

Outpatient parenteral antimicrobial therapy (OPAT) is the process of delivering and administering parenteral antibiotic medications of at least 2 doses to patients in the outpatient setting without the need for intervening acute hospitalization.[1] This is often done in the comfort of the patient's home or in other settings such as a skilled nursing facility (SNF), hemodialysis (HD) unit, or outpatient infusion clinic, and has taken place for more than 4 decades in the United States. It is a complex process that involves multiple stakeholders and care coordination to accomplish, but when properly executed, OPAT is a useful and patient-centered tool that has many opportunities for treatment of complicated infections, improved patient satisfaction, and reduced

[a] Section of Infectious Diseases, Atlanta VA Medical Center, 1670 Clairmont Road, RIM 111, Decatur, GA 30033, USA; [b] Department of Medicine and Biochemistry, Case Western Reserve University School of Medicine, 11100 Euclid Avenue, Cleveland OH 44106, USA
* Corresponding author.
E-mail address: nora.oliver@va.gov

Infect Dis Clin N Am 37 (2023) 123–137
https://doi.org/10.1016/j.idc.2022.09.002
0891-5520/23/© 2022 Elsevier Inc. All rights reserved.

id.theclinics.com

health-care costs by avoiding or reducing acute care resources. In the era of the COVID-19 pandemic, OPAT has played an essential role in freeing acute care hospital resources and reducing the risk of nosocomial SARS-CoV-2 spread. For older adults, the acute care hospital setting can incur risks such as hospital-acquired infections and nosocomial SARS-CoV-2 transmission. With the background of the COVID-19 pandemic, the number of home infusion therapy (HIT) visits for antibiotics in the United States remains high; from April 2020 through March 2021, antibiotic HIT represented about 11% of all HIT service visits, which has tripled in number since 2019.[2]

Outpatient receipt of parenteral antibiotics is generally considered a safe and well-tolerated practice for the patients who appropriately qualify for this type of service. Home administration of parenteral antibiotics confers the most independence for the patient and relies on the patient and/or support of a caregiver to administer the medication to the patient with limited, weekly home nursing support. Settings with more intensive nursing support such as infusion clinics, HD units, and SNFs allow for direct supervision and administration of the antimicrobial agent by a health-care professional. These types of settings may be more applicable to OPAT candidates in which home safety is a concern or additional care cannot be rendered easily at home or autonomously. Determining which OPAT environment is best suited for the individual patient considers a variety of factors, ultimately centered around the safety of the patient.

With the growing number of OPAT use in older adults, there are key issues and challenges this population faces regarding successful participation and completion of OPAT. These include host-related factors, infection-related treatment decisions, and environmental and psychosocial factors. Host-specific factors may include cognitive ability, dexterity, mobility, and personal comfort or willingness to administer parenteral antibiotics. Other individual factors such as comorbidities, polypharmacy, and need for complex care (eg, wound care, physical therapy) may also affect decisions on antibiotic selection and how and where OPAT is delivered. Antibiotic treatment courses are highly variable, depending on underlying infection, and can span from days to weeks. Decisions about length of therapy, coadministration, or substitution with oral antibiotics all play a role in OPAT candidacy and location. Finally, home environmental and psychosocial barriers influence antibiotic selection and OPAT candidacy because administration of parenteral antibiotics and maintenance of venous access demands a safe and clean environment. Successful OPAT also demands participation at some level in the transaction of medications and their administration in exchange for adherence with said medications and accompanying ancillary supportive care.

This article herein reviews the types of infections affecting older adults that may indicate the use of OPAT. We will also discuss the nuanced process of OPAT candidate and location selection for the treatment of those infections. Determining which patient will be successful in the OPAT process is sometimes difficult to clearly define at the start of an OPAT course; success in OPAT hinges on the host, environmental, and disease-specific variables at the time of inpatient discharge or in the outpatient setting. Finally, the COVID-19 pandemic also has had impact on the use of OPAT as a valuable tool to avoid unnecessary acute-care bed utilization as well as keeping vulnerable patients away from health-care settings that could increase the risk of nosocomial COVID-19. OPAT provides many opportunities to deliver the needed care with a patient-centered approach.

Infections Indicating Use of Outpatient Parenteral Antimicrobial Therapy

Intravenous (IV) antimicrobial therapy is often given for severe infections, infections with multidrug-resistant organisms (MDRO), or deep-seated infections with or without source control. IV antimicrobial therapy is used to treat many complex acute and, sometimes, chronic infections affecting older adults. Although this is not an exhaustive review of infections indicating the use of OPAT, reviewed herein are infections with significant impact in older adults: endovascular infections, bacteremias, bone and joint infections, and complicated urinary tract infections (UTI).

Endovascular Infections

Endovascular infections include native valve and prosthetic valve endocarditis (PVE),[3,4] septic thrombophlebitis and endovascular device infections (lead-related endocarditis,[5] central venous catheters (CVCs), and nondriveline, left ventricular assist device infections.[6,7] Persons aged older than 60 years predominantly represent the shifting epidemiology of infectious endocarditis in the past 20 years compared with prior decades.[7,8] Furthermore, older patients with complex cardiovascular disease are more likely to receive implanted devices and prosthetic valves, making this group particularly at the risk for infectious complications necessitating prolonged OPAT. Patients with PVE tend to be older and also incur greater in-hospital mortality compared with native valve infective endocarditis.[9]

Typical pathogens of endovascular infections include skin and gastrointestinal flora such *Staphylococcus aureus*, coagulase-negative staphylococci (CoNs, eg, *Staphylococcus epidermidis*, *Staphylococcus lugdunensis*), beta-hemolytic streptococci, Viridans group streptococci, and enterococci. Other organisms such as fastidious gram-negative pathogens (eg, "HACEK" organisms) as well as more unusual pathogens such as *Abiotrophia* and *Gemella* spp represent a smaller proportion of pathogens.[7,8,10,11] Finally, culture negative endocarditis accounts for 15% to 19% of cases in some studies.[7,8,11,12] There is increasing resistance to antibiotics among CoNS, enterococci, and gram-negative pathogens among *Enterobacterales* and *Pseudomonads*, in particular, necessitating long courses of multiple antibiotics.

Bacteremias

Bacteremias are a common indication of OPAT in older adults. Whether bacteremia occurs more frequently or presents differently in the older adult is still a question but age seems to be a strong risk factor.[13] For example, with each decade more than 60 years, the incidence of *Staphylococcus aureus* bacteremia (SAB) increases dramatically: 100/100,000 persons/y in the sixth decade to the 250/100,000 persons/y in the eighth decade of life.[14] Bacteremia can develop from several sources, if known, including endovascular, odontogenic, gastrointestinal, genitourinary (GU), or respiratory infections. Skin and skin structure infections also account a smaller, but not insignificant proportion of bacteremia, less than 10%.[15]

Bacteremia in older individuals is most commonly related to respiratory and GU sources.[13] Comorbid conditions such as poor dentition, structural lung disease, malignancy, diverticular disease, choledocholithiasis, urinary tract dysfunction (eg, bladder prolapse, neurogenic bladder, benign prostatic hyperplasia), and diabetic foot ulcers all lead to an increased risk of infection and subsequent bacteremia. Occult infections may lead to bacteremia and can be more difficult to diagnose in an older patient with fewer signs or symptoms to guide the clinician. Gram-positive bacteremias with *S aureus*, Enterococcal species, oral streptococci, and fungemias are typically treated with OPAT for extended durations (2–8 weeks) dependent on source and source control and resistance profile of the indicated pathogen. More recent evidence has helped shorten OPAT lengths in uncomplicated gram-negative bacteremia.[16,17]

Musculoskeletal Infections

One of the most common type of infections involves the musculoskeletal system, including septic arthritis of native joints as well as prosthetic joint infections (PJI). The older population is more likely to experience PJI due to the increased likelihood of joint replacement with up to an 8% risk of mortality.[18] Although rare, infections are a feared complication of joint replacement, often requiring source control with explantation of the prosthetic material, and in some cases, prolonged immobilization and OPAT.

The sequelae of chronic diabetes and peripheral vascular disease may manifest as serious bone infections in older adults requiring revascularization, debridement, amputation, and OPAT.[19] Typical bone and joint pathogens include skin flora (S aureus, CoNS, beta-hemolytic streptococci, Cutibacterium acnes), oral streptococci, and less commonly, enteric gram-negative bacteria and enterococci. OPAT can be prolonged, in addition to the other morbidities associated with treatment, for example, deep venous thrombosis, skin and soft tissue infections from prolonged immobilization, and poor tissue healing.

Complicated Urinary Tract Infections

UTI are common in older persons with incidence ranging from 0.05 to 0.13 infections per person year in older men and women.[20] This can be attributed to changes in GU anatomy related to aging such as urinary tract dysfunction secondary to menopause, bladder prolapse, neurogenic bladder, and benign prostatic hyperplasia. Because of these anatomic changes leading to obstruction or poor urine flow, in addition to an increase in immunocompromised states, virtually all UTI in older adults are complicated in nature.[21] In addition, many older persons develop asymptomatic bacteriuria and colonization that beget unnecessary treatment, and consequently MDRO (eg, extended spectrum beta-lactamase [ESBL] producing Enterobacterales, Pseudomonas, and Acinetobacter spp, MRSA, MDR Enterococcus spp). Other risks for infection with MDRO include residence in a long-term care facility.[22] Interestingly, a multivariate study of older men versus younger men with complicated UTI did not show a difference in risk of MDRO associated with age.[23] Bacteremia and sepsis associated with GU infections, as well as infections involving the prostate or with nephrolithiasis will typically require OPAT of some duration. Infections with ESBL producing organisms will also usually necessitate use of OPAT due to limited oral options; however, the length of treatment need not be increased due to the presence of these pathogens.[24]

Outpatient Parenteral Antimicrobial Therapy Candidacy in Older Adults

One of the most critical aspects in a successful OPAT experience is selecting which OPAT setting is most appropriate for each patient, which may include either a SNF, infusion center, home, or HD center in some cases. Many factors must be considered to assure a safe transition to the outpatient environment. Age alone should not be a limiting factor in deciding OPAT eligibility; however, it should be considered in the greater context of the patient's own psychosocial competence and physical ability to participate in OPAT, environmental support, and ambulatory resources to successfully complete OPAT.[1]

Outpatient Parenteral Antimicrobial Therapy Environment

The selection of the OPAT setting is a key aspect of patient-centered care. The home setting is the most independent OPAT location, which thereby requires the most participation by patient or caregiver(s) in the daily OPAT process. Home OPAT typically relies on the patient self-infusing and performing daily care for the venous access in a clean and safe environment. The home must be safe and conducive for receiving weekly home nursing visits for laboratory monitoring and venous catheter care. Despite the onus on the patient, home OPAT is generally very user friendly with the use of elastomeric drug-delivery devices and small, portable infusion pumps, and the selection of medications that be given as an IV push. Patients are often able to carry on with their regular activity inside and outside the home, which lends this to being a highly satisfactory way to receive OPAT compared with receiving OPAT at an SNF or infusion clinic.[25,26]

For older patients who are unable to administer OPAT at home, other alternatives with supervision include infusion clinics and placement at SNFs. Infusion clinics are ambulatory centers where IV antibiotics can be administered by health-care professionals; however, limitations include daily transportation, daily versus multidose antibiotic regimens, and weekend/holiday administration. In our experience, placement at SNF is the least preferred venue for OPAT due to the lack of autonomy and independence available through home or infusion clinic OPAT. Patient satisfaction with quality of services and overall patient happiness while on therapy are lower without any significant return on improved tolerability or fewer problems while on antimicrobial therapy.[25] SNFs are necessary, although, for some older patients who require complicated antimicrobial regimen not amenable for home infusion or circumstances when patients are either unwilling to perform OPAT due to discomfort or fear of self-infusing or are not candidates due to poor psychosocial or physical competency.

For those patients with end-stage renal disease (ESRD) requiring HD, receipt of OPAT at the HD unit is preferred for several reasons, namely convenience. The ability to infuse renally dosed antibiotics using the patient's HD access in a supervised setting, thus, obviates any additional central access. Placing additional CVCs in patients with chronic kidney disease or ESRD should generally be avoided to preserve venous access for future HD needs.[1] However, there may be issues in receiving certain, less common antibiotics that may require special ordering in advance or specific administration by the HD center, which adds to the cost and inconvenience for the patient.

Psycho-Social and Physical Competence

Especially in the older patient, gaining a sense of the patient's competence is important in assessing success of OPAT at home. Aside from the obvious use of cognitive testing to assure competence, the prescribing provider must assess whether the patient understands the nature of their infection, therapeutic plan, and willingness to self-administer antibiotics at home. If a patient is not able to perform these functions, then a reliable caregiver who will be overseeing and providing the OPAT should undergo the same competency assessment. The patient or caregiver must be teachable. Use of techniques such as "teach back" are helpful tools in illuminating a patient's understanding and ability to retain knowledge before embarking in OPAT.[27] This assessment is similar for older patients with active mental health disorders that may impede full participation in OPAT at home.

For those individuals who will truly be self-administering antibiotics in the home, visual acuity and manual dexterity can be assessed through teach back, and if necessary, physical therapy and occupational therapy can be consulted to offer assistance and techniques to improve dexterity. Devices such as elastomeric devices and IV line extenders may also be useful in aiding the older patient. Finally, early and frequent engagement of caregiver support in the OPAT process is critical.

Substance Use Disorder

OPAT in individuals with substance use disorder (SUD) can be challenging to administer, yet SUD remains a risk factor for severe infections such as bacteremia and endovascular infections that predicate prolonged IV antimicrobial therapy. Historically, patients with SUD have conferred bias in health-care providers away from using standard home OPAT for the completion of therapy, rather opting for supervised settings such as prolonged acute care hospitalization, SNF placement, or off-label use of oral therapy or long-acting, extended-interval IV infusions. These medical decisions for alternative, sometimes second-line therapies have been based on provider fear of patient nonadherence with OPAT or misuse of CVC and related medicolegal repercussions.[28,29] A recent literature review of OPAT outcomes in persons who inject drugs (PWID) showed rates of OPAT completion in PWID are high (72%–100%) and no difference in rates of treatment failure, infection relapse, or hospital readmission. PWID also had lower complication rates and greater use of after-hour nursing assistance, suggesting that PWID can independently manage OPAT and seek care when needed.[29] Adverse events related to CVC such as thrombosis and infection were low and similar to persons without injection drug use. Misuse of CVC has also been shown to be infrequent.[29,30]

For those persons with SUD, OPAT and the opportunity for SUD treatment often intersect. OPAT can be an opportunity to engage patients in SUD, mental health, and social services. Administration of opioid partial agonist buprenorphine/naloxone or methadone treatment combined with receipt of OPAT can also be an effective means of increasing adherence and successful treatment of infections in this vulnerable population. This can empower a patient to regain autonomy, avoid stigma, reenter into society, and recover from SUD.[31] Infectious disease clinic teams staffed with nurses, ID pharmacists, social workers, and psychologists are an important resource and advocates for the patient.

Outpatient Parenteral Antimicrobial Therapy Safety in Older Adults

Per the Infectious Disease Society of America (IDSA) OPAT guidelines, there are "many descriptive studies in the adult and pediatric literature documenting the successful administration of OPAT medications at home by patients or family members, with few complications."[1] With respect to age as a risk factor in OPAT, based on 11 observational studies, the IDSA strongly endorsed OPAT for older patients, although it was based on weak evidence using the GRADE analytical approach.[32] Since the publication of these guidelines, 10 additional observational studies including older patient groups have emerged looking at a variety of outcomes in OPAT.[33–42] Most of these studies did not look at age specifically as a risk factor but the subjects ranged in age from 50 to 90s.[33–35,37,40] Five studies looked at age as a risk factor and 2 found worse outcomes in older persons—treatment amendment occurred more frequently in persons aged older than 64.5 years, and increased admissions to adjust OPAT (1.18 RR per decade).[36,38,39,41,42] Overall, careful patient selection, assurance of support in the home setting, laboratory monitoring and oversight by an infectious diseases physician or nurse/pharmacist were factors that assured a favorable outcome.

Duration of Therapy

In most instances, OPAT is administered during several weeks of therapy depending on the clinical syndrome being treated. Per the 2018 IDSA OPAT guidelines, the duration of antimicrobial treatment correlates with increased incidence of adverse drug events (ADE) in both pediatric and adult OPAT.[1,43–45] Complications of OPAT may be directly linked to the duration of therapy (OPAT > 30 days) but these data can also be conflicting (worse outcomes with shorter duration <14 days).[32,35,45] Studies showing worse outcomes associated with shorter length of therapy are possibly confounded by subjects whose OPAT was truncated due to complications versus subjects receiving shorter courses of therapy, for example, cellulitis or UTI. Using an appropriate length of therapy can protect against complications. Opportunities to switch to oral therapies earlier in treatment course or use of long-acting lipoglycopeptide (LA LGP) antibiotics in lieu of daily administration are options to reduce complications relating to length of OPAT.[46]

Adverse Events and Complications

Adverse events are to be anticipated during OPAT treatment in all patients but especially in older patients with increased comorbidities and polypharmacy and for those with severe infections, infections with MDRO, or intensive or prolonged antimicrobial regimens.[36,47] Adverse events including ADE, laboratory abnormalities, noninfectious or non-OPAT-related complications, clinical failure, or disease progression can lead to hospitalization and death. Several studies have tried to assess risk factors for such complications, and one such study interestingly showed older adults were less likely to have adverse outcomes (aOR 0.55) compared with younger patients.[47] Another study looking at nonagenarians compared with controls in the sixth decade of life showed no association with increased risk of OPAT-related admission, emergency room visit, or ADE. However, they had higher risk of death overall from non-OPAT complications.[42] Varying results were seen regarding age but the general consensus is that adverse events are not increased in older adults on OPAT.[36,47,48]

ADE include delayed type hypersensitivity allergic reactions (itching, rash) that can occur with any antibiotic during therapy. Hematologic ADEs include neutropenia, other leukopenias, and thrombocytopenia.[49] Neuropsychiatric complications with encephalopathy and seizures can occur with certain antibiotics such as carbapenems, cefepime, and IV acyclovir. In a review of cefepime included neurotoxicity, neurotoxic side effects have been mostly present in patients aged older than 60 years and also in the setting of underlying renal dysfunction and severe illness.[50] Gastrointestinal ADEs are common and include nausea, vomiting, dysgeusia, diarrhea, *Clostridioides difficile*-associated diarrhea (CDAD), acalculous cholecystitis, liver toxicity, and pancreatitis. Regarding CDAD, older patients especially those in the extreme of age, significantly represent more CDAD-related hospitalization and death.[51] Interestingly, the occurrence of CDAD among OPAT recipients is quite uncommon and has been reported in about less than 1% of patients on OPAT.[52,53]

Renal complications may occur more frequently with certain IV antibiotics or combinations thereof, such as vancomycin, nafcillin, and piperacillin-tazobactam, and must be monitored closely especially in older adults with underlying chronic medical renal disease. Common renal ADE includes acute kidney injury, reduction in tubular secretion of creatinine, and hyperkalemia. One major study in 2017 showed hospitalized patients receiving the combination of vancomycin and piperacillin-tazobactam had an increased risk of AKI (Hazard ratio [HR] 4, $P < .0001$) compared with those receiving vancomycin and cefepime.[54] Patient aged older than 60 years receiving OPAT are more likely to have nephrotoxicity compared with those aged younger than 60 years, probably for a variety of reasons—greater presence of chronic kidney disease, use of nephrotoxic antibiotics, for example.[55]

The IDSA guidelines recommend laboratory monitoring during OPAT but there are insufficient data to recommend specific testing.[1] Laboratory testing should be tailored to the specific side effects of therapy, as well as monitoring drug levels where indicated. Given the high rate of ADEs and DDIs for older patients receiving OPAT, laboratory monitoring is especially important in the outpatient setting.

Drug–Drug Interactions (DDI)/Polypharmacy

Older individuals tend to have increased comorbidities and often are taking a large number of medications in addition to the OPAT regimen. On average, persons aged older than 65 years taking more than 5 drugs is about 44%.[56] Many of these medications are well-known inhibitors or inducers of cytochrome P450 (CYP) 3A4 and other important cytochrome P450 enzymes that mediate drug metabolism. There are also individuals that have particular cytochrome polymorphisms in CYP 219 that can affect individual drug metabolism, for example, hypermetabolizers or low metabolizers of voriconazole.[57] The most common types of medications that interact with antimicrobials are HMG CoA reductase inhibitors (statins), psychiatric medications (eg, selective serotonin reuptake inhibitors), antiarrhythmic medications, direct oral anticoagulants, and warfarin.[58] Particular antibiotics that have increased DDIs are agents in the following classes: fluoroquinolones, macrolides, linezolid, rifamycins, and azoles.[58,59]

Cardiotoxicity is another area of concern in the older patients experiencing polypharmacy with the addition of oral and IV antibiotics during OPAT. This older but very large observational study of nearly 5 million outpatients receiving prescriptions involving medications that influenced QTc showed 22% who filled overlapping prescriptions were aged 65 years or older.[60] As many OPAT regimens often contain a combination of oral antibiotics such as fluoroquinolones or azoles, careful electrocardiogram monitoring may be indicated in some patients with underlying cardiovascular disease or baseline dysrhythmias.

Peripherally Inserted Central Catheter (PICC)/CVC Events

One of the most common issues faced by patients receiving OPAT is malfunction of the CVC. It is estimated that central line thrombosis occurs in 6% to 8% of PICC lines in use or 2.9 to 7/events per 1000 line-days, which increases as a function of time after placement with odds ratio (OR) of 1.25/wk.[33,61–64] Female gender (OR 2.4), number of lumens (2 vs 1; OR 11) and administration of penicillin G (OR 11.6), but not age, were factors related to PICC complications.[65] Other studies also found an association between type of antibiotics administered (eg, penicillins, cephalosporins, and carbapenems) and thrombosis.[66] Administration of thrombolytics in the field to reestablish PICC function is routine practice; however, it must be approached cautiously in the older patient who may be on other blood-thinning agents.

PICC and CVC-associated blood stream infections are also concerns and with increased risk the longer the catheter remains in place.[65–67] Contamination of lines may occur more frequently in individuals with reduced skin compliance and integrity, manual dexterity or cognitive ability if managing infusions alone.[47] A small observational study has shown worse outcomes with midline catheters but a recent large meta-analysis with nearly 11,000 patients suggested that midline catheters have a lower risk of occlusion (2.1 vs 7%) and blood stream infection (0.4% vs 1.6%) when compared with PICC lines.[63] In our experience, midline catheters are suitable options for OPAT use especially when duration of antimicrobial is short (eg, < 2 weeks).

Hospitalization/Readmission

Risk factors for readmission in OPAT include age (1.18 aOR per decade), higher number of comorbidities, endovascular infections, and receipt of OPAT in an SNF.[1,41,68] Studies that looked at readmission rates for self-administered OPAT versus SNF OPAT demonstrate that self-administered OPAT was associated with a lower rate of readmission compared with SNF OPAT.[69] Safety concerns with OPAT in older adults often lead to readmission for adjustment or alteration of antibiotics and monitoring for resolution of complications. It is estimated that 1% to 26% of patients require rehospitalization due to a safety concern with OPAT, with higher percentages of older patients being readmitted.[69] Careful screening of patients' psychosocial risks, comorbidities, administration of test doses of antimicrobials and establishing safety and efficacy in the individual patient are critical in avoiding complications and readmission.[70] Clinic follow-up for older patients is also a helpful practice to prevent 30 day-readmission (OR 0.06, $P < .0001$).[71]

Outpatient Parenteral Antimicrobial Therapy During the COVID-19 Pandemic

The on-going COVID-19 pandemic has caused increased strain on health-care systems globally. Especially during surge periods of infection, hospitalization rates rose to record numbers. During the Delta surge of COVID in 2021, daily hospital admission rate in the United States for patients with confirmed SARS CoV-2 infection exceeded 10,000 and increased to more than 20,000 in January 2022 during the Omicron surge.[72] The pandemic has presented several unique dilemmas in the crossroads of patients requiring long-term antimicrobial therapy and hospital resource utilization. Patients with serious illness but without COVID-19 illness often delayed seeking care either in fear of getting SARS-CoV-2 infection or due to health-care resource lockdowns.[73] Similarly, patients with non-COVID-19 illnesses competed for hospital resources with patients with severe COVID-19. SNFs that often house and provide services for patients needing OPAT demonstrated efficient spread of SARS-CoV-2 within facilities between patients and staff, further lessening the appeal of using these locations for OPAT of patients with and without COVID-19 illness, alike.[74]

Amid the COVID-19 pandemic and stretched hospital resources, necessity for routine long-term antimicrobial therapy turned to opportunities within the OPAT world to continue care for these patients and open hospital resources for patients with COVID-19. One opportunity for growth includes increased use of telemedicine services for OPAT initiation and treatment monitoring. Telemedicine for OPAT delivery and monitoring burgeoned during COVID-19 pandemic but even before COVID, there had been mounting evidence that telemedicine services are effective in managing OPAT care. Prior studies have shown clinical success, minimal drug-related adverse events and few unplanned readmissions, comparable to conventional, nontelemedicine OPAT care.[75,76] Infectious disease (ID)-led OPAT management and follow-up have previously been shown to have lower odds of hospitalization after the initial infection event compared with non-ID-led OPAT (OR 0.661) and lower odds of emergency department admission (OR 0.449). If coupled with telemedicine, ID-led OPAT management not only has the potential to reduce health-care utilization but has also shown promise to reduce health-care costs.[77]

Another area with increased interest is the use of medications that have dosing intervals of greater than 24 hours, such as LA LGP oritavancin and dalbavancin. Furthermore, medications with longer half-lives, may also lend the opportunity to space out therapeutic drug monitoring to longer intervals and avoid CVC insertion all together. LA LGPs have the major advantage of single dose infusions with pharmacokinetic profiles that can extend lengthy periods. For example, 2, once-weekly infusions of dalbavancin can cover an entire course (5–8 weeks) of antimicrobial therapy for common OPAT-indicated infections such as S aureus osteomyelitis.[78] Although these medications carry Food and Drug Administration indication for skin and soft tissue infections, there is growing evidence for the successful use of LA LGP in off-label situations such as bone and joint infections and SAB. The largest study to date looking at real-world data of 134 patients treated with oritavancin for acute osteomyelitis showed majority achieved clinical success with few cases of relapse or persistence of infection (9.7%).[79] Furthermore, a more recent retrospective study comparing dalbavancin with standard of care for SAB showed no difference in clinical failure rate; however, it was able to show much less use of CVC, shorter length of index hospitalization, and thus fewer hospital-acquired infections.[80]

Anecdotally, in our experience, expansion of telemedicine services and increased use of LA LGP at our local institution has provided significant direct and indirect benefits to patients in need of long-term antibiotics for infections. These approaches are patient-centered and work to reduce travel time for the older individuals and time physically spent in health-care settings where they can be exposed to other hospital-acquired infections such as COVID-19 itself. LA LGP has the potential to reduce side effects, pill-burden, and central-venous catheter complications for older adults with complex infections. Finally, these strategies also help to expand home OPAT services to overlooked candidates such as PWID. These approaches are all to reduce health-care exposure and utilization while maintaining safe and successful outcomes of serious infections.

SUMMARY

OPAT can be conducted effectively and safely for older adults with the appropriate supportive care. Age should not be an exclusionary factor for OPAT but rather prompt the OPAT provider to do a thorough candidacy evaluation to ensure the patient will be successful in OPAT regardless of location. Care must be taken in monitoring and evaluating adverse reactions and minimizing DDIs in older adults with underlying polypharmacy. New innovations in OPAT including the use of LA LGP and telemedicine will help bridge OPAT care into a more patient-centered, thoughtful practice. Especially as the COVID-pandemic is among us for the foreseeable future, protecting our older patients from unnecessary health-care exposure and thus health care-associated infections is critical.

CLINICS CARE POINTS

- Older adults with multiple cormorbidities are at risk of severe infections that may require prolonged courses of antibiotics. If intravenous antibiotics are indicated, OPAT is a safe and effective way to deliver the antibiotic course.
- OPAT, especially when given at home, promotes a patient-centered therapeutic plan that fosters patient autonomy and satisfaction.
- The COVID-19 pandemic has spotlighted the role and potential of OPAT as an alternative to delivering antimicrobial therapy outside of the acute care setting. This benefit is two fold – reduce the burden of acute care utilization and avoid unnecessary health care exposure for older patients.

DISCLOSURES

The authors have nothing to disclose.

REFERENCES

1. Norris AH, Shrestha NK, Allison GM, et al. 2018 Infectious Diseases Society of America Clinical Practice Guideline for the Management of Outpatient Parenteral Antimicrobial Therapy. Clin Infect Dis 2019;68(1):e1–35.

2. HIT Monitoring Report. Center for Medicare and Medicaid Services. Available from: www.cms.gov/files/document/hit-monitoring-report-january-2022.pdf. Accessed 25 July, 2022.
3. Chambers HF, Bayer AS. Native-Valve Infective Endocarditis. N Engl J Med 2020; 383(6):567–76.
4. Ivanovic B, Trifunovic D, Petrovic MS, et al. Prosthetic valve endocarditis - A trouble or a challenge? J Cardiol 2019;73(2):126–33.
5. Mohammedzein A, Mozumder A, Milton S. Cardiac implantable electronic device infections-decision-making process in complex patients: report of 3 cases. J Investig Med High Impact Case Rep 2019;7. 2324709619831320.
6. Skalweit MJ. Left Ventricular Assist Device Infections. In: Firstenberg MS, editor. Advanced Concepts in Endocarditis. London: Intech Open; 2018.
7. Hill EH, Herijgers P, Claus P, et al. Infective endocarditis: changing epidemiology and predictors of 6-month mortality: a prospective cohort study. Eur Heart J 2007; 28(2):196–203.
8. Castillo FJ, Anguita M, Castillo JC, et al. Changes in Clinical Profile, Epidemiology and Prognosis of Left-sided Native-valve Infective Endocarditis Without Predisposing Heart Conditions. *Rev Esp Cardiol* (Engl Ed 2015;68(5):445–8.
9. Wang A, Athan E, Pappas PA, et al. Contemporary clinical profile and outcome of prosthetic valve endocarditis. JAMA 2007;297(12):1354–61.
10. Coll PP, Lindsay A, Meng J, et al. The Prevention of Infections in Older Adults: Oral Health. J Am Geriatr Soc 2020;68(2):411–6.
11. Murdoch DR, Corey GR, Hoen B, et al. Clinical presentation, etiology, and outcome of infective endocarditis in the 21st century: the International Collaboration on Endocarditis-Prospective Cohort Study. Arch Intern Med 2009;169(5): 463–73.
12. Skalweit MJ. Culture Negative Endocarditis: Advances in Diagnosis and Treatment. In: Firstenberg MS, editor. Contemporary challenges in endocarditis. London: Intech Open; 2016.
13. Leibovici-Weissman Y, Tau N, Yahav D. Bloodstream infections in the elderly: what is the real goal? Aging Clin Exp Res 2021;33(4):1101–12.
14. Laupland KB, Lyytikainen O, Sogaard M, et al. The changing epidemiology of Staphylococcus aureus bloodstream infection: a multinational population-based surveillance study. Clin Microbiol Infect 2013;19(5):465–71.
15. Gunderson CG, Martinello RA. A systematic review of bacteremias in cellulitis and erysipelas. J Infect 2012;64(2):148–55.
16. Yahav D, Franceschini E, Koppel F, et al. Seven Versus 14 Days of Antibiotic Therapy for Uncomplicated Gram-negative Bacteremia: A Noninferiority Randomized Controlled Trial. Clin Infect Dis 2019;69(7):1091–8.
17. Swamy S, Sharma R. Duration of Treatment of Gram-Negative BacteremiaAre Shorter Courses of Antimicrobial Therapy Feasible? Infect Dis Clin Pract 2016; 24(3):155–60.
18. De Angelis G, Mutters NT, Minkley L, et al. Prosthetic joint infections in the elderly. Infection 2015;43(6):629–37.
19. Uckay I, Holy D, Betz M, et al. Osteoarticular infections: a specific program for older patients? Aging Clin Exp Res 2021;33(3):703–10.
20. Rowe TA, Juthani-Mehta M. Urinary tract infection in older adults. Aging Health 2013;9(5):75–89.
21. Wagenlehner FME, Bjerklund Johansen TE, Cai T, et al. Epidemiology, definition and treatment of complicated urinary tract infections. Nat Rev Urol 2020;17(10): 586–600.

22. Jump RL, Crnich CJ, Mody L, et al. Infectious Diseases in Older Adults of Long-Term Care Facilities: Update on Approach to Diagnosis and Management. J Am Geriatr Soc 2018;66(4):789–803.

23. Smithson A, Ramos J, Niño E, et al. Characteristics of febrile urinary tract infections in older male adults. BMC Geriatr 2019;19(1):334.

24. Fink DL, Collins S, Barret R, et al. Shortening duration of ertapenem in outpatient parenteral antimicrobial therapy for complicated urinary tract infections: A retrospective study. PLoS One 2019;14(9):e0223130.

25. Mansour O, Arbaje AI, Townsend JL. Patient Experiences With Outpatient Parenteral Antibiotic Therapy: Results of a Patient Survey Comparing Skilled Nursing Facilities and Home Infusion. Open Forum Infect Dis 2019;6(12):ofz471.

26. Saillen L, Arensdorff L, Moulin E, et al. Patient satisfaction in an outpatient parenteral antimicrobial therapy (OPAT) unit practising predominantly self-administration of antibiotics with elastomeric pumps. Eur J Clin Microbiol Infect Dis 2017;36(8):1387–92.

27. Yen PH, Leasure AR. Use and Effectiveness of the Teach-Back Method in Patient Education and Health Outcomes. Fed Pract 2019;36(6):284–9.

28. Cortes-Penfield N, Cawcutt K, Alexander BT, et al. A Proposal for Addiction and Infectious Diseases Specialist Collaboration to Improve Care for Patients With Opioid Use Disorder and Injection Drug Use-Associated Infective Endocarditis. J Addict Med 2022;16(4):392–5.

29. Suzuki J, Johnson J, Montgomery M, et al. Outpatient Parenteral Antimicrobial Therapy Among People Who Inject Drugs: A Review of the Literature. Open Forum Infect Dis 2018;5(9):ofy194.

30. Ho J, Archuleta S, Sulaiman Z, et al. Safe and successful treatment of intravenous drug users with a peripherally inserted central catheter In an outpatient parenteral antibiotic treatment service. J Antimicrob Chemother 2010;65(12):2641–4.

31. Serota DP, Chueng TA, Schechter MC. Applying the Infectious Diseases Literature to People who Inject Drugs. Infect Dis Clin North Am 2020;34(3):539–58.

32. Guyatt GH, Oxman AD, Vist GE, et al. GRADE: an emerging consensus on rating quality of evidence and strength of recommendations. BMJ 2008;336(7650):924–6.

33. Briquet C, Cornu O, Servais V, et al. Clinical characteristics and outcomes of patients receiving outpatient parenteral antibiotic therapy in a Belgian setting: a single-center pilot study. Acta Clin Belg 2020;75(4):275–83.

34. Burnett YJ, Spec A, Ahmed MM, et al. Experience with Liposomal Amphotericin B in Outpatient Parenteral Antimicrobial Therapy. Antimicrob Agents Chemother 2021;65(6):e01876–920.

35. Chambers ST, Basevi A, Gllagher K, et al. Outpatient parenteral antimicrobial therapy (OPAT) in Christchurch: 18 years on. N Z Med J 2019;132(1501):21–32.

36. Keller SC, Williams D, Gavgani M, et al. Rates of and Risk Factors for Adverse Drug Events in Outpatient Parenteral Antimicrobial Therapy. Clin Infect Dis 2018;66(1):11–9.

37. Miron-Rubio M, Gonzalez-Ramallo V, Estrada-Cuxart O, et al. Intravenous antimicrobial therapy in the hospital-at-home setting: data from the Spanish Outpatient Parenteral Antimicrobial Therapy Registry. Future Microbiol 2016;11(3):375–90.

38. Ponce Gonzalez MA, Miron-Rubio M, Mujal Martinez A, et al. Effectiveness and safety of outpatient parenteral antimicrobial therapy in acute exacerbation of chronic obstructive pulmonary disease. Int J Clin Pract 2017;71(12).

39. Quirke M, Curran EM, O'Kelly P, et al. Risk factors for amendment in type, duration and setting of prescribed outpatient parenteral antimicrobial therapy (OPAT)

for adult patients with cellulitis: a retrospective cohort study and CART analysis. Postgrad Med J 2018;94(1107):25–31.

40. Suleyman G, Kenney R, Zervos MJ, et al. Safety and efficacy of outpatient parenteral antibiotic therapy in an academic infectious disease clinic. J Clin Pharm Ther 2017;42(1):39–43.

41. Durojaiye OC, Morgan R, Chelaghma N, et al. External validity and clinical usefulness of a risk prediction model for 30 day unplanned hospitalization in patients receiving outpatient parenteral antimicrobial therapy. J Antimicrob Chemother 2021;76(8):2204–12.

42. Shrestha NK, Blaskewicz C, Gordon SM, et al. Safety of Outpatient Parenteral Antimicrobial Therapy in Nonagenarians. Open Forum Infect Dis 2020;7(10): ofaa398.

43. Cunha CB, D'Agata EM. Implementing an antimicrobial stewardship program in out-patient dialysis units. Curr Opin Nephrol Hypertens 2016;25(6):551–5.

44. Hoffman-Terry ML, Fraimow HS, Fox TR, et al. Adverse effects of outpatient parenteral antibiotic therapy. Am J Med 1999;106(1):44–9.

45. Pulcini C, Couadau T, Bernard E, et al. Adverse effects of parenteral antimicrobial therapy for chronic bone infections. Eur J Clin Microbiol Infect Dis 2008;27(12): 1227–32.

46. Krsak M, Morrisette T, Miller M, et al. Advantages of Outpatient Treatment with Long-Acting Lipoglycopeptides for Serious Gram-Positive Infections: A Review. Pharmacotherapy 2020;40(5):469–78.

47. Keller SC, Wang NY, Salinas A, et al. Which Patients Discharged to Home-Based Outpatient Parenteral Antimicrobial Therapy Are at High Risk of Adverse Outcomes? Open Forum Infect Dis 2020;7(6):ofaa178.

48. Keller SC, Williams D, Gavgani M, et al. Environmental Exposures and the Risk of Central Venous Catheter Complications and Readmissions in Home Infusion Therapy Patients. Infect Control Hosp Epidemiol. Infect Control Hosp Epidemiol 2017;38(1):68–75.

49. Cimino C, Allos BM, Phillips EJ. A Review of β-Lactam-Associated Neutropenia and Implications for Cross-reactivity. Ann Pharmacother 2021;55(8):1037–49.

50. Payne LE, Gagnon DJ, Riker RR, et al. Cefepime-induced neurotoxicity: a systematic review. Crit Care 2017;21(1):276.

51. Jump RL. *Clostridium difficile* infection in older adults. Aging health 2013;9(4): 403–14.

52. Wong KK, Fraser TG, Shrestha NK, et al. Low incidence of Clostridium difficile infection (CDI) in patients treated with outpatient parenteral antimicrobial therapy (OPAT). Infect Control Hosp Epidemiol 2015;36(1):110–2.

53. Barr DA, Semple L, Seaton RA. Outpatient parenteral antimicrobial therapy (OPAT) in a teaching hospital-based practice: a retrospective cohort study describing experience and evolution over 10 years. Int J Antimicrob Agents 2012;39(5):407–13.

54. Navalkele B, Pogue JM, Karino S, et al. Risk of Acute Kidney Injury in Patients on Concomitant Vancomycin and Piperacillin-Tazobactam Compared to Those on Vancomycin and Cefepime. Clin Infect Dis 2017;64(2):116–23.

55. Cox AM, MAlani PN, Wiseman SW, et al. Home intravenous antimicrobial infusion therapy: a viable option in older adults. J Am Geriatr Soc 2007;55(5):645–50.

56. Morin L, Johnell K, Laroche ML, et al. The epidemiology of polypharmacy in older adults: register-based prospective cohort study. Clin Epidemiol 2018;10:289–98.

57. Zhang Y, Hao X, Hou Y, et al. Impact of cytochrome P450 2C19 polymorphisms on the clinical efficacy and safety of voriconazole: an update systematic review and meta-analysis. Pharmacogenet Genomics 2022;32(7):257–67.
58. Das B, Ramasubbu SK, Agnihotri A, et al. Leading 20 drug-drug interactions, polypharmacy, and analysis of the nature of risk factors due to QT interval prolonging drug use and potentially inappropriate psychotropic use in elderly psychiatry outpatients. Ther Adv Cardiovasc Dis 2021;15. 17539447211058892.
59. Hale CM, STeele JM, Seabury RW, et al. Characterization of Drug-Related Problems Occurring in Patients Receiving Outpatient Antimicrobial Therapy. J Pharm Pract 2017;30(6):600–5.
60. Curtis LH, Truls Ostby, Sendersky V, et al. Prescription of QT-prolonging drugs in a cohort of about 5 million outpatients. Am J Med 2003;114(2):135–41.
61. Quintens C, Steffens E, Jacobs K, et al. Efficacy and safety of a Belgian tertiary care outpatient parenteral antimicrobial therapy (OPAT) program. Infection 2020; 48(3):357–66.
62. Seo H, Altshuler D, Dubrovskaya Y, et al. The Safety of Midline Catheters for Intravenous Therapy at a Large Academic Medical Center. Ann Pharmacother 2020; 54(3):232–8.
63. Swaminathan L, Flanders S, HOrowitz J, et al. Safety and Outcomes of Midline Catheters vs Peripherally Inserted Central Catheters for Patients With Short-term Indications: A Multicenter Study. JAMA Intern Med 2022;182(1):50–8.
64. Underwood J, Marks M, Collins S, et al. Intravenous catheter-related adverse events exceed drug-related adverse events in outpatient parenteral antimicrobial therapy. J Antimicrob Chemother 2019;74(3):787–90.
65. Lam PW, Graham C, Leis J, et al. Predictors of Peripherally Inserted Central Catheter Occlusion in the Outpatient Parenteral Antimicrobial Therapy Setting. Antimicrob Agents Chemother 2018;62(9):e00900–18.
66. Barr DA, Semple L, Seaton RA. Self-administration of outpatient parenteral antibiotic therapy and risk of catheter-related adverse events: a retrospective cohort study. Eur J Clin Microbiol Infect Dis 2012;31(10):2611–9.
67. Li W, Branley J, Sud A. Outpatient parenteral antibiotic therapy in a suburban tertiary referral centre in Australia over 10 years. Infection 2018;46(3):349–55.
68. Huang V, Ruhe JJ, Lerner P, et al. Risk factors for readmission in patients discharged with outpatient parenteral antimicrobial therapy: a retrospective cohort study. BMC Pharmacol Toxicol 2018;19(1):50.
69. Sriskandarajah S, HObbs J, Roughhead E, et al. Safety and effectiveness of 'hospital in the home' and 'outpatient parenteral antimicrobial therapy' in different age groups: A systematic review of observational studies. Int J Clin Pract 2018;19: e13216.
70. Barnes A, Nunez M. Diabetic Foot Infection and Select Comorbidities Drive Readmissions in Outpatient Parenteral Antimicrobial Therapy. Am J Med Sci 2021; 361(2):233–7.
71. Palms DL, Jacob JT. Close Patient Follow-up Among Patients Receiving Outpatient Parenteral Antimicrobial Therapy. Clin Infect Dis 2020;70(1):67–74.
72. COVID Data Tracker Weekly Review. 2022. Available from: www.cdc.gov/coronavirus/2019-ncov/covid-data/covidview/index.htm. Accessed 28 July, 2022.
73. Anderson KE, McGinty EE, Presskreischer R, et al. Reports of Forgone Medical Care Among US Adults During the Initial Phase of the COVID-19 Pandemic. JAMA Netw Open 2021;4(1):e2034882.
74. Barnett ML, Hu L, Martin T, et al. Mortality, Admissions, and Patient Census at SNFs in 3 US Cities During the COVID-19 Pandemic. JAMA 2020;324(5):507–9.

75. Tan SJ, Ingram PR, Rothnie AJ, et al. Successful outpatient parenteral antibiotic therapy delivery via telemedicine. J Antimicrob Chemother 2017;72(10): 2898–901.
76. Sheridan KR, Abdel-Massih R, Gupta N, et al. Tele-OPAT Outcomes at Two Community Hospitals. Open Forum Infect Dis 2020;7(Suppl 1):S373–4.
77. Shah A, Petrak R, Fliegelman R, et al. Infectious Diseases Specialty Intervention Is Associated With Better Outcomes Among Privately Insured Individuals Receiving Outpatient Parenteral Antimicrobial Therapy. Clin Infect Dis 2019; 68(7):1160–5.
78. Cojutti PG, Rinaldi M, Zamparini E, et al. Population pharmacokinetics of dalbavancin and dosing consideration for optimal treatment of adult patients with staphylococcal osteoarticular infections. Antimicrob Agents Chemother 2021; 65(5):e02260–320.
79. Van Hise NW, Chundi V, Didwania V, et al. Treatment of Acute Osteomyelitis with Once-Weekly Oritavancin: A Two-Year, Multicenter, Retrospective Study. Drugs Real World Outcomes 2020;7(Suppl 1):41–5.
80. Molina KC, Lunow C, Lebin M, et al. Comparison of Sequential Dalbavancin With Standard-of-Care Treatment for *Staphylococcus aureus bloodstream infections*. Open Forum Infect Dis 2022;9(7):ofac335.

Considering Patient, Family, and Provider Goals and Expectations in a Rapidly Changing Clinical Context: A Framework for Antimicrobial Stewardship at the End of Life

Jeffrey Larnard, MD[a],*, Wendy Stead, MD[a],
Westyn Branch-Elliman, MD, MMSc, FSHEA[b,c]

KEYWORDS

• Antibiotics • End of life • Hospice • Palliative care

KEY POINTS

- Antibiotic use is a common component of end-of-life (EOL) medical care across different care settings and underlying diseases.
- The effectiveness of antimicrobials for improving quantity or quality of life, for example, by reducing discomfort from the symptoms of infection, in the EOL population is unclear and likely context- and disease-specific.
- Providers may be influenced by patients and/or family members when making decisions about antimicrobial administration during the EOL period.
- In addition to providing typical antimicrobial use guidance about appropriate choice and duration of therapy, antimicrobial stewardship providers can have a role in this population by providing guidance in how effective antimicrobials may be at achieving specified goals of care, potential adverse effects of antimicrobials, and adjusting recommendations in real time to meet the individual needs of the EOL patient.

INTRODUCTION

End of life (EOL) is a loosely defined term in clinical medicine that often encompasses the final days or weeks of life but may also be used to describe a substantially longer time horizon.[1] Although patients at EOL are often older adults, this is a heterogenous

[a] Division of Infectious Disease, Beth Israel Deaconess Medical Center, Harvard Medical School, 110 Francis Street, Suite GB, Boston, MA 02215, USA; [b] Department of Medicine, Section of Infectious Diseases, VA Boston Healthcare System, 1400 VFW Parkway, West Roxbury, MA 02132, USA; [c] Department of Medicine, Harvard Medical School
* Corresponding author.
E-mail address: jclarnar@bidmc.harvard.edu

Infect Dis Clin N Am 37 (2023) 139–151
https://doi.org/10.1016/j.idc.2022.09.003
0891-5520/23/© 2022 Elsevier Inc. All rights reserved.

id.theclinics.com

population with different underlying disease states and different expected benefits from antimicrobial therapy, as well as prognoses, expectations, and belief processes. All of these different factors interact in complex ways to ultimately determine a patient or caregiver's goals of care, which itself can be nebulous and evolve with time and changes in clinical status and context. The focus of this review is on antimicrobial prescribing for the treatment of diagnosed infections among patients with a known terminal but noncritical illness and a life expectancy of 6 months or less.

Patients at EOL are often more susceptible to infection due to host factors such as immobility, malnutrition, failure of host barriers, and the use of foreign bodies.[2–5] Infections in the EOL population range from critical and life-threatening, such as severe pneumonia and sepsis, to mild, such as lower urinary tract infections (UTIs). However, accurate diagnosis of infection in this population is often difficult; patients may not be able to express their own symptoms and presentation of infections may be subtle.[5–7] In addition, diagnostics may be limited by care setting or patient preferences. Because antimicrobials in patients at the EOL are used for a variety of purposes ranging from extending the duration of life (eg, for treatment of pneumonia or sepsis in the intensive care unit [ICU]) to symptom relief (eg, treatment of a lower UTI), factors that drive antimicrobial prescribing and potential stewardship interventions that may improve antimicrobial use at the EOL are also varied.

Patient and family preferences and shared decision-making about treatment may also be an important factor in EOL care,[8,9] thus the roles and responsibilities of antimicrobial stewardship providers (ASPs) and infectious disease providers can be different than in other clinical contexts, where the focus is on achieving clinical cure while minimizing long-term harms of antimicrobial use, including antimicrobial resistance. In the context of EOL care, patients and/or family members often have more clearly defined expectations, and additional specialists, such as palliative care physicians and geriatricians, may also have an active role in medical decision-making. This is a setting often filled with emotion, but lacking in certainties and thus goals and expectations can change rapidly. ASP operating in this milieu may find what would otherwise be a straightforward recommendation to be far more complex and driven by different factors than those that impact decision-making and recommendations in other clinical settings.

Defining End of Life

As above, this review defines the EOL population as patients with a terminal illness with a prognosis of 6 months or less that is not due to an acute critical illness. Most of the published literature in this population is composed of studies of patients with advanced cancer or advanced dementia, but this population also encompasses patients with other terminal illnesses, such as chronic obstructive pulmonary disease (COPD) and heart failure.[1] There is still significant heterogeneity within this group. Clinical care needs to account for the specific context of each patient and infection. A patient living at home with terminal cancer on palliative chemotherapy who develops a lower UTI without systemic symptoms suggests a different clinical approach than if that the same patient is intubated for hypoxic respiratory failure from the progression of their lung malignancy. We will use patient prognosis, as well as the goals of antibiotic therapy, to guide a framework for antimicrobial decision-making among EOL patients.

Recommendations for End-of-Life Antimicrobial Stewardship Providers from Guideline-Issuing Bodies

Because antimicrobials are often a part of EOL care and also a potential driver of antimicrobial resistance, the Infectious Diseases Society of America and the Society for

Healthcare Epidemiology of America (SHEA) recommended in 2016 that antimicrobial stewardship programs "provide support to clinical care providers in decisions relating to antimicrobial therapy" for terminally ill patients (good practice recommendation).[10] In a subsequent survey of antimicrobial stewardship programs in the SHEA research network in 2018, most respondents reported monitoring antimicrobial use at the EOL; however, only 8% reported that antimicrobial stewardship provided guidelines for EOL antimicrobial use.[11] In long-term care facilities, a meta-analysis of antimicrobial stewardship programs showed a reduction in overall antimicrobial use.[12] However, although observational data were promising, a subsequent cluster randomized trial at nursing homes in Massachusetts to promote goal-directed care for UTIs and lower respiratory tract infections (LRTI) in nursing home residents with advanced dementia failed to demonstrate a reduction in days of therapy.[13] ASPs in all settings have a role in assisting with delineating active infections from bacterial colonization that does not require treatment, antimicrobial selection for different clinical scenarios, and in recommending duration of treatment based on the type and severity of infection. At EOL, ASPs and infectious disease specialists can also have a role in determining whether the treatment of true infections will help to achieve the patient's and families' goals of care. Specifically, ASP has a role in EOL care by providing support to prescribers to help delineate whether there is an infection present and to frame the potential benefits and harms of the desired antimicrobial in the specific clinical scenario. ASP can also assist with providing verbal scripts to prescribers to guide the discussion of potential benefits and harms of antimicrobials with patients and families, who may overestimate the benefit of antimicrobial therapy.[14]

Defining Patient, Family, and Provider Goals

ASPs should take time to delineate the patient and/or family goals and the goals of the treating clinician. Defining the goals of antimicrobial therapy, as well as the goals of care in general, is essential for advising on antimicrobial decision-making at EOL. ASPs can then provide support to prescribers (and subsequently patients and families) by commenting on the probability that antimicrobial therapy could help to achieve identified goals. In addition, they can provide guidance on the potential harms of antimicrobial therapy—including harms that may be detrimental to the overall goals of care. For example, for patients whose main goal is to spend as much time as possible with loved ones at home, antimicrobial use in the hospital could potentially delay discharge, particularly if intravenous antimicrobials are needed to achieve clinical cure of the infection.[15]

Antimicrobial Use at the End of Life: Frequency and Drivers of Practice

Current clinical guidelines highlight the importance of ASP activities in all patients, including those at EOL. Current evidence supports the need for ASP specifically focused in this setting and on this population. For example, a recent systematic review found that antimicrobials are commonly prescribed among patients at the EOL, irrespective of underlying disease and across care settings.[1] Studies investigating antimicrobial use at EOL were separated by underlying diseases: advanced cancer, advanced dementia, and mixed populations. For all three groups, most of the studies found over 50% of patients received antimicrobials during the period of study.[1]

In acute care hospitals, many patients receive antimicrobials during terminal hospitalization with rates as high as 90% cited in the literature.[15–20] Although some of this high use is attributable to critically ill patients in intensive care settings, many patients continue to receive antimicrobials even after transition to comfort-focused care.[16,17]

Underscoring the frequency of antimicrobial use in EOL patients outside of critical care settings, rates of antimicrobial prescribing have been reported between 8% and 21% among patients being transferred from acute care hospitals to hospice care.[21,22] A national sample of patients enrolled in hospice care found that about a quarter of patients received at least one antimicrobial during the final week of life.[23] In addition, antimicrobial use was found to be common in patients with advanced dementia residing at long-term care facilities.[24]

Although there is robust evidence to support that antimicrobial use at the EOL is common, research explaining the reasons for the practice is limited. In one study examining the rationale for antimicrobials prescribed for patients discharged to hospice, only a small minority of the antimicrobials prescribed in this setting was prescribed for palliative reasons. In this study, which focused on patients who were not critically ill, antimicrobials were more commonly prescribed to cure, prevent, or suppress an infection.[8] However, a survey study of internal medicine and pediatric physicians at academic medical centers found that the desire to palliate symptoms was an important factor when deciding to continue antimicrobials at EOL.[9] Patient and family influence has also been seen as an important factor in antimicrobial decision-making in survey studies.[9,25] We suspect that given the heterogenous nature of this population, the rational for antimicrobial prescribing is likely variable based on the prescriber, clinical scenario, and patient/family preference. Moreover, patients and/or families may want antimicrobials to be continued for very different reasons, whether it is for symptom palliation or to not be perceived as "giving up." In **Fig. 1**, we outline the potential drivers of antimicrobial prescribing at EOL as well as potential actions ASP can take.

POTENTIAL BENEFITS OF ANTIMICROBIALS AT THE END OF LIFE
Palliation of Symptoms

The potential benefits of antimicrobials at EOL remain ambiguous and context-specific, with observational data demonstrating substantial variability in symptom reduction. The only systematic review on the effectiveness of antimicrobials for

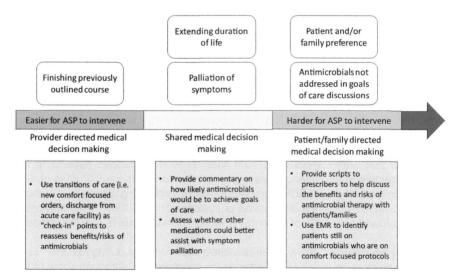

Fig. 1. Potential drivers of antimicrobial prescribing at EOL, appropriateness of ASP involvement, and potential ASP interventions.

symptom management in this population noted significant limitations in the available data, including a lack of comparison groups of patients not receiving antimicrobial therapy as well as heterogeneity in measurement of symptom reduction. The investigators of the systematic review also provide helpful tables detailing the individual studies that investigated the palliative effect of antimicrobials and estimated effect sizes of treatment.[26] A subsequent retrospective study of patients hospitalized in the last 14 days of life showed symptom relief in only 23% of patients (most of whom had pneumonia or intra-abdominal infection)[18]; in contrast, a retrospective study of patients enrolled in home hospice found that 60% of patients whose antimicrobials met a minimum use criterion had symptom resolution. In the latter study, UTI and LRTI were the most common infections treated.[27]

Observational studies have generally shown antimicrobials prescribed for UTI to be more effective for palliating symptoms than antimicrobials for treatment of other infections at EOL.[27-30] The rates of symptom improvement for lower respiratory infections are more varied, although some of the variation is due to treatment directed at viral, rather than bacterial infections. Impact on symptom control was more promising in an observational study limited to those whose included prescriptions met appropriate use criteria; in this smaller cohort, the rate of symptom response was similar to UTI.[27] Studies investigating at the effectiveness of antimicrobials at improving comfort in patients with pneumonia and underlying dementia are mixed,[31,32] though note should be made of the prospective study by Givens and colleagues, which adjusted for more variables and found that antimicrobial use was associated with greater *discomfort*.[31] In observational studies looking at the resolution of fever, the rate of symptom improvement after receipt of antimicrobial therapy directed toward a diagnosed bacterial infection was generally around 50%.[27,33,34]

A substantial proportion of the variability in the effectiveness of antimicrobials in improving symptoms seen in the available literature is likely due at least in part to the heterogenous nature of the EOL population. In a patient with terminal cancer and weeks to months to live, antimicrobials could undoubtedly help relieve dysuria from a UTI or pain from a cellulitis around a central venous catheter. However, in the same patient who is subsequently hospitalized with hypoxic respiratory failure and a prognosis of hours to days, antimicrobials would likely be of minimal help in relieving symptoms related to a possible LRTI. Data from an observational study underscore that the palliative effects of antimicrobials are likely to be lower in the last week of life.[35] Thus, when providing advice about potential benefits of antimicrobial use in patients for whom palliation is the goal, ASP should discuss how benefits vary depending on the expected duration of remaining life and specifically provide council that antimicrobials are likely to be less effective for achieving palliation during the very EOL.

ASP should also consider whether antimicrobials are the best way to help the patient achieve symptom relief. In the above example—a patient with terminal cancer admitted with hypoxic respiratory failure and extremely limited prognosis, antimicrobials are likely not the most effective treatment for achieving palliation of the patient's dyspnea. As patients and/or family members are often more involved in care decisions at EOL, care should be taken to give an accurate representation of the anticipated benefits of antimicrobials, particularly in relation to other symptom directed therapy. For example, administration of intravenous antimicrobials can worsen edema and fluid overload, given high salt and volume loads. Thus, in this clinical scenario, a primary focus on diuresis and fluid removal to improve the comfort of breathing may be more effective than antimicrobials for alleviating symptoms—and antimicrobials may in fact worsen the patient's clinical symptoms by worsening fluid overload.

However, it should be also noted that other symptom-directed therapies have their own set of side effects, which may be undesirable for patients and/or families. The clinical management strategy needs to balance risks, benefits, and patient and family goals and expectations.

Extending Duration of Life

The effectiveness of antimicrobials for extending duration of life is also uncertain and depends on the specific clinical context. Some observational data suggested no survival benefit from antimicrobial therapy at EOL,[28,29] whereas others have found that antimicrobial therapy was associated with increased duration of life; differences in these studies can at least be partially explained by the different patient populations and expected life expectancy included in these investigations.[2,31,34] A prospective study by Givens and colleagues found that treating pneumonia in patients with advanced dementia led to increased duration of life, but also that antimicrobial administration lead to a concurrent worsening of comfort scores. This finding underscores the importance of clearly defining goals and expectations as antimicrobial prescribing may have divergent impacts on different clinical goals—specifically, extending life may worsen comfort.[31] Another observational study found that antibiotics were actually hazardous to patient survival if administered in the 2 days before death.[36] In certain cases, continuing antimicrobials may be desired by patients and families to achieve a short-term goal (ie, extending life so that a patient can be discharged from an acute care hospital to a hospice setting). If discharge to home or hospice is the goal, ASP should provide input into whether antimicrobial administration is likely to help achieve that goal.

POTENTIAL HARMS OF ANTIMICROBIALS AT THE END OF LIFE

There is a relative paucity of data examining the adverse effects of antimicrobials specifically in EOL populations, but antimicrobial harms can be divided into short-term direct impacts of antimicrobials on the EOL patient, such as allergic reactions and gastrointestinal impacts, short-term indirect impacts, such as the pain caused by intravenous infusions, and long-term impacts, which are unlikely to directly impact the comfort and longevity of the EOL patient, such as antimicrobial resistance. Investigations into the incidence of direct, short-term harms among patients at the EOL are limited, but in one retrospective study of patients with advanced cancer who died while hospitalized, 5.6% of the 126 patients who received antimicrobials developed *Clostridioides difficile* infection.[16] In another retrospective study from a palliative care center in Sweden, the overall rate of adverse events among patients receiving antimicrobials was only 3.8%, primarily diarrhea and nausea.[37] Studies of the indirect potential adverse effects of antimicrobials, including discomfort associated with peripheral and/or central line placement,[38] are even more limited, and thus providing an estimate of these risks is not possible. However, if an EOL experiences indirect harms, such as intravenous (IV) infiltration or fluid overload, it is reasonable to reassess the value of intravenous antimicrobials in particular for achieving the patient's goals and to consider discontinuing the medication or switching to an oral antibiotic to minimize discomfort.

Antimicrobial use in EOL populations has been associated with acquisition of resistant organisms[39] and increased length of stay.[15] Nonbeneficial antimicrobial use can also contribute to health care costs at EOL, which are already substantial.[6,40,41] Prescribers, patients, and families may be more or less motivated by the potential adverse effects of antimicrobials that do not directly impact the patient at the EOL, such as the long-term risk of antimicrobial resistance, but taking these factors into consideration are another role of ASP in this population.

APPROACHING DIAGNOSTICS AT THE END OF LIFE

Compounding the challenges of optimizing antimicrobial use at the EOL, infection diagnosis in this population can be particularly challenging. Although patients at EOL are often at high risk of infection, it is often still difficult to distinguish between active infection and colonization with bacterial organisms, particularly when patients may be limited in their ability to verbalize symptoms and symptoms may be nonspecific.[5–7] The difficulties with diagnosis in this population are underscored by prior studies, which have found that patients receiving antimicrobials at EOL frequently do not have a documented infectious diagnosis.[17,23] For example, Clark and colleagues applied an appropriate use criterion to antimicrobials prescribed among a cohort of patients admitted to an outpatient hospice service and found that only 42% of prescriptions met the appropriateness criteria.[27]

Adding to the diagnostic challenges, certain diagnostics may not be available and/ or within the goals of care of the EOL patient and may be impacted by the specific clinical context. For example, in a patient receiving hospice care at home, obtaining a chest radiograph to evaluate for pneumonia may not be feasible or appropriate. However, for a patient with advanced dementia in a skilled nursing facility, it may be a feasible and appropriate minimally invasive diagnostic test to help determine whether a new cough is attributable to an LRTI or to other treatable conditions, such as volume overload from heart failure.

Even when diagnostics are available and within the patient's goals of care, the benefits of accurate diagnosis must be balanced against the potential discomfort and/or anxiety associated with that diagnostic procedure. Even procedures that are perceived as minor (ie, peripheral line insertion) may be associated with patient discomfort.[38] Other procedures such as MRI, may not necessarily cause discomfort, but can provoke anxiety.[42] In addition, any risk posed by invasive diagnostics must also be considered—as an example, pulmonary hemorrhage can occur after 4% to 27% of percutaneous lung biopsies.[43] Diagnostic and treatment decisions at the EOL should also be fluid—if a diagnostic is recommended but the patient's quality of life is worsened by the intervention, it is reasonable to shift goals and expectations to meet the specific goals of the EOL patient as their goals and expectations evolve. ASP should be adaptable in these circumstances and shift their recommendations to align with those of the patient and their caregivers.

ASP can help prescribers by providing guidance on whether additional diagnostics should be pursued. For example, if a prescriber has decided to treat a hospital acquired pneumonia in concert with patient/family wishes, obtaining methicillin-resistant *Staphylococcus aureus* (MRSA) nasal swab may be a helpful tool to de-escalate vancomycin and prevent potential harms associated with continued anti-MRSA therapy.[44,45] In the right clinical scenario, sending a biomarker, such as procalcitonin, may provide reassurance to a prescriber or patient/family that an LRTI has been adequately treated, thus facilitating discontinuation of antimicrobial therapy.[46] In other circumstances, the antimicrobial steward can also provide diagnostic stewardship in discouraging tests that may be unnecessary and lead to harm. Discouraging blood cultures in patients with low pretest probability of having bacteremia, for example, can help avoid false positive results which, in turn, can prevent additional unnecessary antibiotics and longer length of stay.[47] This is of particular importance for patients at EOL who have goals of care that are comfort oriented.

ETHICAL CONSIDERATIONS OF ANTIMICROBIAL PRESCRIBING AT THE END OF LIFE

In the setting of limited evidence to guide antimicrobial decision-making at EOL, as well as the influence of patients and families on antimicrobial decision-making, the ASP may find themselves struggling with several ethical considerations. At EOL, and especially among patients who are in the active dying process, ASP and pre-scribers alike may be concerned that antimicrobials may be prolonging the dying process and accompanying suffering.[48,49] As a theoretic example, in a patient with terminal malignancy, treating an infection may lead to an incremental increase in the duration of life but at the cost of continued suffering from the underlying ma-lignancy.[48] ASP and prescribers should not feel obligated to treat a reversible infec-tious condition that would not have a measurable impact on quantity or quality of life.[48,49]

In addition, focusing on infection management rather than the underlying terminal illness can also delay addressing the underlying disease, which could in turn delay transition to more comfort-oriented care. The focus on a potentially reversible con-dition such as infection may promote the belief that a patient's overall condition is curable.[48] In other cases, clinicians may wish to continue antimicrobials so they are not perceived as "giving up" or to avoid burdening families with additional decisions at EOL.[25,49] Advanced care directives can help both clinicians and ASPs navigate medical decision-making at EOL. A specified preference for limited antimicrobials on a Physician Orders for Life-Sustaining Treatment (POLST) form that was filled out greater than 30 days before death was found to be associated with less inpatient antimicrobial use in the last 30 days of life.[20] However, antimicro-bials are not always addressed in POLST forms,[20] and patient/families may be ill equipped to consider the potential hypothetical benefits and harms of antimicro-bials at EOL.

As discussed in prior sections, ASPs are likely all too aware of the societal implica-tions of unnecessary antimicrobial use such as community antimicrobial resistance and increasing health care costs, but patients and/or their family members, who are focused primarily on the comfort of their loved ones, may understandably not share these concerns.[48] ASP and prescribers may feel uncomfortable with prescribing anti-microbials perceived to be unnecessary or even harmful, particularly in the context of the aforementioned larger societal effects. An unanswered and uncomfortable ques-tion looms large—is the societal cost of short periods of antimicrobials deemed futile or unnecessary in patients at EOL significant enough to more firmly influence the with-drawal of antibiotics?[50]

PUTTING THE PIECES TOGETHER: A FRAMEWORK FOR CONSIDERING THE UNIQUE ASPECTS OF ANTIMICROBIAL STEWARDSHIP AT THE END OF LIFE

Although the ultimate destination of antimicrobial stewardship—right drug, right time, right dose, and right duration[51]—remains the same at EOL as with other circum-stances, the journey to get there may be starkly different, and recommendations and goals may change rapidly depending on the patient's clinical condition, comfort, and experience. The goals of antimicrobial therapy may not be to cure the infection, but rather to palliate symptoms, and antimicrobial decision-making may be more likely to be shared between patient and prescriber. The priorities of different stakeholders may be different—ASPs often focus on long-term, population harms of antimicrobial overuse and antimicrobial resistance, whereas patients, family members, and direct health care providers are more focused on short-term potential positive impacts at the level of the individual patient. Because the focus on the individual patient is so strong at the EOL, stewardship strategies implemented in this population should focus on whether patients are likely to benefit from antimicrobials—either in terms of symptom relief or life extension—and how any potential benefits are weighed against any potential for harm.

ASPs are unlikely to interface with patients and/or family members directly, but they should be aware of the influence they might have on prescribers. Survey and observational clinical data have shown that patient and family preference is an important factor in antimicrobial decision-making at EOL.[8,9,25] However, antimicrobials are not always discussed in goals of care meetings, and some providers may be concerned about overwhelming patients and families with decisions at EOL.[25] Other literature has additionally demonstrated that health care proxies were infrequently aware of infections in nursing home patients with advanced dementia.[52]

The influence of patients and families on antimicrobial decision-making at EOL presents both challenges and opportunities for ASP. ASP should be prepared to take into account the goals and preferences of patients and families when providing guidance. ASP can also help prescribers assess the realistic potential benefits and harms of the desired antimicrobial and provide framing in which to discuss antimicrobials with patients and families and to adjust recommendations based on goals that can change rapidly. This is of paramount importance as not only will patients and families likely overestimate the potential benefit of antimicrobials,[14] but prescribers as well may not be cognizant of the potential risks associated with antimicrobial therapy.[25] Although the exact likelihood of benefits and harms of antimicrobials therapy may be often uncertain, stewardship providers can at least try to offer impartial insight to help prescribers and patients/families with antimicrobial decision-making.

Overall, the heterogenous nature of the EOL population does not lend itself to an algorithmic approach to antimicrobial decision-making. However, the prognosis of the patient can help stratify the general approach of the ASP.[53] We have outlined three different overarching clinical scenarios based on the prognosis and goals of care with a general approach and questions for ASP to consider (**Fig. 2**). However, with such a heterogenous population and innumerable potential specific circumstances, ASP will need to approach each case separately.

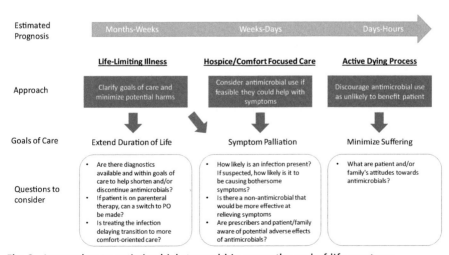

Fig. 2. Approaches to antimicrobial stewardship across the end-of-life spectrum.

SUMMARY

Antimicrobial use is often a part of EOL care and ASP should be prepared to be involved in antimicrobial decision-making in this population. ASP can play a critical role at EOL by supporting clinicians in assessing the potential benefits and harms of antimicrobials for patients at the EOL and also providing a "big picture" view that takes into account the larger societal costs of unnecessary antimicrobial use. Given that patients and families may be more influential in medical decision-making in this population, antimicrobial stewards should also be prepared to guide clinicians in how best to discuss antimicrobial decision-making with patients and families and to adjust recommendations based on clinical contexts that can change quickly. Despite the unfamiliar milieu, the principal goal of antimicrobial stewardship remains the same—right drug, right time, right dose, and right duration.[49] With care taken to use a holistic approach of the factors leading to antimicrobial use, ASP can help to achieve these goals and improve the quality of life for patients at the EOL.

CLINICS CARE POINTS

- Antibiotic use is a common component of end-of-life (EOL) medical care across different care settings and underlying diseases
- The effectiveness of antimicrobials for improving quanity or quality of life in the EOL population is unclear and likely context- and disease-specific
- Providers may be influenced by patients and/or family members when making decisions about antimicrobials during the EOL period

DISCLOSURE

W. Branch-Elliman reports research grants from the VA Health Services Research and Development Service, United States and support from the VA Boston Cooperative Studies Program. W. Branch-Elliman was the site PI for a study funded by Gilead Sciences, United States (funds to institution).

REFERENCES

1. Marra AR, Puig-Asensio M, Balkenende E, et al. Antibiotic use during end-of-life care: A systematic literature review and meta-analysis. Infect Control Hosp Epidemiol 2021;42(5):523–9.
2. Vitetta L, Kenner D, Sali A. Bacterial infections in terminally ill hospice patients. J Pain Symptom Manage 2000;20(5):326–34.
3. Pereira J, Watanabe S, Wolch G. A retrospective review of the frequency of infections and patterns of antibiotic utilization on a palliative care unit. J Pain Symptom Manage 1998;16(6):374–81.
4. Chen JH, Lamberg JL, Chen YC, et al. Occurrence and treatment of suspected pneumonia in long-term care residents dying with advanced dementia. J Am Geriatr Soc 2006;54(2):290–5.
5. Macedo F, Nunes C, Ladeira K, et al. Antimicrobial therapy in palliative care: an overview. Support Care Cancer 2018;26(5):1361–7.
6. Baghban A, Juthani-Mehta M. Antimicrobial Use at the End of Life. Infect Dis Clin North Am 2017;31(4):639–47.

7. Bentley DW, Bradley S, High K, Schoenbaum S, Taler G, Yoshikawa TT, American Geriatrics Society, Gerontological Society of America, Clinical Medicine Section;; Infectious Diseases Society of America;; Society for Healthcare Epidemiology of America. Practice guideline for evaluation of fever and infection in long-term care facilities. Clin Infect Dis 2000 Sep;31(3):640–53.

8. Servid SA, Noble BN, Fromme EK, et al. Clinical Intentions of Antibiotics Prescribed Upon Discharge to Hospice Care. J Am Geriatr Soc 2018;66(3):565–9.

9. Gaw CE, Hamilton KW, Gerber JS, et al. Physician Perceptions Regarding Antimicrobial Use in End-of-Life Care. Infect Control Hosp Epidemiol 2018;39(4): 383–90.

10. Barlam TF, Cosgrove SE, Abbo LM, et al. Implementing an Antibiotic Stewardship Program: Guidelines by the Infectious Diseases Society of America and the Society for Healthcare Epidemiology of America. Clin Infect Dis 2016;62(10): e51–77.

11. Datta R, Topal J, McManus D, et al. Perspectives on antimicrobial use at the end of life among antibiotic stewardship programs: A survey of the Society for Healthcare Epidemiology of America Research Network. Infect Control Hosp Epidemiol 2019;40(9):1074–6.

12. Wu JHC, Langford BJ, Daneman N, et al. Antimicrobial Stewardship Programs in Long-Term Care Settings: A Meta-Analysis and Systematic Review. J Am Geriatr Soc 2019;67(2):392–9.

13. Mitchell SL, D'Agata EMC, Hanson LC, et al. The Trial to Reduce Antimicrobial Use in Nursing Home Residents With Alzheimer Disease and Other Dementias (TRAIN-AD): A Cluster Randomized Clinical Trial. JAMA Intern Med 2021; 181(9):1174–82.

14. Yao CA, Hsieh MY, Chiu TY, et al. Wishes of Patients With Terminal Cancer and Influencing Factors Toward the Use of Antibiotics in Taiwan. Am J Hosp Palliat Care 2015;32(5):537–43.

15. Datta R, Zhu M, Han L, et al. Increased Length of Stay Associated With Antibiotic Use in Older Adults With Advanced Cancer Transitioned to Comfort Measures. Am J Hosp Palliat Care 2020;37(1):27–33.

16. Thompson AJ, Silveira MJ, Vitale CA, et al. Antimicrobial use at the end of life among hospitalized patients with advanced cancer. Am J Hosp Palliat Care 2012;29(8):599–603.

17. Merel SE, Meier CA, McKinney CM, et al. Antimicrobial Use in Patients on a Comfort Care Protocol: A Retrospective Cohort Study. J Palliat Med 2016;19(11): 1210–4.

18. Tagashira Y, Kawahara K, Takamatsu A, et al. Antimicrobial prescribing in patients with advanced-stage illness in the antimicrobial stewardship era. Infect Control Hosp Epidemiol 2018;39(9):1023–9.

19. Taverner J, Ross L, Bartlett C, et al. Antimicrobial prescription in patients dying from chronic obstructive pulmonary disease. Intern Med J 2019;49(1):66–73.

20. Kates OS, Krantz EM, Lee J, et al. Association of Physician Orders for Life-Sustaining Treatment With Inpatient Antimicrobial Use at End of Life in Patients With Cancer. Open Forum Infect Dis 2021;8(8):ofab361.

21. Lantz TL, Noble BN, McPherson ML, et al. Frequency and Characteristics of Patients Prescribed Antibiotics on Admission to Hospice Care. J Palliat Med 2022; 25(4):584–90.

22. Furuno JP, Noble BN, Horne KN, et al. Frequency of outpatient antibiotic prescription on discharge to hospice care. Antimicrob Agents Chemother 2014;58(9): 5473–7.

23. Albrecht JS, McGregor JC, Fromme EK, et al. A nationwide analysis of antibiotic use in hospice care in the final week of life. J Pain Symptom Manage 2013;46(4): 483–90.
24. D'Agata E, Mitchell SL. Patterns of antimicrobial use among nursing home residents with advanced dementia. Arch Intern Med 2008;168(4):357–62.
25. Datta R, Topal J, McManus D, et al. Education needed to improve antimicrobial use during end-of-life care of older adults with advanced cancer: A cross-sectional survey. Palliat Med 2021;35(1):236–41.
26. Rosenberg JH, Albrecht JS, Fromme EK, et al. Antimicrobial use for symptom management in patients receiving hospice and palliative care: a systematic review. J Palliat Med 2013;16(12):1568–74.
27. Clark MD, Halford Z, Herndon C, et al. Evaluation of Antibiotic Initiation Tools in End-of-Life Care. Am J Hosp Palliat Care 2022;39(3):274–81.
28. White PH, Kuhlenschmidt HL, Vancura BG, et al. Antimicrobial use in patients with advanced cancer receiving hospice care. J Pain Symptom Manage 2003;25(5): 438–43.
29. Reinbolt RE, Shenk AM, White PH, et al. Symptomatic treatment of infections in patients with advanced cancer receiving hospice care. J Pain Symptom Manage 2005;30(2):175–82.
30. Clayton J, Fardell B, Hutton-Potts J, et al. Parenteral antibiotics in a palliative care unit: prospective analysis of current practice. Palliat Med 2003;17(1):44–8.
31. Givens JL, Jones RN, Shaffer ML, et al. Survival and comfort after treatment of pneumonia in advanced dementia. Arch Intern Med 2010;170(13):1102–7.
32. Van Der Steen JT, Pasman HRW, Ribbe MW, et al. Discomfort in dementia patients dying from pneumonia and its relief by antibiotics. Scand J Infect Dis 2009;41(2):143–51.
33. Oh DY, Kim JH, Kim DW, et al. Antibiotic use during the last days of life in cancer patients. Eur J Cancer Care (Engl) 2006;15(1):74–9.
34. Chen LK, Chou YC, Hsu PS, et al. Antibiotic prescription for fever episodes in hospice patients. Support Care Cancer 2002;10(7):538–41.
35. Nakagawa S, Toya Y, Okamoto Y, et al. Can anti-infective drugs improve the infection-related symptoms of patients with cancer during the terminal stages of their lives? J Palliat Med 2010;13(5):535–40.
36. Chih AH, Lee LT, Cheng SY, et al. Is it appropriate to withdraw antibiotics in terminal patients with cancer with infection? J Palliat Med 2013 Nov;16(11):1417–22.
37. Helde-Frankling M, Bergqvist J, Bergman P, et al. Antibiotic Treatment in End-of-Life Cancer Patients-A Retrospective Observational Study at a Palliative Care Center in Sweden. Cancers (Basel) 2016;8(9):E84.
38. Morrison RS, Ahronheim JC, Morrison GR, et al. Pain and discomfort associated with common hospital procedures and experiences. J Pain Symptom Manage 1998;15(2):91–101.
39. Levin PD, Simor AE, Moses AE, et al. End-of-life treatment and bacterial antibiotic resistance: a potential association. Chest 2010;138(3):588–94.
40. Khandelwal N, Benkeser D, Coe NB, et al. Patterns of Cost for Patients Dying in the Intensive Care Unit and Implications for Cost Savings of Palliative Care Interventions. J Palliat Med 2016;19(11):1171–8.
41. Angus DC, Barnato AE, Linde-Zwirble WT, et al. Use of intensive care at the end of life in the United States: an epidemiologic study. Crit Care Med 2004;32(3): 638–43.
42. Brennan SC, Redd WH, Jacobsen PB, et al. Anxiety and panic during magnetic resonance scans. Lancet 1988;2(8609):512.

43. Winokur RS, Pua BB, Sullivan BW, et al. Percutaneous lung biopsy: technique, efficacy, and complications. Semin Intervent Radiol 2013;30(2):121–7.

44. Paonessa JR, Shah RD, Pickens CI, et al. Rapid Detection of Methicillin-Resistant Staphylococcus aureus in BAL: A Pilot Randomized Controlled Trial. Chest 2019; 155(5):999–1007.

45. Jones BE, Ying J, Stevens V, et al. Empirical Anti-MRSA vs Standard Antibiotic Therapy and Risk of 30-Day Mortality in Patients Hospitalized for Pneumonia. JAMA Intern Med 2020;180(4):552–60.

46. Schuetz P, Wirz Y, Sager R, et al. Procalcitonin to initiate or discontinue antibiotics in acute respiratory tract infections. Cochrane Database Syst Rev 2017;10: CD007498.

47. Fabre V, Klein E, Salinas AB, et al. A Diagnostic Stewardship Intervention To Improve Blood Culture Use among Adult Nonneutropenic Inpatients: the DISTRIBUTE Study. J Clin Microbiol 2020;58(10):e01053–120.

48. Ford PJ, Fraser TG, Davis MP, et al. Anti-infective therapy at the end of life: ethical decision-making in hospice-eligible patients. Bioethics 2005;19(4):379–92.

49. Vaughan L, Duckett AA, Adler M, et al. Ethical and Clinical Considerations in Treating Infections at the End of Life. J Hosp Palliat Nurs 2019;21(2):110–5.

50. Broom J, Broom A, Good P, et al. Why is optimisation of antimicrobial use difficult at the end of life? Intern Med J 2019;49(?):269–71.

51. Dryden M, Johnson AP, Ashiru-Oredope D, et al. Using antibiotics responsibly: right drug, right time, right dose, right duration. J Antimicrob Chemother 2011; 66(11):2441–3.

52. Givens JL, Spinella S, Ankuda CK, et al. Healthcare Proxy Awareness of Suspected Infections in Nursing Home Residents with Advanced Dementia. J Am Geriatr Soc 2015;63(6):1084–90.

53. Sinert M, Stammet Schmidt MM, Lovell AG, et al. Guidance for Safe and Appropriate Use of Antibiotics in Hospice Using a Collaborative Decision Support Tool. J Hosp Palliat Nurs 2020;22(4):276–82.

Update in Human Immunodeficiency Virus and Aging

Jason R. Faulhaber, MD[a],*, Anthony W. Baffoe-Bonnie, MD[a],
Krisann K. Oursler, MD[b], Shikha S. Vasudeva, MD[b]

KEYWORDS

- HIV • Aging • Antiretroviral therapy

KEY POINTS

- With earlier initiation of effective antiretroviral therapy (ART), more people with human immunodeficiency virus (HIV) (PWH) survive longer and face similar age-related comorbidities and risks as their peers without HIV.
- The aging process in PWH is complex and affected by several factors, leading to increased risk for certain age-related comorbidities.
- Heightened awareness and surveillance of long-term consequences of ART, polypharmacy, and cancers are required for providing care to aging PWH.
- A multidisciplinary team approach could prove beneficial in identifying the challenges encountered in PWH and subsequently strategizing targeted management plans for them.

INTRODUCTION

Over the last 40 years, the journey of people with human immunodefiency virus (HIV) (PWH) has moved a long way from a near-certain mortality resulting from destruction of the immune system and its devastating consequences, to a much longer life span and the challenges of old age and consequent comorbidities. The clinical presentation of HIV infection before the advent of highly effective combination antiretroviral therapy (ART) was driven by the impact on the immune system, including increased risk of specific cancers associated with viral coinfections. Opportunistic infections and rare cancers were responsible for most of the deaths in PWH. Age-related diseases such as shingles and tuberculosis in younger individuals occurred because of impaired immune function. As ART evolves to be more efficacious, PWH are living longer, thus widening the age spectrum. Age-related comorbidity and geriatric syndromes

[a] Virginia Tech Carilion School of Medicine, Carilion Clinic, Division of Infectious Diseases, 213 McClanahan St SW, Roanoke, VA 24014, USA; [b] Virginia Tech Carilion School of Medicine, VA Salem Healthcare System, 1970 Roanoke Boulevard Salem, VA 24153-6404, USA
* Corresponding author.
E-mail address: jrfaulhaber@carilionclinic.org

Infect Dis Clin N Am 37 (2023) 153–173
https://doi.org/10.1016/j.idc.2022.11.006
0891-5520/23/© 2022 Published by Elsevier Inc.

id.theclinics.com

constitute the primary clinical challenges of PWH receiving ART today. However, the problem is more than just a shift in age demographics. Aging is a progressive, inevitable loss of physiologic reserves that is gauged by disease and impaired function and affected by both genetic and environmental factors. The body of literature points toward an accelerated aging process in PWH, even with fully suppressed viral loads, compared with matched uninfected peers. The objective of this review is to discuss the various changes in PWH as they age, review potential long-term effects of ART and their impact on comorbidities, and develop clinical approaches to managing aging PWH and those who acquire HIV later in life.

EPIDEMIOLOGY

The Joint United Nations Programme on HIV/AIDS (UNAIDS) estimates that globally there are 8.1 million people aged 50 years and older living with HIV accounting for one-fifth of persons living with HIV in 2020.[1] Worldwide, the number of people aged 50 years and older living with HIV is increasing, especially in high-income countries such as the United States, where more than half of the people with HIV in 2018 were aged 50 years and older.[2] From 2014 through 2018 the United States saw a large percentage increase (51%) in the rate of persons with diagnosed HIV infection (per 100,000 population) among persons aged 65 years and older (from 130.0 in 2014 to 196.6 in 2018).[3] This new finding is thought to be primarily due to improved survival with the advent of highly active ART and the continued new acquisition of HIV in older age groups.[4,5] The death rate of PWH has uniformly decreased across race, gender, and ethnicity and decreased by nearly half from 2010 to 2017, leading to "graying" of the HIV epidemic.[6]

BIOLOGICAL AGING IN PEOPLE WITH HUMAN IMMUNODEFICIENCY VIRUS

The physiology of aging in PWH is complex and extends beyond simple biological aging processes. Our current understanding remains limited due to the scarcity of longitudinal cohort studies and relatively narrow observational outcomes and limited serial tissue sampling. Cross-sectional research based on individuals who represent different age groups may not necessarily characterize the effect of aging, a process that occurs over time.[7] Although these challenges in gerontology are not unique to PWH, the complex interactions across HIV infection, ART, and environmental/lifestyle factors complicate clinical research and make conclusions on causal factors challenging at best.

Several excellent recent reviews discuss various mechanisms of biological aging in PWH, including diverse cellular processes and organ functions.[8,9] Because the latter is discussed in detail later, the focus here is cellular pathophysiology of aging with HIV. Geroscience is an approach to the biology of aging with the central theme that distinct biological mechanisms (termed "hallmarks" or "pillars") combine to create global susceptibility to diseases and loss of physiologic reserve.[10] The geroscience approach to HIV is a subtle but important shift to viewing aging as a process of increasing multimorbid risk due to loss in homeostatic control of hallmarks. Montano and colleagues[11] recently provided a comprehensive review of HIV and biological aging in the context of geroscience and several key hallmarks, including DNA instability, mitochondrial dysfunction, cellular senescence, and inflammation.

DNA instability broadly encompasses genomic modifications (eg, point mutations, insertions/deletions), epigenetic changes (DNA methylation), telomere shortening, and certain mitochondrial functions. Research has shifted from the putative effects of early nucleoside reverse transcriptase inhibitors (NRTIs) on DNA damage response to DNA methylation captured by epigenetic clocks, which provide a direct estimate of age acceleration in PWH.[12] Further work is needed to differentiate the effects of ART and HIV infection on DNA methylation as well as the predictive value for clinical outcomes beyond HIV-associated neurocognitive disorder (HAND) and all-cause mortality.[13] Alternatively, shorter telomere length in PWH seems to be independent of ART.[14] Whether these changes are amplified in PWH compared with age-matched controls with similar risk factors remains an important question.

Mitochondrial dysfunction, a well-established hallmark of aging in diverse patient populations, is multifactorial, due to accumulation of mutations in mitochondrial DNA (mtDNA), mitophagy, and reduced oxidative function. Early in the HIV epidemic, mitochondrial dysfunction garnered attention due to toxicity of initial ART and decreased oxidative phosphorylation from mutations in skeletal muscle mtDNA.[15] Contemporary NRTIs (eg, abacavir and tenofovir) may still adversely affect mitochondrial function.[16] Mitochondrial DNA haplogroup in PWH independently predicted accelerated decline in gait speed, a driver of age-related disability.[17] Tissue biopsy of the quadricep muscle in older PWH demonstrated reduced oxidative function compared with age-/race-/sex-matched controls without HIV that correlated with cardiorespiratory fitness.[18] Thus, mitochondrial dysfunction is a hallmark in aging and HIV that drives determinants of the healthspan, healthy aging with minimal disease and disability.

Cellular senescence has been linked to age-related comorbidities in PWH and affects several key hallmarks, such as mitochondrial dysfunction, stem cell exhaustion, and inflammation. Given this potential broad impact, improvement in cellular senescence with drug therapy is a possible avenue to improve healthspan in PWH.[19] The extracellular modulators that characterize the senescence-associated secretory phenotype[20] supports chronic systemic inflammation in PWH as a primary hallmark of accelerated aging.

"Inflammaging" refers to the complex interplay between immune dysregulation, cytokine upregulation, drug toxicities, comorbidities, chronic infections, substance use, and low-grade inflammation.[21] Although inflammaging is not unique to HIV-associated aging, in vitro studies of individual mechanisms supported the original concept of accelerated aging versus accentuated aging in PWH.[22] However, at the population level, differences between HIV infection and aging are introduced by several factors: (1) variability in the latency period, potency, and toxicity of ART; (2) coinfections; and (3) increased substance abuse and smoking.[23,24] Given the recent paradigm shift in treatment, which involves earlier initiation of more potent and less toxic ART, the role of inflammaging in aging with chronic HIV infection may change. Some early studies already point toward a decreased impact of inflammation on systemic manifestations.[25–27]

Several pathways of inflammaging play a central role in PWH, such as the gut microbiota.[28] During acute HIV infection there is disruption of gut mucosa by rapidly replicating virus causing the destruction of gut-associated lymphatic tissue, decreases in CD_4 cells, increase in epithelial barrier permeability and epithelial apoptosis. There is also a shift in gut microbiota toward bacterial compositional taxa that are proinflammogenic.[26,29,30] This dysbiosis affects biochemical pathways (eg, activation of kynurenine/indoleamine 2,3-dioxygenase, changes in tryptophan pathways) that lead to proinflammatory cytokine production further breaching the gut mucosa.[31] Elevated levels of gut injury markers such as lipopolysaccharide-binding protein, zonulin, soluble CD14 (sCD14), and citrulline support this hypothesis in PWH.[31]

Products of microbial translocation, such as lipopolysaccharide (LPS), activate monocytes and macrophages that possess pattern recognition receptors, initiating a metabolic cascade to produce proinflammatory molecules. Surface proteins CD14 and CD163, markers of activated monocytes, are elevated in virally suppressed PWH.[32] Other metabolic processes are reprogrammed to produce a proglycolytic proinflammatory state that persists despite viral suppression and dampens the T-cell response. A perpetual cycle of gut mucosal damage with leaching of microbial products and LPS into circulation and activation of inflammatory pathways leading to further gut breach becomes established. This dysbiosis is restored partially with ART; but gut inflammation marker myeloperoxidase and Th17 cells did not change post-ART, providing evidence of ongoing inflammation.[26] Newer evidence suggests natural killer (NK) cells might have a protective role.[33] The gut proinflammatory cytokines access the liver through the portal vein, leading to liver dysfunction by activating Kupffer cells and hepatic stellate cells (HSC).[34] The proinflammatory and profibrogenic cytokines thence released by these cells alter coagulation synthetic function, leading to an imbalance between anticoagulants and procoagulants in favor of the latter. This state of persistent low-level coagulopathy and altered chemokine receptor expression recruits more monocytes to atherosclerotic plaques and promotes lipid oxidation by oxidative stress pathways in all organ systems but especially in the vascular system (Fig. 1).[35] C-X-C motif chemokine ligand 10, sCD163, neopterin, and other biomarkers of monocyte activation are increased in PWH and were only partially ameliorated by viral suppression.[36] NK cell function is disrupted by the depletion of T cells, thereby affecting fibrosis by killing activated HSCs and thus creating a profibrotic state.[34] Coinfection with hepatitis B virus (HBV) and/or hepatitis C virus (HCV) enhances the profibrotic effects.

Elevated plasma biomarkers of systemic inflammation, D-dimer, high-sensitivity C-reactive protein, and interleukin-6, in PWH are associated with increased cardiovascular events and link inflammation and coagulopathy in the genesis of atherosclerotic disease. Monocytes migrate into the intima and accumulate lipid droplets to form foam cells, leading to the initiation of atherosclerotic plaques that can progress and

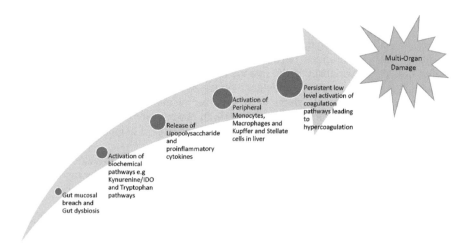

Fig. 1. Pathway of chronic inflammation in PWH. The figure provides an overview of downstream effects of dysbiosis on systemic inflammation and end organ damage. Products of microbial translocation such as lipopolysaccharide (LPS) initiate a metabolic cascade to produce proinflammatory molecules; this causes activation of monocytes and macrophages, which in turn leads to release of more proinflammatory and profibrogenic cytokines, causing activation of coagulation pathways that contribute to end organ damage.

subsequently rupture.[32] A summary of these factors in accelerated aging is provided in **Fig. 2.**

LONG-TERM EFFECTS OF ANTIRETROVIRAL THERAPY

Although ART has prolonged the lives of PWH, there are notable negative effects. Short-term and long-term effects have been identified with all available antiretrovirals (**Box 1** and **Table 1**). Earlier generation ART has been associated with more severe long-term effects, including mitochondrial toxicity, peripheral neuropathy, and changes in fat distribution. Long-term use of ART has been linked to an increased risk of chronic kidney disease (CKD) and diabetes mellitus (DM).[37–40] With effective ART, PWH are using antiretroviral medications over a much longer period of time. The potential cumulative toxicity from prolonged ART exposure is not fully understood yet. Polypharmacy (discussed later) may also factor in with toxicities and drug-drug interactions. Long-term toxicities may lead to an overall poor health status and a diminished quality of life. Reducing the number of ARVs taken (eg, 2-drug regimen vs 3-drug regimen) might reduce the potential cumulative toxicities without sacrificing control of viral suppression.[41]

The high prevalence of age-related comorbid conditions in PWH[42,43] contributes to a greater pill burden that may result in other complications.[44,45] Common comorbidities in older PWH include cardiovascular disease (CVD), liver disease, renal and metabolic disorders, central nervous system disorders, and osteoporosis with consequent risk of fracture[41] (**Box 2**).

EFFECTS OF HUMAN IMMUNODEFICIENCY VIRUS AND ANTIRETROVIRAL THERAPY BASED ON ORGAN SYSTEM
Central Nervous System

The study of cognitive impairment in PWH continues to evolve. Study methods and choice of neurocognitive measurement methods and outcomes are varied, thus

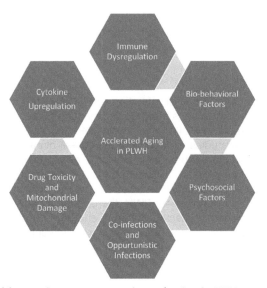

Fig. 2. Interplay of factors that promote accelerated aging in PWH.

Box 1
Potential long-term effects of antiretroviral therapy

Potential Long-term ART Effects
  Weight gain
  Dyslipidemia
  Bone mineral density loss
  Kidney impairment
  Insulin resistance/Diabetes
  Depression

---

affecting the ability to analyze the data in a systematic fashion. The Frascati criteria for describing the stages of HAND has more recently been widely adopted, allowing for a better systematic review of the literature in this field. The stages include asymptomatic neurocognitive impairment, mild neurocognitive disorder, and HIV-associated dementia (HAD).[46]

In virologically suppressed individuals, HAD is rare.[47] Although effective at suppressing viral replication, ART may not offer complete protection against neurocognitive impairment.[47] Consistent with other studies, the CNS Antiretroviral Therapy Effects Research (CHARTER) study[48] identified a higher decline in the milder forms of cognition in a cohort of older persons living with HIV and on ART for a mean duration of 15 years when compared with individuals of the same age without HIV. Decline was associated with the presence of certain comorbid conditions in the HIV group: chronic lung disease, diabetes, and hypertension (HTN). Speed of processing, working memory, motor function, and verbal fluency seemed to be the affected cognitive domains.[49]

This decline is postulated to be due to host factors such as persistent inflammation that occurs in PWH, which further increases their risk for age-related comorbidities such as vascular disease and diabetes. Other studies have identified a possible direct effect of HIV on the central nervous sytem being associated with poorer global cognitive performance.[50] Overall, the risk of dementia among PWH aged older than 50 years, although decreasing, remains elevated when compared with non-HIV–infected persons with similar age and comorbidities.[51] In virologically suppressed PWH, strategies to prevent or optimally manage chronic comorbidities will likely have salutary effects on neurocognition.

Cardiovascular System

Excessive risk of acute myocardial infarction (AMI), heart failure, pulmonary HTN, ischemic stroke, and deep venous thrombosis has been observed in PWH.[52] Earlier studies indicated a greater risk of AMI in HIV-infected individuals compared with uninfected; however, later studies, notably after the advent of early ART initiation, have shown a closing of the gap, approaching similar rates of those uninfected.[25,36] In a study of virologically suppressed PWH with a low Framingham risk score, a higher prevalence of carotid atherosclerosis was found compared with uninfected individuals with similar score.[52] In suppressed PWH there is an increased plaque burden compared with a matched uninfected cohort. Computed tomography angiography also demonstrates a plaque morphology that is more vulnerable to rupture.[53] The reasons for elevated risks might be multifold, including both HIV-related inflammation and increased prevalence of traditional risk factors.

Traditional risk factors of HTN, dyslipidemia, and obesity are compounded by the increased prevalence of substance abuse and smoking, fat distribution, metabolic

Table 1
Common adverse effects of antiretroviral therapy by class

NRTIs	NNRTIs	PIs	INSTIs	Entry Inhibitors
Peripheral neuropathy	Hepatotoxicity	Hyperlipidemia	Headache	Nausea
Lactic acidosis	Rash	Insulin resistance	Weight gain	Site reactions (with injectables)
Hepatic steatosis	QTc prolongation	Lipodystrophy	Insomnia	Increased risk of infections
Pancreatitis	Neuropsychiatric	Elevated liver enzymes	Elevated CK	Elevated liver enzymes
Lipoatrophy		Nephrolithiasis	—	—

Abbreviations: CK, creatine kinase; INSTIs, integrase strand transfer inhibitors; NNRTIs, nonnuclecside reverse transcriptase inhibitors; NRTIs, nucleoside reverse transcriptase inhibitors; PIs, protease inhibitors; QTc, corrected Q-T interval.

Box 2
Common comorbidities in older people with human immunodeficiency virus

Common Comorbidities

Mental health:

Bipolar, depression

Metabolic:

DM, dyslipidemia

Heart disease

Hepatitis B and/or C

Hypertension

Osteoporosis

Substance use:

Alcohol, tobacco, illicit

Cancer

Sexually transmitted infections

Frailty

Macular degeneration

Hearing loss

Arthritis

Abbreviation: DM, diabetes mellitus.

---

syndrome, insulin resistance, and renal insufficiency from ART or HIV nephropathy, leading to elevated CVD risk. Traditional risk calculators consistently underestimate CVD risk in HIV. There is no validated risk calculator for CVD for PWH. Predictor models that include CD_4 counts, ART use, protease inhibitor use, viremia, and clinical signs of lipodystrophy still fail to give an accurate assessment of CVD risk.[54,55] In one study coronary artery calcification score greater than 100 was associated with higher incidence of MI,[56] but a recent metanalysis showed that PWH have higher prevalence of noncalcified coronary plaques but similar prevalence of coronary artery calcium compared with HIV-negative individuals.[57] In 2019, the American Heart Association did not recommend specific imaging for enhancing cardiovascular care in PWH but more aggressive risk modifications was recommended.[58] The Randomized Trial to Prevent Vascular Events in HIV (REPRIEVE) is evaluating primary prevention of CVD in low-to-moderate risk PWH.[59]

Respiratory System

Chronic obstructive pulmonary disease (COPD) is the most common noninfectious pulmonary disease in PWH since the advent of ART.[60] Overall, PWH are more likely to have pulmonary diseases compared with individuals who do not have HIV, even when other factors (eg, age, sex, race, alcohol, or drug use) are taken into account. HIV is an independent risk factor for emphysema, even in the absence of injection drug use, smoking, age, race, or alcohol abuse.[61] Emphysema may result from a direct infection of alveolar macrophages with HIV and upregulation of matrix metalloproteases in adjacent macrophages that are not infected.[62] There are synergistic effects between HIV and smoking on the development of emphysematous changes. At baseline, the incidence of emphysematous changes in nonsmoking PWH is 15%; with smoking, the incidence increases to 37%.[63]

Fischer and colleagues[64] describe a "pathogenic triad" of COPD: persistent inflammation, oxidative stress, and protease-antiprotease imbalance. Although ART restores immune function, the immune system does not return to normal preinfection levels and chronic immune activation persists. This low-grade immune activation is also present in lung immune cells (lymphocytes, alveolar macrophages, and neutrophils), leading to airway inflammation and tissue remodeling.[65,66] Among PWH, early and rapid decline in lung function is common and cannot be explained by smoking and other traditional risk factors alone, thus implicating ART and/or HIV.[60,61,67–72] Smoking, however, continues to be the major risk factor for disease severity and progression in PWH. Smoking cessation is therefore a critical component of COPD management and prevention in the general population, PWH, and those who are not living with HIV.[67]

Gastrointestinal System

HIV can affect the liver in several ways. It directly causes liver damage and can lead to fibrosis. Opportunistic infections, alcohol abuse, nonalcoholic fatty liver disease (NAFLD), ART, and coinfection with hepatitis viruses all contribute to liver damage. In a retrospective study out of China, mortality was 42%, 65%, and 123% higher in those coinfected with HBV, HCV, and both, respectively.[73] Liver cirrhosis, liver failure, and hepatocellular carcinoma (HCC) have accounted for 20% to 25% mortality in HCV-HIV coinfection.[74,75] In a study by Berenguer, HCV cure led to reduction in the frequency of death, HIV progression, and liver-related events and possibly even a decreased incidence of DM and chronic renal failure.[73] HBV infection negatively affects HIV outcomes. Chung and colleagues[76] found a higher rate of AIDS or death despite having drugs active against HBV as part of their ART regimen. In one study, the prevalence of NAFLD, nonalcoholic steatohepatitis, and fibrosis in HIV monoinfection was 35%, 42%, and 22%, respectively,[77] with NAFLD being the single most common cause of cirrhosis in PWH. Evaluation and treatment of metabolic processes should be undertaken in all patients with NAFLD as well as promotion of lifestyle modification and pharmacotherapy initiation as needed.

Earlier ARVs were often associated with transaminitis; however, there is conflicting evidence regarding the effects of newer ARVs.[78] Even with older ARVs the hepatotoxicity was often limited to transaminitis. Liver toxicity is limited with current standard of care ART.[79]

The Kidneys

Kidney disease is the fourth most common cause of non-AIDS–related mortality in PWH (after oncologic, cardiac, and liver disorders, respectively).[80,81] HIV infection can result in diverse renal pathology including, but not limited to, HIV-associated nephropathy (HIVAN), HIV-associated immune complex kidney disease, and thrombotic microangiopathy–related renal disease.[82] HIV actively replicates in kidney cells, and even low levels of viremia have been associated with impaired renal function.[83] HIVAN, once a common condition, has been primarily seen in PWH of African descent, partly related to the genetic susceptibility of the apolipoprotein L1 gene.[84] Although the incidence of HIVAN has decreased in the era of effective ART, the number of PWH with comorbidities associated with kidney disease (eg, HTN, DM) has increased namely due to the prolonged longevity resulting from effective ART.[85,86]

The prevalence of CKD in PWH varies in different populations. A study of military veterans living with HIV identified 0.2% had CKD at baseline, with 1.7% later developing end-stage renal disease.[87] A cohort from the Women's Interagency HIV Study found about one-third of the women had proteinuria at baseline.[88] A cross-sectional study in the Multicenter AIDS Cohort Study (MACS) determined 5% to 7% of men living with HIV had CKD.[89] There are myriad risk factors implicated in the development of CKD in PWH. Traditional risk factors include DM and HTN. Risk factors related to HIV include low CD_4 lymphocyte count, elevated plasma HIV level, certain ARVs as well as other drugs (eg, trimethoprim-sulfamethoxazole), and coinfection with HCV. A cross-sectional retrospective case-control study found that PWH had a higher prevalence of both renal failure and DM compared with HIV-uninfected controls, especially among those aged older than 60 years.[90]

Musculoskeletal System

The 2 primary age-related disorders of the musculoskeletal system that affect the healthspan of PWH are low bone mineral density (BMD) and age-related loss of skeletal muscle and strength (sarcopenia). The link between skeletal muscle and bone, a basic gerontologic tenet, is established in middle-aged PWH[91] and has important implications for the essential role of strength training for healthy aging with HIV.[92] Osteopenia and osteoporosis, the clinical diagnoses of low BMD, are more prevalent in PWH and translate to increased risk of frailty fractures.[93] A large cross-sectional study found that the prevalence of fractures in a single health care system was higher in PWH compared with HIV-uninfected patients among men and women, and the differences widened as age increased.[94] Low BMD in aging PWH is complicated by long-term toxicity of ARVs, notably tenofovir disoproxil fumarate, that independently predicted fractures in a longitudinal study.[95] Because the putative effects of HIV infection and ART toxicity are complex and may vary, a screening dual-energy x-ray absorptiometry (DXA) scan is recommended for men aged 50 years or older and postmenopausal women regardless of ART and HIV disease status.[96] Clinical assessment for sarcopenia is more difficult to quantify, as clinically performed DXA scans do not include body composition, presenting therefore in a more advanced stage as frailty syndrome.[97]

AGE-RELATED SYSTEMIC CONDITIONS
Geriatric Syndromes

Multisystem dysfunction in older individuals, compounded frequently by decreased physical function, are portrayed by geriatric syndromes. Among these, frailty has been widely studied in PWH as both a frailty phenotype and frailty index. Using the Fried phenotype, the AIDS Linked to the IntraVenous Experience (ALIVE) cohort demonstrated that increased comorbidity and viral load are strongly associated with both increased frailty progression and reduced frailty recovery.[98] Results confirmed that frailty is associated with increased mortality in PWH but also emphasized the dynamic nature of a frail state over time, raising the question of effective interventions. Interventions for frailty in the general population focus on improving components of the frailty phenotype (eg slow gait, weakness, weight loss) through increased exercise or physical activity and improved diet.[99] Falls and bone fractures are geriatric syndromes related to frailty.[100] The Veterans Aging Cohort Study (VACS) Index is a measure of physiologic frailty that predicts falls and bone fractures in PWH.[101] Sarcopenia is a common element in each of these geriatric syndromes, underscoring the urgent need in PWH for effective strategies to increase muscle mass and strength and improve function.[92]

Age-Related Cancers

Although there has been a significant decrease in cancer incidence in PWH since the advent of ART,[102] PWH still have a higher risk for cancer than the general population.[103] One in six deaths among PWH in the United States from 2011 to 2015 was due to cancer, exceeding cancer-related deaths in the general population.[104] AIDS-related cancers such as non-Hodgkin lymphoma, Kaposi sarcoma, and cervical cancer have seen a decline, whereas there has been an increase in anal, liver, and lung cancers, which are non-AIDS defining and more likely associated with ongoing inflammation.[105,106] The high rate of lung cancer in PWH is thought to be due to chronic inflammation and the higher prevalence of tobacco use in PWH.[107] Strategies aimed at early identification of the patient who smokes, along with interventions to improve smoking cessation and adherence to annual lung cancer screening protocols for the general population, are recommended to address the high rate of lung cancer in PWH.[108,109]

People with HIV also have a markedly increased risk of anal cancer than the general population.[110] The highest incidence is in men who have sex with men. There is a strong causal relationship of anal cancers and the human papilloma virus (HPV), particularly types 16 and 18. Anal intercourse and a high number of sexual partners increase the risk of HPV acquisition. Vaccination for HPV, use of condoms, and early identification of precancerous lesions via annual anal cytology with follow-up high-resolution anoscopy and biopsy of suspicious lesions has been suggested as a good strategy to reduce the incidence of anal cancer in PWH.[111,112]

Liver cancer is the fourth most common non-AIDS–related cancer in the United States,[104] with a 4-fold increased risk of HCC compared with the general population, and the second highest cause of non-AIDS–related cancer deaths in PWH between 1995 and 2009, accounting for 0.9% of deaths.[113] Patients with cirrhosis due to chronic hepatitis C, alcohol-associated liver disease (AALD), NAFLD, and hepatitis B are more likely to develop HCC when coinfected with HIV. Treatment of viral hepatitis has been shown to decrease the risk of progression to HCC,[114] whereas abstaining from continued alcohol use and optimal management of obesity and dyslipidemia have beneficial effects for both AALD and NAFLD.[115] In patients with cirrhosis, HCC monitoring every 6 months is recommended.

In general, all persons with HIV should receive their age-appropriate cancer screening during routine visits, with a focus on identifying risk factors for cancers that are being increasingly observed as the population matures.

PRIMARY CARE OF OLDER ADULTS WITH HUMAN IMMUNODEFICIENCY VIRUS

Primary care for an adult living with HIV is complex and challenges clinicians, whether they are traditional primary care providers (Internists and Family Medicine) or infectious diseases (ID) specialists. Frequently ID clinicians assume the duties of primary care, long-term prevention, and treatment of disease, given the potential for multiple coinfections, atypical disease manifestation, and both toxicity and drug interactions of ARVs.[116] Our discussion of the multiorgan effects of aging in PWH highlights the importance of incorporating principles of geriatrics into the HIV chronic care model to maintain and improve patients' quality of life despite the presence of multimorbidity and polypharmacy.[117,118] Fortunately, the need for multidisciplinary care is becoming increasingly recognized. Recently updated primary care guidelines from The Infectious Diseases Society of America (IDSA) recommends routine screening for age-related comorbidities and providing appropriate vaccinations.[119] Recommendations from the US Preventive Services Task Force (USPSTF) for malignancy screening should be followed.[120–122] With age-related diseases as the leading cause of death in PWH on ART, all the usual principles of evidence-based primary and secondary prevention apply. In addition, monitoring for HAND and mental health screening should be conducted routinely.

Several geriatric syndromes are more prevalent in PWH and warrant consideration as part of routine clinical care. Polypharmacy, defined as the concurrent use of at least 5 medications, has a prevalence of about 14% in PWH.[42] Many studies have established increasing adverse event rates with increasing pill burden including organ system injury, hospitalization, decreased medication adherence, decreased cognition, and mortality.[123,124] The mean number of events per patient increased by 10% for each additional medication in one study[125] and another identified a 5% increased risk in falls for each additional medication added[126]; this underscores the importance of frequent medication reconciliation and the involvement of a pharmacist as part of the multidisciplinary team. Other geriatric syndromes require screening or testing procedures that are not commonplace in HIV clinics. The DXA is a standard screening test for certain high-risk geriatric patient groups that is more widely recommended in PWH.[96,118,119] The clinic-based geriatric assessment in PWH is a subject of ongoing research that is complicated by potential different thresholds for screening tests to identify high-risk individuals as well as variability in clinical resources. There is no one-size-fits-all approach, and various models with outpatient referral to a geriatrician, a multidisciplinary team embedded in the HIV clinic, geriatric trained ID provider, and online support have been used in providing enhanced care based on available resources logistics and feasibility.[127] The domains of geriatric assessments of special interest for PWH are functioning (physical and cognitive), frailty (including sarcopenia), nutritional status, social network (including disclosure of HIV), safe housing (including fall risk), and polypharmacy. Although the need for HIV specific guidelines and geriatric tools is debated, a systematic approach to identifying, prioritizing, and coordinating care is needed.

Based on our experience in HIV clinics in the university and VA health care settings, we have summarized our approach to care of older PWH in **Fig. 3**. Specific social, biobehavioral, and mental health issues for older PWH lead to health care barriers, disengagement with care, and poor adherence.[119] Although these important topics are beyond the scope of this review, we acknowledge the importance of providing a stigma-free, respectful, caring environment that leads to a long-term trusting relationship with the primary provider of PWH.

The general approach to HIV care is essentially the same, regardless of age. However, there are additional considerations for older individuals who are newly diagnosed. Although it is recommended that all PWH should be on ART, with few exceptions, initiating ART as soon as possible in older adults becomes more important, given immune senescence and impaired recovery with age. Selecting an appropriate antiretroviral regimen may be affected by comorbid conditions (eg, dyslipidemia, DM, CVD) and polypharmacy and drug-drug interactions.

SUMMARY

The landscape of HIV infection has changed dramatically over the past 40 years, resulting in people living longer with HIV. The focus has shifted from preventing death due to the lethality of the infection to prevention and management of age-related conditions, including comorbidities and geriatric syndromes such as frailty fractures and polypharmacy. We have gained significant insight into pathophysiological processes leading to accelerated biological aging, which is being translated into a heightened

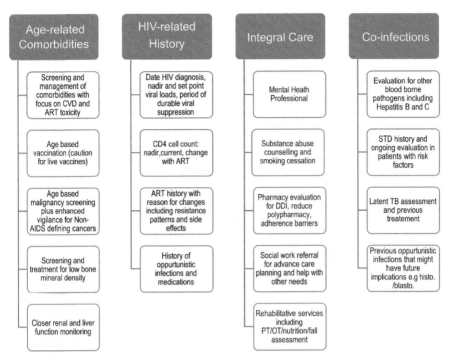

Fig. 3. Primary care of PWH.

awareness of clinical syndromes in PWH that are more prevalent than their uninfected peers. The need for a multidisciplinary approach is even more evident for this patient population group than the general geriatric population, given the complexities of their past medical histories, concurrent infections, polypharmacy, socioenvironmental factors, and accelerated biological aging. This need is being recognized and multiple models for care of PWH are being developed. However, the increasing number of older PWH is outpacing the advances in research and clinical care. The role of inflammation has been expanded to the construct of inflammaging, but a more systematic approach that targets the key drivers of aging in PWH needs to be developed. Longitudinal studies that include older PWH are investigating acceleration of aging but differentiating effects of ART remains a challenge, especially as older individuals may have had longer exposure to early generation ARVs. Best practices based specifically on studies in PWH need to be developed. On the clinical level, more resources are needed to provide a multidisciplinary approach to a very complex group of aging people whose sociopsychological and biobehavioral needs may be more prominent than their uninfected peers. And lastly, patient-driven clinical priorities may vary more in older PWH compared with other disease-specific patient populations, given our experience with the HIV Care Continuum.[128] There is a great need for studies that consider locally relevant factors while designing aging studies. Translation of these studies into meaningful goals to increase both lifespan and health span of PWH will need carefully balanced priorities with local policies and solutions.

CLINICS CARE POINTS

- Despite effective antiretroviral therapy, people with human immunodeficiency virus (HIV) (PWH) have greater risk of age-related comorbidities compared to people without HIV.

- Traditional risk calculators for cardiovascular disease (CVD) underestimate the risk of CVD in PWH and more aggressive prevention and treatment strategies are needed.
- Prolonged exposure to antiretrovirals may be associated with toxicities and cellular damage that impact organ system function contributing to the development of certain disease states, such as diabetes mellitus and chronic kidney disease.
- Increasing physician awareness and risk mitigation with age-appropriate cancer screening is needed to decrease mortality from non-AIDS-related malignancies.
- A multidisciplinary approach, including management of polypharmacy and multimorbidity, would improve the care of PWH.

DISCLOSURE

The authors have nothing to disclose.

REFERENCES

1. The lancet healthy longevity. Ageing with HIV. Lancet Heal Longev 2022;3(3): e119.
2. National Institutes of Health. HIV and older people. Available at: https://hivinfo.nih.gov/understanding-hiv/fact-sheets/hiv-and-older-people. Accessed August 21, 2022.
3. Centers for Disease Control and Prevention. HIV surveillance report. 2018. Available at: http://www.cdc.gov/hiv/library/reports/hiv-surveillance.html. Accessed August 21, 2022.
4. Vance D, McGuiness T, Musgrove K, et al. Successful aging and the epidemiology of HIV. Clin Interv Aging 2011;181. https://doi.org/10.2147/CIA.S14726.
5. Centers for Disease Control and Prevention. National profile. Available at: https://www.cdc.gov/hiv/library/reports/hiv-surveillance/vol-33/content/national-profile.html. Accessed August 20, 2022.
6. Bosh KA, Johnson AS, Hernandez AL, et al. Vital signs: deaths among persons with diagnosed HIV Infection, United States, 2010–2018. MMWR Morb Mortal Wkly Rep 2020. https://doi.org/10.15585/mmwr.mm6946a1.
7. Oursler KK, Sorkin JD. HIV and aging. Int J Infect Dis 2016;53:59–60.
8. Gabuzda D, Jamieson BD, Collman RG, et al. Pathogenesis of aging and age-related comorbidities in people with HIV: highlights from the HIV ACTION Workshop. Pathog Immun 2020;5(1):143–74.
9. Montano M, Bhasin S, D'Aquila RT, et al. Harvard HIV and aging workshop: perspectives and priorities from claude D. Pepper Centers and Centers for AIDS Research. AIDS Res Hum Retroviruses 2019;35(11–12):999–1012.
10. Kennedy BK, Berger SL, Brunet A, et al. Geroscience: linking aging to chronic disease. Cell 2014;159(4):709–13.
11. Montano M, Oursler KK, Xu K, et al. Biological ageing with HIV infection: evaluating the geroscience hypothesis. Lancet Heal Longev 2022;3(3):e194–205.
12. Horvath S, Lin DTS, Kobor MS, et al. HIV, pathology and epigenetic age acceleration in different human tissues. GeroScience 2022. https://doi.org/10.1007/s11357-022-00560-0.
13. Titanji BK, Gwinn M, Marconi VC, et al. Epigenome-wide epidemiologic studies of human immunodeficiency virus infection, treatment, and disease progression. Clin Epigenetics 2022;14(1):8.

14. Zanet DL, Thorne A, Singer J, et al. Association between short leukocyte telomere length and HIV infection in a cohort study: no evidence of a relationship with antiretroviral therapy. Clin Infect Dis 2014;58(9):1322–32.

15. Hunt M, Payne BAI. Mitochondria and ageing with HIV. Curr Opin HIV AIDS 2020;15(2):101–9.

16. McComsey GA, Daar ES, O'Riordan M, et al. Changes in fat mitochondrial DNA and function in subjects randomized to abacavir-lamivudine or tenofovir DF-emtricitabine with atazanavir-ritonavir or efavirenz: AIDS Clinical Trials Group study A5224s, substudy of A5202. J Infect Dis 2013;207(4):604–11.

17. Sun J, Brown TT, Samuels DC, et al. The Role of Mitochondrial DNA Variation in Age-Related Decline in Gait Speed among Older Men Living with Human Immunodeficiency Virus. Clin Infect Dis 2018;67(5). https://doi.org/10.1093/cid/ciy151.

18. Ortmeyer HK, Ryan AS, Hafer-Macko C, et al. Skeletal muscle cellular metabolism in older HIV-infected men. Physiol Rep 2016;4(9). https://doi.org/10.14814/phy2.12794.

19. Masters MC, Landay AL, Robbins PD, et al. Chronic HIV Infection and Aging: Application of a Geroscience-Guided Approach. J Acquir Immune Defic Syndr 2022;89(Suppl 1):S34–46.

20. Han X, Lei Q, Xie J, et al. Potential regulators of the senescence-associated secretory phenotype during senescence and ageing. J Gerontol A Biol Sci Med Sci 2022. https://doi.org/10.1093/gerona/glac097.

21. Franceschi C, Garagnani P, Parini P, et al. Inflammaging: a new immune–metabolic viewpoint for age-related diseases. Nat Rev Endocrinol 2018. https://doi.org/10.1038/s41574-018-0059-4.

22. Pathai S, Bajillan H, Landay AL, et al. Is HIV a model of accelerated or accentuated aging? J Gerontol - Ser A Biol Sci Med Sci 2014;69(7). https://doi.org/10.1093/gerona/glt168.

23. De Socio GV, Pasqualini M, Ricci E, et al. Smoking habits in HIV-infected people compared with the general population in Italy: a cross-sectional study. BMC Public Health 2020;20(1):734.

24. Shiau S, Arpadi SM, Yin MT, et al. Patterns of drug use and HIV infection among adults in a nationally representative sample. Addict Behav 2017. https://doi.org/10.1016/j.addbeh.2017.01.015.

25. Klein DB, Leyden WA, Xu L, et al. Declining relative risk for myocardial infarction among HIV-positive compared with HIV-negative individuals with access to care. Clin Infect Dis 2015. https://doi.org/10.1093/cid/civ014.

26. Mak G, Zaunders JJ, Bailey M, et al. Preservation of gastrointestinal mucosal barrier function and microbiome in patients with controlled HIV infection. Front Immunol 2021. https://doi.org/10.3389/fimmu.2021.688886.

27. Tarr PE, Ledergerber B, Calmy A, et al. Subclinical coronary artery disease in Swiss HIV-positive and HIV-negative persons. Eur Heart J 2018. https://doi.org/10.1093/eurheartj/ehy163.

28. Sortino O, Phanuphak N, Schuetz A, et al. Impact of acute HIV infection and early antiretroviral therapy on the human gut microbiome. Open Forum Infect Dis 2020. https://doi.org/10.1093/ofid/ofz367.

29. Lozupone CA, Li M, Campbell TB, et al. Alterations in the gut microbiota associated with HIV-1 infection. Cell Host Microbe 2013. https://doi.org/10.1016/j.chom.2013.08.006.

30. Dinh DM, Volpe GE, Duffalo C, et al. Intestinal Microbiota, microbial transloca-tion, and systemic inflammation in chronic HIV infection. J Infect Dis 2015. https://doi.org/10.1093/infdis/jiu409.

31. Alzahrani J, Hussain T, Simar D, et al. Inflammatory and immunometabolic con-sequences of gut dysfunction in HIV: Parallels with IBD and implications for reservoir persistence and non-AIDS comorbidities. EBioMedicine 2019;46: 522–31.

32. Angelovich TA, Hearps AC, Maisa A, et al. Viremic and virologically suppressed HIV infection increases age-related changes to monocyte activation equivalent to 12 and 4 years of aging, respectively. J Acquir Immune Defic Syndr 2015. https://doi.org/10.1097/QAI.0000000000000559.

33. Psomas CK, Waters L, Barber T, et al. Highlights of the 10th International AIDS Society (IAS) Conference on HIV Science, 21-25 July 2019, Mexico City, Mexico. J Virus Eradication 2019. https://doi.org/10.1016/S2055-6640(20)30035-2.

34. Kardashian A, Peters MG, Tien PC, et al. The Pathogenesis of Liver Disease in People Living With Human Immunodeficiency Virus: The Emerging Role of the Microbiome. Clin Liver Dis 2020. https://doi.org/10.1002/cld.880.

35. Jaworowski A, Hearps AC, Angelovich TA, et al. How monocytes contribute to increased risk of atherosclerosis in virologically-suppressed HIV-positive indi-viduals receiving combination antiretroviral therapy. Front Immunol 2019. https://doi.org/10.3389/fimmu.2019.01378.

36. Froiberg MS, Chang CCH, Kuller LH, et al. HIV infection and the risk of acute myocardial infarction. JAMA Intern Med 2013. https://doi.org/10.1001/jamainternmed.2013.3728.

37. Scherzer R, Estrella M, Li Y, et al. Association of tenofovir exposure with kidney disease risk in HIV infection. Aids 2012;26(7):867–75.

38. Scherzer R, Gandhi M, Estrella MM, et al. A chronic kidney disease risk score to determine tenofovir safety in a prospective cohort of HIV-positive male veterans. Aids 2014;28(9):1289–95.

39. Mocroft A, Kirk O, Reiss P, et al. Estimated glomerular filtration rate, chronic kid-ney disease and antiretroviral drug use in HIV-positive patients. Aids 2010; 24(11):1667–78.

40. Tien PC, Schneider MF, Cole SR, et al. Antiretroviral therapy exposure and insu-lin resistance in the women's interagency HIV study. J Acquir Immune Defic Syndr 2008;49(4):369–76.

41. Chawla A, Wang C, Patton C, et al. A Review of Long-Term Toxicity of Antiretro-viral Treatment Regimens and Implications for an Aging Population. Infect Dis Ther 2018;7(2):183–95.

42. Hasse B, Ledergerber B, Furrer H, et al. Morbidity and aging in HIV-infected persons: The swiss HIV cohort study. Clin Infect Dis 2011;53(11):1130–9.

43. Mata-Marín JA, Martínez-Osio MH, Arroyo-Anduiza CI, et al. Comorbidities and polypharmacy among HIV-positive patients aged 50 years and over: A case-control study. BMC Res Notes 2019;12(1):1–6.

44. Krentz HB, Cosman I, Lee K, et al. Pill burden in HIV infection: 20 Years of expe-rience. Antivir Ther 2012;17(5):833–40.

45. Zhou S, Martin K, Corbett A, et al. Total daily pill burden in HIV-infected patients in the Southern United States. AIDS Patient Care STDS 2014;28(6):311–7.

46. Matchanova A, Woods SP, Kordovski VM. Operationalizing and evaluating the Frascati criteria for functional decline in diagnosing HIV-associated neurocogni-tive disorders in adults. J Neurovirol 2020;26(2):155–67.

47. Brew BJ, Chan P. Update on HIV Dementia and HIV-Associated Neurocognitive Disorders. Curr Neurol Neurosci Rep 2014;14(8):468.
48. Letendre S, Ellis R, Tang B. 12-year cognitive decline is associated with lung disease, diabetes and depression. Abstr Virtual 2021;29(1):483, 2021 Conf Retroviruses Opportunistic Infect Top Antivir Med.
49. Ances BM, Anderson AM, Letendre SL. CROI 2021: neurologic complications of HIV-1 infection or COVID-19. Top Antivir Med 2021;29(2):334–43.
50. Wing EJ. HIV and aging. Int J Infect Dis 2016;53:61–8.
51. Lam JO, Hou CE, Hojilla JC, et al. Comparison of dementia risk after age 50 between individuals with and without HIV infection. AIDS 2021;35(5):821–8.
52. León R, Reus S, López N, et al. Subclinical atherosclerosis in low Framingham risk HIV patients. Eur J Clin Invest 2017. https://doi.org/10.1111/eci.12780.
53. Lo J, Abbara S, Shturman L, et al. Increased prevalence of subclinical coronary atherosclerosis detected by coronary computed tomography angiography in hiv-infected men. AIDS 2010. https://doi.org/10.1097/QAD.0b013e328333ea9e.
54. Triant VA, Perez J, Regan S, et al. Cardiovascular risk prediction functions underestimate risk in HIV infection. Circulation 2018. https://doi.org/10.1161/CIRCULATIONAHA.117.028975.
55. Feinstein MJ, Nance RM, Drozd DR, et al. Assessing and refining myocardial infarction risk estimation among patients with human immunodeficiency virus: A study by the Centers for AIDS Research Network of Integrated Clinical Systems. JAMA Cardiol 2017. https://doi.org/10.1001/jamacardio.2016.4494.
56. Raggi P, Zona S, Scaglioni R, et al. Epicardial adipose tissue and coronary artery calcium predict incident myocardial infarction and death in HIV-infected patients. J Cardiovasc Comput Tomogr 2015. https://doi.org/10.1016/j.jcct.2015.08.002.
57. Soares C, Samara A, Yuyun MF, et al. Coronary artery calcification and plaque characteristics in people living with hiv: A systematic review and meta-analysis. J Am Heart Assoc 2021. https://doi.org/10.1161/JAHA.120.019291.
58. Feinstein MJ, Hsue PY, Benjamin LA, et al. Characteristics, prevention, and management of cardiovascular disease in people living with HIV: a scientific statement from the american heart association. Circulation 2019. https://doi.org/10.1161/CIR.0000000000000695.
59. Hoffmann U, Lu MT, Olalere D, et al. Rationale and design of the mechanistic substudy of the randomized trial to prevent vascular events in HIV (REPRIEVE): effects of pitavastatin on coronary artery disease and inflammatory biomarkers. Am Heart J 2019;212:1–12.
60. Crothers K, Huang L, Goulet JL, et al. HIV infection and risk for incident pulmonary diseases in the combination antiretroviral therapy era. Am J Respir Crit Care Med 2011;183(3):388–95.
61. Crothers K, Butt AA, Gibert CL, et al. Increased COPD among HIV-positive compared to HIV-negative veterans. Chest 2006;130(5):1326–33.
62. Yearsley MM, Diaz PT, Knoell D, Nuovo GJ. Correlation of HIV-1 Detection and Histology in AIDS-Associated Emphysema. Diagnostic Molecular Pathology. 2005;14(1):48–52.
63. Diaz PT, King MA, Pacht ER, et al. Increased susceptibility to pulmonary emphysema among HIV-seropositive smokers. Available at: https://annals.org. Accessed August 24, 2022.
64. Fischer BM, Pavlisko E, Voynow JA. Pathogenic triad in COPD: Oxidative stress, protease-antiprotease imbalance, and inflammation. Int J COPD 2011;6(1):413–21.

65. Deeks SG, Tracy R, Douek DC. Systemic Effects of Inflammation on Health during Chronic HIV Infection. Immunity 2013;39(4):633–45.
66. Cribbs SK, Crothers K, Morris A. Pathogenesis of hiv-related lung disease: Immunity, infection, and inflammation. Physiol Rev 2020;100(2):603–32.
67. Byanova K, Kunisaki KM, Vasquez J, et al. Chronic obstructive pulmonary disease in HIV. Expert Rev Respir Med 2021;15(1):71–87.
68. Sussenbach AE, Van Gijzel SWL, Lalla-Edward ST, et al. The influence of smoking and HIV infection on pulmonary function. South Afr J HIV Med 2022; 23(1):1–7.
69. Petrache I, Diab K, Knox KS, et al. HIV associated pulmonary emphysema: A review of the literature and inquiry into its mechanism. Thorax 2008;63(5):463–9.
70. Drummond MB, Merlo CA, Astemborski J, et al. NIH Public Access 2014;27(8): 1303–11. https://doi.org/10.1097/QAD.0b013e32835e395d.
71. Gingo MR, George MP, Kessinger CJ, et al. Pulmonary function abnormalities in HIV-infected patients during the current antiretroviral therapy era. Am J Respir Crit Care Med 2010;182(6):790–6.
72. Varkila MRJ, Vos AG, Barth RE, et al. The association between HIV infection and pulmonary function in a rural African population. PLoS One 2019;14(1):1–12.
73. Jia J, Zhu Q, Deng L, et al. Treatment outcomes of HIV patients with hepatitis B and C virus co-infections in Southwest China: an observational cohort study. Infect Dis Poverty 2022;11(1):1–7.
74. Chammartin F, Lodi S, Logan R, et al. Risk for non-AIDS-defining and AIDS-defining cancer of early versus delayed initiation of antiretroviral therapy: A multinational prospective cohort study. Ann Intern Med 2021;174(6):768–76.
75. Kronfli N, Bhatnagar SR, Hull MW, et al. Trends in cause-specific mortality in HIV-hepatitis C coinfection following hepatitis C treatment scale-up. Aids 2019;33(6): 1013–22.
76. Chun HM, Roediger MP, Hullsiek KH, et al. Hepatitis B virus coinfection negatively impacts HIV outcomes in HIV seroconverters. J Infect Dis 2012. https://doi.org/10.1093/infdis/jir720.
77. Maurice JB, Patel A, Scott AJ, et al. Prevalence and risk factors of nonalcoholic fatty liver disease in HIV-monoinfection. AIDS 2017. https://doi.org/10.1097/QAD.0000000000001504.
78. Bakasis AD, Androutsakos T. Liver fibrosis during antiretroviral treatment in hiv-infected individuals. Truth or tale? Cells 2021. https://doi.org/10.3390/cells10051212.
79. Neff GW, Jayaweera D, Sherman KE. Drug-induced liver injury in HIV patients. Gastroenterol Hepatol 2006.
80. Chaudhary SR, Workeneh BT, Montez-Rath ME, et al. Trends in the outcomes of end-stage renal disease secondary to human immunodeficiency virus-associated nephropathy. Nephrol Dial Transplant 2015;30(10):1734–40. https://doi.org/10.1093/ndt/gfv207.
81. Adnani H, Agrawal N, Khatri A, et al. Impact of Antiretroviral Therapy on Kidney Disease in HIV Infected Individuals – A Qualitative Systematic Review. J Int Assoc Provid AIDS Care 2022;21. https://doi.org/10.1177/23259582221089194.
82. Lener MS. 乳鼠心肌提取 HHS Public Access. Physiol Behav 2016;176(1): 139–48.
83. Choi AI, Shlipak MG, Hunt PW, et al. HIV-infected persons continue to lose kidney function despite successful antiretroviral therapy. AIDS 2009;23(16): 2143–9.

84. Papeta N, Sterken R, Kiryluk K, et al. The molecular pathogenesis of HIV-1 associated nephropathy: Recent advances. J Mol Med 2011;89(5):429–36.

85. Samji H, Cescon A, Hogg RS, et al. Closing the gap: Increases in life expectancy among treated HIV-positive individuals in the United States and Canada. PLoS One 2013;8(12):6–13.

86. Röling J, Schmid H, Fischereder M, et al. HIV-associated renal diseases and highly active antiretroviral therapy-induced nephropathy. Clin Infect Dis 2006; 42(10):1488–95.

87. Jotwani V, Li Y, Grunfeld C, et al. Risk factors for ESRD in HIV-infected individuals: Traditional and HIV-related factors. Am J Kidney Dis 2012;59(5):628–35.

88. Szczech LA, Gange SJ, Van Der Horst C, et al. Predictors of Proteinuria and Renal Failure among Women with HIV Infection. Kidney International 2002;61(1):195–202.

89. Estrella MM, Parekh RS, Astor BC, et al. Chronic Kidney Disease and Estimates of Kidney Function in HIV Infection: A Cross-Sectional Study in the Multicenter AIDS Cohort Study. Available at: http://www.statepi.jhsph.edu/macs/macs.html. Accessed August 21, 2022.

90. Guaraldi G, Orlando G, Zona S, et al. Linked references are available on JSTOR for this article : UIHUm MAJOR ARTICLE Premature Age-Related Comorbidities Among HIV-infected Persons Compared With the. Gen Popul 2018;53(11). 1120–6.

91. Oursler KK, Iranmanesh A, Jain C, et al. Low Muscle Mass Is Associated with Osteoporosis in Older Adults Living with HIV. AIDS Res Hum Retroviruses 2019.

92. Montoya JL, Jankowski CM, O'Brien KK, et al. Evidence-informed practical recommendations for increasing physical activity among persons living with HIV. AIDS 2019;33(6):931–9.

93. Starup-Linde J, Rosendahl SB, Storgaard M, et al. Management of Osteoporosis in Patients Living With HIV-A Systematic Review and Meta-analysis. J Acquir Immune Defic Syndr 2020;83(1):1–8.

94. Triant VA, Brown TT, Lee H, et al. Fracture prevalence among human immunodeficiency virus (HIV)-infected versus non-HIV-infected patients in a large U.S. healthcare system. J Clin Endocrinol Metab 2008;93(9):3499–504.

95. Borges ÁH, Hoy J, Florence E, et al. Antiretrovirals, Fractures, and Osteonecrosis in a Large International HIV Cohort. Clin Infect Dis 2017;64(10):1413–21.

96. Brown TT, Hoy J, Borderi M, et al. Recommendations for evaluation and management of bone disease in HIV. Clin Infect Dis 2015;60(8):1242–51.

97. Hawkins KL, Zhang L, Ng DK, et al. Abdominal obesity, sarcopenia, and osteoporosis are associated with frailty in men living with and without HIV. AIDS 2018;32(10):1257–66.

98. Piggott DA, Bandeen-Roche K, Mehta SH, et al. Frailty transitions, inflammation, and mortality among persons aging with HIV infection and injection drug use. AIDS 2020;34(8):1217–25.

99. Erlandson KM, Piggott DA. Frailty and HIV: moving from characterization to intervention. Curr HIV/AIDS Rep 2021;18(3):157–75.

100. Hawkins KL, Brown TT, Margolick JB, et al. Geriatric syndromes: new frontiers in HIV and sarcopenia. Aids 2017;31(February):S137–46.

101. Justice AC, Tate JP. Strengths and limitations of the veterans aging cohort study index as a measure of physiologic frailty. AIDS Res Hum Retroviruses 2019; 35(11–12):1023–33.

102. Park LS, Tate JP, Sigel K, et al. Time trends in cancer incidence in persons living with HIV/AIDS in the antiretroviral therapy era: 1997-2012. AIDS 2016;30(11): 1795–806.
103. Veyri M, Lavolé A, Choquet S, et al. Do people living with HIV face more secondary cancers than general population: From the French CANCERVIH network. Bull Cancer 2021;108(10):908–14.
104. Horner MJ, Shiels MS, Pfeiffer RM, et al. Deaths Attributable to Cancer in the US Human Immunodeficiency Virus Population During 2001–2015. Clin Infect Dis 2021;72(9):e224–31.
105. Altekruse SF, Shiels MS, Modur SP, et al. Cancer burden attributable to cigarette smoking among HIV-infected people in North America. AIDS 2018;32(4): 513–21.
106. Rihana N, Nanjappa S, Sullivan C, et al. Malignancy Trends in HIV-Infected Patients Over the Past 10 Years in a Single-Center Retrospective Observational Study in the United States. Cancer Control 2018;25(1). https://doi.org/10.1177/1073274818797955. 1073274818797955.
107. Ledgerwood DM, Yskes R. Smoking cessation for people living with HIV/AIDS: a literature review and synthesis. Nicotine Tob Res 2016;18(12):2177–84.
108. Smith RA, Andrews KS, Brooks D, et al. Cancer screening in the United States, 2019: a review of current American Cancer Society guidelines and current issues in cancer screening. CA Cancer J Clin 2019;69(3):184–210.
109. Stanton CA, Papandonatos GD, Shuter J, et al. Outcomes of a tailored intervention for cigarette smoking cessation among latinos living with HIV/AIDS. Nicotine Tob Res 2015;17(8):975–82.
110. Stewart DB, Gaertner WB, Glasgow SC, et al. The american society of colon and rectal surgeons clinical practice guidelines for anal squamous cell cancers (Revised 2018). Dis Colon Rectum 2018;61(7):755–74.
111. Revollo B, Videla S, Llibre JM, et al. Routine screening of anal cytology in persons with human immunodeficiency virus and the impact on invasive anal cancer: a prospective cohort study. Clin Infect Dis 2020;71(2):390–9.
112. New York State Department of Health AIDS Institute. Screening for anal dysplasia and cancer in patients with HIV. Available at: https://www.hivguidelines.org/hiv-care/anal-dysplasia-cancer.
113. Engels EA, Yanik EL, Wheeler W, et al. Cancer-attributable mortality among people with treated human immunodeficiency virus infection in North America. Clin Infect Dis 2017;65(4):636–43.
114. Ioannou GN, Green PK, Beste LA, et al. Development of models estimating the risk of hepatocellular carcinoma after antiviral treatment for hepatitis C. J Hepatol 2018;69(5):1088–98.
115. Loomba R, Lim JK, Patton H, et al. AGA Clinical Practice Update on Screening and Surveillance for Hepatocellular Carcinoma in Patients With Nonalcoholic Fatty Liver Disease: Expert Review. Gastroenterology 2020;158(6):1822–30.
116. Lakshmi S, Beekmann SE, Polgreen PM, et al. HIV primary care by the infectious disease physician in the United States - extending the continuum of care. AIDS Care - Psychol Socio-Medical Asp AIDS/HIV 2018;30(5):569–77.
117. Singh HK, Del Carmen T, Freeman R, et al. From One Syndrome to Many: Incorporating Geriatric Consultation Into HIV Care. Clin Infect Dis 2017;65(3):501–6.
118. Erlandson KM, Karris MY. HIV and Aging: Reconsidering the Approach to Management of Comorbidities. Infect Dis Clin North Am 2019;33(3):769–86.
119. Thompson MA, Horberg MA, Agwu AL, et al. Primary Care Guidance for Persons with Human Immunodeficiency Virus: 2020 Update by the HIV Medicine

Association of the Infectious Diseases Society of America. Clin Infect Dis 2021. https://doi.org/10.1093/cid/ciaa1391.

120. Home page | United States Preventive Services Taskforce. Available at: https://www.uspreventiveservicestaskforce.org/uspstf/. Accessed August 24, 2022.

121. HIV Infection and Cancer Risk - NCI. Available at: https://www.cancer.gov/about-cancer/causes-prevention/risk/infectious-agents/hiv-fact-sheet. Accessed August 24, 2022.

122. Coghill AE, Pfeiffer RM, Shiels MS, et al. Excess mortality among HIV-infected individuals with cancer in the United States. Cancer Epidemiol Biomarkers Prev 2017;26(7):1027–33.

123. Edelman EJ, Gordon KS, Glover J, et al. The next therapeutic challenge in HIV: Polypharmacy. Drugs and Aging 2013;30(8):613–28.

124. Ware D, Palella FJ, Chew KW, et al. Prevalence and trends of polypharmacy among HIV-positive and -negative men in the Multicenter AIDS Cohort Study from 2004 to 2016. PLoS One 2018;13(9):1–14.

125. Gandhi TK, Hussar DA, Minsk AG. Adverse drug events in ambulatory care prescriptions for improvement. Med Crossfire 2003;5(7):21–4.

126. Erlandson KM, Allshouse AA, Jankowski CM, et al. Risk factors for falls in HIV-infected persons. J Acquir Immune Defic Syndr 2012;61(4):484–9.

127. Davis AJ, Greene M, Siegler E, et al. Strengths and Challenges of Various Models of Geriatric Consultation for Older Adults Living With Human Immunodeficiency Virus. Clin Infect Dis 2022;74(6):1101–6.

128. Kay ES, Batey DS, Mugavero MJ. The HIV treatment cascade and care continuum: updates, goals, and recommendations for the future. AIDS Res Ther 2016; 13:35.

Acute and Chronic Infectious Prostatitis in Older Adults

Tyler J. Brehm, MD[a], Barbara W. Trautner, MD, PhD[b,c], Prathit A. Kulkarni, MD[d,e],*

KEYWORDS

• Prostatitis • Acute bacterial prostatitis • Chronic bacterial prostatitis
• Infectious prostatitis • Urinary tract infection

KEY POINTS

• Acute bacterial prostatitis should be considered in all male patients with sepsis from an acute urinary tract infection.
• Prostate-specific antigen is not sufficiently sensitive or specific to rule in or rule out a diagnosis of acute bacterial prostatitis.
• Chronic bacterial prostatitis typically has an indolent clinical presentation without systemic symptoms, and patients are rarely hospitalized.
• Diagnosis of chronic bacterial prostatitis is most commonly made with the two-glass test in clinical practice, although the four-glass test has been the historical gold standard.
• Evidence regarding how to diagnose and manage acute and chronic infectious prostatitis in older patients is scant, and increased clinician awareness of these conditions will ideally drive future research in this field.

INTRODUCTION

Prostatitis is a clinically significant entity with a prevalence ranging from 2.2% to 9.7% in adult males. This prevalence estimate includes all forms of prostatitis.[1] Prostatitis is particularly relevant to the older adult population, with one study showing a lifetime reported rate of prostatitis of ~25% in patients over the age of 65.[2] A new classification system for prostatitis was proposed in 1999 and remains the standard for defining prostatitis at the present time (**Table 1**).[3]

This review will focus specifically on National Institutes of Health (NIH) categories I and II—acute bacterial prostatitis (ABP) and chronic bacterial prostatitis (CBP), respectively.

[a] Department of Medicine, Section of General Internal Medicine, Baylor College of Medicine, Houston, TX 77030, USA; [b] Center for Innovations in Quality, Effectiveness and Safety (IQuESt), Michael E. DeBakey Veterans Affairs Medical Center, Houston, TX 77030, USA; [c] Department of Medicine, Section of Health Services Research, Baylor College of Medicine, Houston, TX 77030, USA; [d] Medical Care Line, Michael E. DeBakey Veterans Affairs Medical Center, Houston, TX 77030, USA; [e] Department of Medicine, Infectious Diseases Section, Baylor College of Medicine, Houston, TX 77030, USA
* Corresponding author. Michael E. DeBakey Veterans Affairs Medical Center, 2002 Holcombe Boulevard, MCL-111, Houston, TX 77030.
E-mail address: pakulkar@bcm.edu

Infect Dis Clin N Am 37 (2023) 175–194
https://doi.org/10.1016/j.idc.2022.09.004
0891-5520/23/Published by Elsevier Inc.

id.theclinics.com

Table 1 National Institutes of Health classification of prostatitis	
Classification	**Definition**
Category I—Acute bacterial prostatitis	Acute bacterial infection of the prostate gland
Category II—Chronic bacterial prostatitis	Chronic (>3 mo) infection of the prostate gland
Category III—Chronic pelvic pain syndrome	Chronic pelvic pain consistent with prostatitis but without pathogenic bacterial growth in the urine
IIIA—Inflammatory	Elevated level of white blood cells (WBCs) in post-prostatic massage urine and prostatic fluid samples
IIIB—Noninflammatory	No WBC elevation in post-prostatic massage urine and prostatic fluid samples
Category IV—Asymptomatic inflammatory prostatitis	Absence of genitourinary symptoms but presence of elevated WBCs in post-prostatic urine and prostatic fluid samples

J.Curtis Nickel, Leroy M Nyberg, Mike Hennenfent, Research guidelines for chronic prostatitis: consensus report from the First National Institutes of Health International Prostatitis Collaborative Network11A complete list of the contributing participants of the first meeting of the International Prostatitis Collaborative Network is given in the Appendix., Urology, 54 (2), 1999, 229-233, https://doi.org/10.1016/S0090-4295(99)00205-8.

ABP is an acute infection of the prostate gland. It is generally caused by organisms known to cause urinary tract infections (UTIs), most commonly *Escherichia coli*. Patients with ABP have an acute onset of genitourinary (GU) symptoms and are typically quite ill, often meeting clinical criteria by Sepsis-2[4] (two or more systemic inflammatory response syndrome [SIRS] criteria plus suspected or confirmed infection) and/or Sepsis-3[5] (increase in the sequential organ failure assessment score by 2 or more over time plus an infection) definitions. SIRS criteria include fever or hypothermia, tachycardia, tachypnea, and leukocytosis or leukopenia. Conversely, CBP is defined by the presence of chronic and/or recurrent urogenital symptoms in the setting of infection of the prostate. CBP, by definition, has an indolent course. Patients are typically not ill-appearing, and management primarily occurs in the outpatient setting.

The purpose of this review is to provide clinicians with a practical overview of ABP and CBP, including diagnostic and treatment approaches for these conditions.

Prostatitis in the Older Adult

As this review article will address, the available evidence related to the diagnosis and management of both ABP and CBP has numerous gaps. As a result, much of this review relies on data from all adults (including but not limited to adults > 65 year old) because studies conducted only in older adult populations or comparing age groups are not as common. However, there are still several key takeaways that can be highlighted for the older age group.

First, older adults have a higher lifetime risk of acquiring antibiotic-resistant bacteria[6,7] and can suffer significant morbidity and mortality from infections due to such bacteria.[8] Thus, a review of prior culture data is imperative when choosing empiric regimens for ABP in this patient population. In addition, obtaining cultures before the administration of antibiotics is crucial in both ABP and CBP. Second, diagnosis of ABP and CBP might be especially challenging in older adults if they are nonverbal or have acute or chronic encephalopathy (eg, due to delirium or dementia). Finally, older adults are particularly susceptible to both ABP and CBP, as they have increased prevalence of many of the risk factors for these diseases, including but not limited to diabetes mellitus,[9] benign prostatic hyperplasia (BPH),[10] and prostate cancer.[11]

Acute Bacterial Prostatitis

When to suspect acute bacterial prostatitis

ABP should be considered in a male patient with acute UTI causing significant illness with the patient lacking clinical evidence of another urinary source of infection, such as pyelonephritis. The condition typically results in such a significant inflammatory reaction that patients require hospitalization. Patients will frequently meet clinical criteria for sepsis (either by Sepsis-2[4] and/or Sepsis-3[5] guidelines, as outlined above), but will typically lack classical signs and symptoms of acute pyelonephritis, such as flank or back pain, nausea, and vomiting. One large retrospective cohort study noted a distribution of the prevalence of different signs and symptoms as follows:[12]

- Abnormal digital rectal examination (DRE)—83%[a] (painful prostate—63%)
- Fever—80%
- Urinary symptoms[b]—72%
- Pelvic pain—43%

ABP, therefore, should specifically be suspected when a male patient has an acute UTI resulting in a serious illness causing a sepsis-like syndrome, but does not have clinical evidence of pyelonephritis or another infectious urinary source by history, physical examination, or radiographic imaging. In theory, it is possible that a man could have pyelonephritis, cystitis, and prostatitis concurrently, but literature is not available to define the frequency of these infections occurring together. Our point is that in male patients who seem more ill than might be warranted by cystitis alone and who do not seem to have pyelonephritis to explain their symptoms, the clinician should consider ABP in the differential diagnosis because the duration of antibiotic therapy would differ from that typically prescribed for acute cystitis. Importantly, DRE should be included as part of the physical examination in this scenario when there is no clinical suspicion of another urinary source of infection causing severe illness.

CLINICAL CARE POINTS

- An abnormal (painful) digital rectal examination is a clinical clue to diagnosing acute bacterial prostatitis.
- Acute bacterial prostatitis should be considered in all male patients with sepsis from a urinary tract infection.

Risk Factors for Acute Bacterial Prostatitis

Any condition which predisposes a male patient to UTI also increases the risk of ABP. Risk factors include:

- Anatomic abnormalities (eg, urethral strictures, BPH)
- Diabetes mellitus

---

[a] Abnormal DRE is defined as a painful prostate, prostate hypertrophy, or prostate irregularity.

[b] Urinary symptoms are defined as burning micturition, dysuria, frequency, bladder outlet obstruction, or macroscopic hematuria.

- Urogenital instrumentation (eg, prostate biopsy, intermittent catheterization, chronic indwelling urinary catheters)[13–15]
- Immunosuppression, particularly in persons with HIV, even if not advanced[16,17]

Diagnosis of Acute Bacterial Prostatitis

Diagnosis of ABP is clinical and is supported by physical examination, laboratory studies, and imaging findings, as described below.

Physical Examination

DRE can provide supportive clinical evidence for the diagnosis of ABP. Although there is theoretic concern for causing bacteremia with vigorous prostate examination, the authors of this review believe a brief, gentle examination to identify acute tenderness or any gross abnormalities (eg, fluctuance) is diagnostically useful and limits the theoretic downside. Bacteremia is a well-documented and undesirable outcome of prostate biopsy in men with bacteriuria,[18–20] but prostate biopsy breaches the mucosa, unlike DRE. No literature was identified to address a possible link between DRE and bacteremia, but in the interest of caution, we recommend against prostatic massage or any attempt to express prostatic secretions in the acute setting.[21,22] Current clinical practice does not typically include DRE in an older male patient with sepsis suspected to be due to an acute UTI, but it is possible that increased awareness of ABP may drive increased DRE testing, in particular when evidence for another urinary source of infection is lacking.

Laboratory Data

Urinalysis and urine culture

Urinalysis (UA) and urine culture are useful in the diagnosis of ABP, and are particularly important for guiding antibiotic therapy. In one study, urine cultures were positive in 65% of patients, with the majority (58%) of sterile cultures occurring in patients who received antibiotics before cultures were obtained.[23] Importantly, even among patients with sterile cultures, a majority (68%) still had significant pyuria on UA. Without a gold standard for the diagnosis of ABP, it is difficult to determine how sensitive and specific these urine tests are for diagnosis.

Blood cultures

Blood cultures are not inherently required for the diagnosis of ABP. In one retrospective cohort study, blood cultures contributed to the microbiological diagnosis of ABP in only 5% of patients.[23] However, a febrile, ill-appearing patient has a strong indication for blood cultures, and given possible diagnostic uncertainty early in the clinical presentation of ABP, most clinicians would justifiably acquire blood cultures. Blood cultures drawn at the initial point of care (such as the Emergency Department) might detect a causative pathogen if the urine culture is obtained after antibiotics have been administered.

Prostate-specific antigen

The role of prostate-specific antigen (PSA) measurement in ABP is ill-defined, although an association between PSA elevation and ABP seems intuitive. PSA elevation has been reported in 60% to 100% of cases of ABP across various studies,[23–25] with the wide range likely explained by variations in sample size and inclusion criteria. Studies have additionally shown a decrease in PSA levels with antibiotic treatment for ABP.[24,26] However, PSA elevation has also been noted in studies investigating complicated UTIs in up to 83% of male patients.[26] In the presence of urinary tract inflammation, it can be difficult to differentiate prostatic inflammation as a secondary effect of urinary infection versus the prostate being the primary source of UTI. Therefore, PSA can be used in conjunction with other clinical data for diagnosing or excluding ABP, but PSA has not shown sufficient sensitivity or specificity to be used in isolation.

Erythrocyte sedimentation rate and C-Reactive protein
Erythrocyte sedimentation rate (ESR) and C-reactive protein (CRP) are commonly elevated in ABP (95% and 96%, respectively, in one cohort).[23] However, there are no studies showing that the degree of elevation or monitoring trends of these laboratory studies has an impact on clinical practice or outcomes. Because of this, routine use of these nonspecific markers in suspected ABP is likely unnecessary.

Imaging

Imaging is not required for the initial diagnosis of ABP, although it might help contribute to making a diagnosis if there is clinical uncertainty or in identifying alternative pathology (eg, pyelonephritis).

Both computed tomography (CT) scanning of the pelvis (with intravenous iodinated contrast) and transrectal ultrasound of the prostate have been utilized in diagnosing ABP, although there are few studies defining their sensitivity or specificity for the identification of prostatic inflammation or edema. In one prospective cohort study conducted from 1996 to 1998, only 46% of patients had identifiable lesions on the transrectal ultrasound, and only 61.1% of lesions improved or resolved with treatment.[27]

Radiographic imaging can be useful for the identification of prostatic abscesses. Transrectal ultrasound of the prostate has a high sensitivity of 80% to 100% for prostatic abscesses,.[28–30] CT or MRI of the pelvis can also be used. However, routine evaluation for abscesses is not recommended, as studies have shown low (0%–2.7%) rates of prostatic abscesses in ABP.[23,27] Thus, imaging to evaluate for prostatic abscess should primarily be obtained in patients refractory to antibiotic therapy. A timeframe for when to order imaging is not well-defined, but it would be reasonable to consider imaging if patients have not clinically improved after 48 hours of appropriate antibiotic treatment.[31] To note, as a practical matter, in routine clinical practice, many male patients with febrile UTI might have already undergone an imaging study early during their clinical course to evaluate for GU tract abnormalities. CT might also be able to show that the patient has pyelonephritis, for example,

Indium-labeled white-blood cell (WBC) scintigraphy might also be of benefit in ABP. A small prospective study reported scintigraphy to be effective in differentiating ABP from non-prostate-including UTIs and in demonstrating clearance of infection after treatment.[32] However, additional studies are needed before this can be recommended as part of routine evaluation for ABP.

CLINICAL CARE POINTS

- Gentle digital rectal examination can be helpful in diagnosing acute bacterial prostatitis.
- Prostatic massage to express secretions is discouraged in the setting of suspected acute bacterial prostatitis.
- Prostate-specific antigen is not sufficiently sensitive or specific to rule in or rule out a diagnosis of acute bacterial prostatitis, but can be used in conjunction with other data.
- Radiographic imaging cannot be used to rule in or rule out acute bacterial prostatitis, but can be used in conjunction with other aspects of the overall clinical picture.

Treatment of Acute Bacterial Prostatitis

ABP should be treated with antibiotics. The route, specific drug, and duration of therapy can vary from case to case, and are detailed below.

Bacteriology

The etiologic organisms which typically cause ABP are important in guiding empirical antibiotic regimens. ABP is most often caused by organisms known to cause UTIs more generally:[12,21,33–36]

- *E coli* (>50% of cases)
- *Proteus* species
- Other *Enterobacterales,* including *Klebsiella, Serratia,* and *Enterobacter spp*
- *Pseudomonas aeruginosa*
- *E spp*

Specific antibiotic choices to treat these organisms are discussed below, but importantly, clinicians should use local and regional antimicrobial resistance data to guide initial empiric antibiotic therapy.

Of note, other less frequently encountered organisms can sequester in the prostate and cause acute prostatitis. These include mycobacteria *(eg, Mycobacterium abscessus, Mycobacterium tuberculosis)*[37,38] and fungi (eg, *Cryptococcus, Coccidloides, and Histoplasma).*[39,40] Patients with infections due to these organisms often have historical exposure or manifestations of the infection at other anatomic sites that can serve as a clue to the diagnosis. For example, prior receipt of bacille Calmette-Guérin treatment for bladder cancer can be a clue to suspect mycobacterial infection of the prostate.

Parenteral Antibiotics

IV therapy is not inherently required to treat ABP but is warranted in patients with:

- Sepsis
- Hemodynamic instability
- Inability to tolerate oral antibiotics
- High risk for multi-drug resistant (MDR) organisms unlikely to be susceptible to oral antibiotics

Because most patients with ABP will be seriously ill at presentation, we recommend initiating IV therapy with a plan for step-down to oral therapy when clinically appropriate.

The classes of IV agents most commonly used for UTIs are acceptable antibiotics for initial empiric therapy for ABP. These include:

- Penicillins (eg, piperacillin-tazobactam, ampicillin-sulbactam)
- Cephalosporins
- Carbapenems
- More rarely (for Gram-positive organisms): vancomycin, daptomycin
- If critically ill: can consider short-term addition of an aminoglycoside until further microbiological data are available

In the case of ABP following a urologic procedure, such as prostate biopsy, it is reasonable to start coverage for multidrug-resistant organisms as these patients have often received preprocedural antibiotics. Post-procedural infections are, therefore, more likely to be due to resistant organisms.[35]

In ABP, the inflamed prostate is believed to allow for increased penetration of antibiotics that would otherwise not reach therapeutic levels. Tissue penetration becomes a more important concern during prolonged oral antibiotic courses, when prostatic inflammation has decreased.

Oral Antibiotics

For oral step-down antimicrobial therapy, fluoroquinolones and trimethoprim-sulfamethoxazole (TMP-SMX) have classically been used for ABP because of their excellent oral bioavailability, prostatic penetration, and historical data on clinical effectiveness.[41]

Agents which have not been as extensively evaluated in the treatment of ABP include fosfomycin and cephalosporins. Fosfomycin has good prostatic tissue penetration,[42] but evidence of clinical effectiveness for the treatment of ABP is sparse. One recent review article noted only three reported cases of successful treatment of ABP with fosfomycin.[43] Oral cephalosporins have not been thoroughly evaluated in the treatment of ABP, and there are concerns about the oral bioavailability of some medications in this class.[44] Although not studied in the setting of ABP, macrolides, and tetracyclines have good prostatic tissue penetration and might be effective for susceptible isolates. Finally, nitrofurantoin, although often used for the treatment of cystitis, does not have good prostatic tissue penetration and should not be used for ABP.

Duration of Antimicrobial Therapy

Well-designed, randomized controlled trials for the duration of treatment of ABP are lacking. Expert opinion has historically recommended 2 to 4 weeks,[45,46] with which the authors of this review concur. This range of treatment duration affords room for clinical judgment based on severity of infection and rapidity of clinical improvement.

To note, if a patient with an indwelling urinary catheter develops sepsis from suspected acute UTI, ABP can be considered. However, if the indwelling catheter is chronic and cannot be removed, a longer course of antibiotics is likely not justified because of the possibility of recolonization after completion of antimicrobial therapy and unnecessary promotion of antimicrobial resistance because of increased antibiotic exposure.

Surgical Intervention

Routine surgical intervention is not required in the management of ABP, but a procedure by urology or interventional radiology for management might be necessary for complications such as a prostatic abscess. However, randomized controlled trials evaluating surgical vs. antimicrobial-only management for prostatic abscess are lacking. Historically, surgical intervention has been pursued in cases of prostatic abscess > 1 cm, or if ≤1 cm, with failure to respond to antimicrobial therapy.[47,48] For patients with urinary retention and suspected ABP, urology consultation might be necessary for assistance with the placement of a urinary catheter. Some urologists might choose a suprapubic approach, whereas others might proceed with transurethral catheter placement. In either scenario, expert placement of a catheter with as little trauma as possible provides patient-centered care.

CLINICAL CARE POINTS

- Because patients with acute bacterial prostatitis are often severely ill at presentation, it is recommended to start with IV antimicrobial therapy with a plan for step-down to oral therapy when clinically appropriate.

- Fluoroquinolones and trimethoprim-sulfamethoxazole are first-line step-down oral therapy for the treatment of acute bacterial prostatitis.
- The recommended total duration of therapy is 2 to 4 weeks.

Clinical Outcomes and Follow-up

The extant literature has a varying amount of evidence for different clinical outcomes and follow-up of ABP. Certain outcomes, such as progression to CBP and chronic prostatitis, are relatively well-defined, whereas information about other outcomes, such as mortality, is lacking.

One cohort study showed that 1.3% of patients with ABP had progression to CBP, and another 10.5% of patients progressed to inflammatory chronic pelvic pain syndrome.[49] Other studies reported progression from ABP to chronic prostatitis in general (encompassing NIH class II, class IIIa, and class IIIb prostatitis) in 4.2%[49] and 8.1%[50] of patients. Overall, across studies, approximately 90% of patients consistently had complete symptom resolution without progression to chronic prostatitis of any type at 12-month follow-up.

Mortality outcomes from ABP are not well-defined in the literature, but would presumably be similar to other acute, complicated UTIs. For example, acute pyelonephritis has reported 30-day mortality rates as high as 4.7%.[51] Another study of male patients older than 60 with febrile UTI showed in-hospital mortality rates of up to 4.3%.[52]

Urology follow-up is recommended in nearly all causes of ABP, as there is a high prevalence of intervenable pathologies (~25%) in males with a history of a febrile UTI.[53] Intervenable pathologies include severe BPH potentially requiring resection, urethral stricture, bladder stones, renal calyceal stones, and previously unrecognized GU malignancies. Regarding the need for follow-up urine culture as a "test of cure", in the absence of clear data, we recommend monitoring patients clinically for any signs or symptoms of treatment failure rather than obtaining routine urine culture after completion of antimicrobial therapy. Follow-up imaging and laboratory studies could be required if the patient had a prostatic abscess and/or underwent surgical intervention. In such scenarios, expert consultation is advised.

CLINICAL CARE POINTS

- At 12 months post-ABP treatment, up to 10% of patients will have chronic prostatitis (encompassing NIH classes II, IIIa, and IIIb).
- Patients with acute bacterial prostatitis do not require routine follow-up laboratory studies or imaging.
- Outpatient urology follow-up is recommended in nearly all cases of acute bacterial prostatitis.

Chronic Bacterial Prostatitis

When to suspect chronic bacterial prostatitis

The hallmark of CBP is chronicity, classically described as recurrent UTIs caused by the same organism. However, historically, this pattern of recurrent UTI has been documented in only 25% to 43% of cases diagnosed and treated as CBP.[54] Clinical symptoms of CBP include those typically associated with UTIs, such as dysuria, urinary frequency, and urgency, but also include pain (lower abdominal, perineal, penile, or testicular), hematospermia, and dysorgasmia. By definition these symptoms occur over a prolonged period (greater than 3 months at minimum). *A diagnosis of CBP should be considered in all male patients with chronic GU symptoms.*

Risk Factors

The same risk factors which apply to ABP also apply to CBP (see Risk Factors above). ABP itself is also a risk factor for progression to CBP (1.4% of patients in one study). A retrospective study of 480 men with ABP in Korea found that the following factors were associated with the subsequent onset of CBP: diabetes mellitus, prior urologic manipulation, urethral catheterization, and lack of cystostomy (for bladder drainage during the episode of ABP).[55] Prostatic calculi are also a risk factor for CBP.[56]

CLINICAL CARE POINTS

> • Chronic bacterial prostatitis typically has an indolent presentation without systemic symptoms, and patients are rarely hospitalized.

Diagnosis of Chronic Bacterial Prostatitis

The gold standard for diagnosis of CBP is presence of elevated concentrations of bacteria in prostatic fluid when compared with bladder or urethral specimens. However, in clinical practice, the diagnosis is instead often made via a combination of suggestive clinical history and other microbiological data and is sometimes augmented through additional laboratory tests and imaging. Suggestive clinical history includes recurrent UTI with the same causative organism and chronic lower abdominal or pelvic pain without another explanation.

Physical Examination

Physical examination in CBP is often unrevealing. The prostate might be normal, boggy, nodular, or tender. Systemic symptoms are typically absent, and patients are rarely hospitalized for CBP.

Laboratory and Microbiological Data

Urinalysis and urine culture

Classically, the Meares-Stamey four-glass test was used for the diagnosis of CBP. This test requires the collection of four samples in this order: the first 5 to 10 mL of voided urine, a midstream urine sample, post-prostatic massage secretions, and a sample of the first 5 to 10 mL of urine post-prostatic massage.[57] However, this approach has fallen out of favor, with one survey of 504 urologists registered with the American Medical Association reporting 80% rarely or never used this test. Further, in this same study, ~40% of patients referred for chronic prostatitis were treated with antibiotics regardless of whether the urologist reported using the four-glass test or not.[58]

Instead, the two-glass test is often the preferred alternative in today's urologic practice. This method compares a post-prostatic massage urine sample with a pre-massage urine sample. The two-glass method has 100% positive predictive value and 96% negative predictive value when compared with the four-glass method.[59] When utilizing the two-glass method, $\geq$ 12 WBCs/high-powered field (HPF) in the post-massage sample is suggestive of chronic prostatitis, whereas $\geq$20 WBCs/HPF is considered diagnostic.[60] These thresholds only apply when the pre-massage urine sample does not show pyuria. In addition, a 10-fold increase in bacterial concentration between pre- and post-prostatic massage urine samples is also considered diagnostic of CBP. Importantly, the two-glass test should be performed > 72 hours from the last ejaculation because ejaculation can temporarily elevate the leukocyte count in prostatic fluid.[61]

Semen culture
The utility of semen culture in the diagnosis of CBP is controversial. Several studies have reported increased sensitivity in diagnosing CBP with use of semen cultures or the 5-glass method (semen culture with the four-glass method) when compared with the traditional four-glass or two-glass methods.[62–64] However, a drawback of utilizing semen cultures is an increase in false-positive findings, especially when Gram-positive organisms are detected.[62] This problem could theoretically be rectified by repeating cultures and only treating for CBP in the case of persistent isolation of the same bacterial species. Overall, semen culture could be useful for the diagnosis of CBP, especially in otherwise culture-negative prostatitis (via 2- or four-glass methods), although its utility is not firmly established. In the case of non-traditional uropathogen isolates, however, repeat culture and consultation with an infectious diseases physician are warranted before initiating treatment.

Prostate-specific antigen
PSA levels do not factor into the diagnosis of CBP. Only 25% of participants with CBP have an elevated PSA.[65] There are some data suggesting a correlation between decrease in PSA levels and microbiological clearance, but the clinical utility of this finding has yet to be shown.

Miscellaneous laboratory testing in atypical cases
In patients with signs and symptoms suggestive of CBP, but who have persistently negative urine cultures, it is reasonable to test for Chlamydia trachomatis.[66–68] Cases involving mycobacterial or fungal infections are also described in the literature (particularly in immunosuppressed populations), although diagnosis in these cases can be challenging and should be managed with appropriate specialist assistance.[37,40]

Imaging
Imaging (ultrasound, CT, and MRI) does not play a role in the diagnosis of CBP. One study of transrectal ultrasound showed no difference in findings between category II, IIIa, or IIIb prostatitis,[69] with most imaging having been reported as normal. CT and MRI are similarly unreliable for the diagnosis of CBP. In addition, even if abnormalities are detected, imaging findings present in CBP have significant overlap with other etiologies such as prostate cancer, and are therefore nonspecific.[70]

CLINICAL CARE POINTS

- Diagnosis of chronic bacterial prostatitis in clinical practice is commonly made with the two-glass test, although the four-glass test is the reported gold standard in the extant literature.
- Prostate-specific antigen levels have no demonstrated benefit in the diagnosis of chronic bacterial prostatitis.

- There is no demonstrated benefit for use of imaging in the diagnosis of chronic bacterial prostatitis.

Treatment of Chronic Bacterial Prostatitis

Treatment of CBP should ideally be initiated after culture susceptibility data are available, as CBP is indolent by nature and does not require urgent treatment. However, in cases where appropriate diagnostic testing (2-, 4-, or 5-glass tests) is unable to be performed expeditiously, empiric regimens are chosen based on the incidence of typical causative pathogens. Of note, the unique environment of the prostate has a significant impact on tissue penetration of certain antibiotics when compared with other UTIs, thereby limiting available treatment options.

Organisms

A wide range of organisms cause CBP, although they tend to correlate with usual uropathogens:[46]

- *E coli* (50%–80%)
- *Enterobacterales* such as *Klebsiella* and *Proteus* (10%–30%)
- *E spp* (5%–10%)
- Non-lactose-fermenting Gram-negative bacilli such as *Pseudomonas* (<5% of cases)

Gram-positive organisms other than *Enterococcus* are rare. Although staphylococci and streptococci are potential etiologic causes of CBP, identification of these bacteria should prompt consideration of dissemination from another anatomic site.

In addition, atypical infections caused by *Chlamydia, Cryptococcus, Blastomyces,* and mycobacterial species have been described previously. The incidence of these organisms varies greatly among different populations based on risk factors related to sexual history, immunocompromised status, etc.

Oral Antibiotics

Fluoroquinolones

Fluoroquinolones are considered first-line therapy for the treatment of both initial and recurrent CBP, particularly if the isolate is susceptible to fluoroquinolones. Most studies have shown no appreciable difference in therapeutic response or adverse effects between different specific fluoroquinolones.[71–74] Suggested regimens include:

- Levofloxacin 500 mg PO daily for 4 to 6 weeks
- Ciprofloxacin 500 mg PO every 12 hours for 4 to 6 weeks

Shorter durations are not recommended due to higher rates of relapse.[75]

Trimethoprim-sulfamethoxazole

Trimethoprim-sulfamethoxazole (TMP-SMX) is often the first alternative therapy used to treat CBP. A review of several studies reported excellent prostatic penetration of this drug, particularly the trimethoprim component.[44] However, data supporting its therapeutic use is sparse, and mainly comes from older studies with smaller numbers of patients and longer treatment courses (90 days).[76–79] Although there have been no head-to-head randomized control trials comparing TMP-SMX to fluoroquinolones for the treatment of CBP, one cost-analysis study did find a benefit for fluoroquinolones over TMP-SMX.[80] If TMP-SMX is used to treat CBP, a suggested regimen is as follows (depending upon renal function):

- 1 Double-Strength Tablet PO every 12 hours for 6 weeks (many older studies involving TMP/SMX for treatment of CBP from the 1970s[76–78] evaluated 90 days of treatment, but a duration of 6 weeks seems reasonable in the absence of clear evidence)

Macrolides and tetracyclines

Macrolides and tetracyclines (minocycline and doxycycline specifically) penetrate the prostate well.[44] However, they have limited use in CBP because many GU organisms might not be susceptible to them. If prior culture data show susceptibility, and antibiotics with a stronger evidence base (ie, fluroquinolones or TMP-SMX) are otherwise contraindicated (eg, due to allergies, resistance, concern for tendinopathy or other side effects, etc.), macrolides and tetracyclines are a reasonable alternative choice.[79,81]

An exception to the above is in the case of CBP specifically due to C trachomatis, Mycoplasma spp, or Ureaplasma urealyticum. Azithromycin has been shown to be superior to ciprofloxacin in patients with C trachomatis.[82] For these particular pathogens, the suggested antimicrobial regimen is as follows:

- Azithromycin 500 mg PO once weekly for 3 weeks (based on one trial of azithromycin vs ciprofloxacin for CBP caused by C trachomatis)[82]
- Tetracycline, doxycycline, minocycline—no specific dosing recommendations are available for prostatitis

Fosfomycin

Fosfomycin is a newer alternative agent for the treatment of CBP.[42] Having good prostatic penetration, it has effectively been used to treat CBP in several studies.[83–85] It is less studied than fluoroquinolones but would be reasonable to prescribe in patients with a fluoroquinolone-resistant infection. A suggested regimen as follows:

- Fosfomycin 3g PO every 48 hours for 6 weeks (can consider extending to 12 weeks if prostatic calcifications are noted on imaging, as was done in one study)[84]

Oral cephalosporins

There are no robust clinical data demonstrating the efficacy of oral cephalosporins for the treatment of CBP, as these agents tend to have poor penetration into the prostate. In the case where the above therapies have failed and there is an isolate with known susceptibility to an oral cephalosporin, it might be reasonable to pursue a prolonged course with close monitoring for recurrence and relapse. Regimens should be selected only with appropriate specialist assistance.

Nitrofurantoin

Although commonly used for lower acute UTIs, nitrofurantoin is not recommended for the treatment of CBP, as it has poor prostatic tissue penetration[44] and a potentially unfavorable safety profile with extended durations of treatment.

Parenteral Antibiotics

In general, use of IV antibiotics for the treatment of CBP is not recommended when oral options are available. In cases of CBP where oral antibiotic options are not available, expert Infectious Diseases consultation is advised.

Another route of therapy under investigation is the direct injection of antibiotics into the prostate. One small, randomized control trial of 50 patients showed improved cure rates from 5% to 33% with intramuscular vs. prostatic injection of amikacin.[86] However, overall evidence for this approach is lacking, as is availability for referral for this type of treatment.

Duration

The recommended duration of antibiotic therapy varies by the specific antimicrobial agent prescribed, as noted above. The extant literature on how long to treat CBP varies with recommendations ranging from 4 to 12 weeks. The 2015 consensus guidelines from the Prostatitis Expert Reference Group in the United Kingdom,[87] one of the more recent evidence summaries, recommends a treatment duration of 4 weeks for fluoroquinolones, TMP-SMX, or doxycycline (other antimicrobial agents were not discussed). This shorter duration for CBP is in line with current trends in many infectious syndromes to attempt a shorter course of antibiotics compared with historical recommendations, for reasons related to the known side effects of long-term antibiotics and risk of antimicrobial resistance. Although in cases of recurrence or relapse a longer course is typically pursued, there are little data to support an optimal regimen or duration in this situation. Similarly, although long-term antibiotic suppression might also be considered, there are no robust data to support such an approach. If chronic antibiotic suppression is considered, expert consultation is advised.

Recurrence/Relapse

Recurrence and relapse are common in CBP, with some studies showing rates as high as 25% to 50% at 6 to 24 months.[72,88] In general, fluoroquinolones remain the treatment of choice for recurrent CBP, even if used for the initial treatment regimen. In cases where a fluoroquinolone was previously used, the treatment course is usually extended to a minimum of 6 weeks. There are no guidelines for when antibiotics other than fluoroquinolones should be used for recurrent CBP.

Non-Antibiotic Medications

Evidence is overall lacking for non-antimicrobial medications for the treatment of CBP. One study showed decreased recurrence of CBP (95% vs 76% for microbiological clearance) with use of alpha-blockers concurrently with antibiotics,[89] but this has not been investigated further. Non-steroidal anti-inflammatory drugs (NSAIDs) have been historically prescribed, but as discussed in a recent guideline, the evidence is scant, and NSAIDs likely only provide short-term benefit.[87] In general, the focus of clinical management, in addition to antimicrobial therapy, should be on risk-factor optimization (eg, diabetes mellitus, BPH) within the usual standard of care.

Surgical Intervention

A recent systematic review highlighted the dearth of available data related to the surgical management of CBP.[90] Investigated therapies include transurethral resection of the prostate and prostatectomy. Available studies show an overall cure rate of 70%. For the other 30%, half had improved symptoms, and the other half had unchanged symptomatology. Radical prostatectomy was evaluated in 6 case series and showed an overall cure rate of 95%.

Based on this data, we agree with Schoeb and colleagues[90] that surgical intervention can be considered in certain clinical scenarios. However, given the well-established risks of prostatectomy (urinary incontinence, erectile dysfunction, strictures), we recommend discussing this option with a urologic specialist in situations of:

- Frequently recurrent CBP
- CBP from resistant bacterial species with limited to no available antimicrobial therapies
- Uncertainty related to the diagnosis of CBP

CLINICAL CARE POINTS

- Oral fluoroquinolones are first-line therapy for chronic bacterial prostatitis if bacterial isolates are susceptible.
- Duration of treatment varies by antibiotic, but usually ranges from 4 to 12 weeks.
- Up to 25% to 50% of patients with chronic bacterial prostatitis will have microbiologic or symptomatic recurrence by 24 months posttreatment.

Clinical Outcomes and Follow-up

Clinical outcomes

There are limited data on overall morbidity and mortality related to CBP, and treatment response rates vary by drug choice, duration of therapy, and study. However, reported response rates for fluoroquinolones (first-line therapy) are highlighted in **Table 2**:[71–73,91]

Table 2 is a combination of data from four studies investigating response rates of patients with CBP to fluoroquinolones (ciprofloxacin, levofloxacin, prulifloxacin, and lomefloxacin). "Response rate" is heterogeneous among studies and can refer to cure, symptomatic improvement, and/or microbiological eradication.

For TMP-SMX, studies showed initial cure rates as low as 32%[77] and as high as 100%.[76] However, even the most robust initial responses were followed by high relapse rates of up to 67% by 18 months of follow-up.[76]

Overall, in the management of CBP, initial responses to treatment are positive, but enduring clinical resolution remains a challenge.

Follow-up

Follow-up of patients treated for CBP is warranted for a variety of reasons, including the high rate of treatment failure and relapse, and for monitoring of adverse drug events, which become more prevalent with prolonged antibiotic courses. No guidelines exist for specific follow-up intervals, although it would be reasonable to re-evaluate a patient soon after completion of antimicrobial therapy, and if symptoms have resolved, at 6 to 12 months thereafter.

There are no data supporting the routine use of follow-up laboratory or imaging studies. One study did show a correlation between a decrease in PSA and microbiological eradication of bacterial pathogens,[65] but the clinical significance of this finding remains to be shown. In the case of persistent or recurrent symptoms, patients should be evaluated diagnostically utilizing the same approach as during the initial episode.

Table 2 Time from end of fluoroquinolone therapy				
Duration from End of Therapy	**< 2 wk**	**1 mo**	**3 mo**	**6 mo**
Response rate (%)	73–98	77–90	66–89	62–89

(Data from Refs[71–73,91])

Adverse Effects of Therapy

A detailed, extensive review of the adverse effects of the multitude of antibiotics recommended for the treatment of CBP is beyond the scope of this review. However, given the first-line recommendation of fluoroquinolones, it is pertinent to point out the higher rates of complications from prolonged courses of this antibiotic class. In particular, tendinopathy is a relevant concern in the older population (men > 60 years old) or those taking concurrent glucocorticoids, and a patient-centered conversation discussing the relevant risks and benefits of different therapies is recommended before initiating a therapeutic regimen.

Specialty Referral

Urology

When CBP is suspected but the diagnosis is not yet confirmed, referral to urology specialists can be beneficial. Although the two-glass method can theoretically be executed by any clinician capable of performing prostatic massage, studies demonstrating its efficacy were performed by experienced urologists. Urology referral is additionally recommended when surgical treatment may be indicated (see "Surgical Interventions" above).

Infectious Diseases

Infectious diseases referral is not required for uncomplicated CBP, but may be beneficial in the following scenarios:

- Recurrent or refractory CBP
- Causative organism resistant to oral treatment options
- Before surgical treatment of CBP (as part of a holistic review of available alternatives)
- When the diagnosis of CBP is uncertain

CLINICAL CARE POINTS

- Six-month response rates for fluoroquinolones in the treatment of chronic bacterial prostatitis range from 62% to 89%.
- There are no data supporting routine use of laboratory or imaging studies for follow-up of chronic bacterial prostatitis.
- Prolonged courses of antimicrobial therapy used for chronic bacterial prostatitis increase the incidence of adverse drug effects. These possibilities should be discussed with patients before initiating a treatment regimen.

SUMMARY

ABP and CBP are prevalent and clinically relevant conditions that the practicing clinician should be able to recognize, diagnose, treat, and follow-up effectively.

ABP represents an acute infection of the prostate gland. It should be suspected in a male patient who becomes significantly ill from an acute UTI in whom a different urinary source is not suspected and another infectious source is not established. Diagnosis relies heavily upon history and examination (in particular DRE) but can be augmented by labs and imaging. Initial treatment is often empiric IV antibiotics followed by a course of oral step-down therapy. Approximately 90% of individuals completely return to baseline without any residual effects by 6 months posttreatment.

CBP has a much more indolent clinical presentation, and should be suspected in any male patient with greater than 3 months of GU symptoms or who has recurrent UTIs caused by the same organism. Diagnosis should be made via the 2-, 4-, or 5-glass tests. Treatment should be tailored according to microbiologic susceptibilities, with a 4 to 6 week course of a fluoroquinolone (depending upon susceptibilities) as the antibiotic regimen of choice. Follow-up is recommended in all cases due to the high rates of recurrence and relapse in management of CBP.

Several questions remain related to optimal diagnosis and treatment of ABP and CBP, and there is a need for more large-scale randomized controlled trials and prospective cohort studies. Increased awareness of ABP and CBP as diagnostic considerations may fuel additional investigations to provide essential, currently missing evidence about how best to diagnose and treat these common and important conditions in older men.

DISCLOSURE

Dr Barbara W. Trautner has received research funding from Genentech, United States. Dr Prathit A. Kulkarni has received research funding from Vessel Health, Inc.

REFERENCES

1. Krieger JN, Lee SWH, Jeon J, et al. Epidemiology of prostatitis. Int J Antimicrob Agents 2008;31(Suppl 1):S85–90.
2. Daniels NA, Ewing SK, Zmuda JM, et al. Osteoporotic Fractures in Men (MrOS) Research Group. Correlates and prevalence of prostatitis in a large community-based cohort of older men. Urology 2005;66(5):964–70.
3. Krieger JN, Nyberg L, Nickel JC. NIH consensus definition and classification of prostatitis. JAMA 1999;282(3):236–7.
4. Dellinger RP, Levy MM, Rhodes A, et al. Surviving Sepsis Campaign: International Guidelines for Management of Severe Sepsis and Septic Shock, 2012. Intensive Care Med 2013;39(2):165–228.
5. Rhodes A, Evans LE, Alhazzani W, et al. Surviving Sepsis Campaign: International Guidelines for Management of Sepsis and Septic Shock: 2016. Intensive Care Med 2017;43(3):304–77.
6. Detweiler K, Mayers D, Fletcher SG. Bacteriuria and Urinary Tract Infections in the Elderly. Urol Clin North Am 2015;42(4):561–8.
7. Esposito S, Leone S, Noviello S, et al. Antibiotic resistance in long-term care facilities. New Microbiol 2007;30(3):326–31.
8. Nelson RE, Hyun D, Jezek A, et al. Mortality, Length of Stay, and Healthcare Costs Associated With Multidrug-Resistant Bacterial Infections Among Elderly Hospitalized Patients in the United States. Clin Infect Dis Soc Am 2022;74(6):1070–80.
9. Wilson PW, Anderson KM, Kannel WB. Epidemiology of diabetes mellitus in the elderly. The Framingham Study. Am J Med 1986;80(5A):3–9.
10. Egan KB. The Epidemiology of Benign Prostatic Hyperplasia Associated with Lower Urinary Tract Symptoms: Prevalence and Incident Rates. Urol Clin North Am 2016;43(3):289–97.
11. Bell KJL, Del Mar C, Wright G, et al. Prevalence of incidental prostate cancer: A systematic review of autopsy studies. Int J Cancer 2015;137(7):1749–57.
12. Etienne M, Chavanet P, Sibert L, et al. Acute bacterial prostatitis: heterogeneity in diagnostic criteria and management. Retrospective multicentric analysis of 371 patients diagnosed with acute prostatitis. BMC Infect Dis 2008;8:12.

13. Wyndaele JJ. Complications of intermittent catheterization: their prevention and treatment. Spinal Cord 2002;40(10):536–41.
14. Mosharafa AA, Torky MH, El Said WM, et al. Rising incidence of acute prostatitis following prostate biopsy: fluoroquinolone resistance and exposure is a significant risk factor. Urology 2011;78(3):511–4.
15. Ozden E, Bostanci Y, Yakupoglu KY, et al. Incidence of acute prostatitis caused by extended-spectrum beta-lactamase-producing Escherichia coli after transrectal prostate biopsy. Urology 2009;74(1):119–23.
16. Breyer BN, Van den Eeden SK, Horberg MA, et al. HIV status is an independent risk factor for reporting lower urinary tract symptoms. J Urol 2011;185(5):1710–5.
17. Lee LK, Dinneen MD, Ahmad S. The urologist and the patient infected with human immunodeficiency virus or with acquired immunodeficiency syndrome. BJU Int 2001;88(6):500–10.
18. Grabe M, Forsgren A, Hellsten S. The effect of a short antibiotic course in transurethral prostatic resection. Scand J Urol Nephrol 1984;18(1):37–42.
19. Grabe M, Forsgren A, Hellsten S. The effectiveness of a short perioperative course with pivampicillin/pivmecillinam in transurethral prostatic resection: clinical results. Scand J Infect Dis 1986;18(6):567–73.
20. Grabe M. Antimicrobial agents in transurethral prostatic resection. J Urol 1987; 138(2):245–52.
21. Coker TJ, Dierfeldt DM. Acute Bacterial Prostatitis: Diagnosis and Management. Am Fam Physician 2016;93(2):114–20.
22. Matsumoto M, Yamamoto S. AAUS guideline for acute bacterial prostatitis 2021. J Infect Chemother 2021;27(9):1277–83.
23. Etienne M, Pestel-Caron M, Chapuzet C, et al. Should blood cultures be performed for patients with acute prostatitis? J Clin Microbiol 2010;48(5):1935–8.
24. Gamé X, Vincendeau S, Palascak R, et al. Total and free serum prostate specific antigen levels during the first month of acute prostatitis. Eur Urol 2003;43(6):702–5.
25. Pansadoro V, Emiliozzi P, Defidio L, et al. Prostate-specific antigen and prostatitis in men under fifty. Eur Urol 1996;30(1):24–7.
26. Ulleryd P, Zackrisson B, Aus G, et al. Prostatic involvement in men with febrile urinary tract infection as measured by serum prostate-specific antigen and transrectal ultrasonography. BJU Int 1999;84(4):470–4.
27. Horcajada JP, Vilana R, Moreno-Martínez A, et al. Transrectal prostatic ultrasonography in acute bacterial prostatitis: findings and clinical implications. Scand J Infect Dis 2003;35(2):114–20.
28. Bhagat SK, Kekre NS, Gopalakrishnan G, et al. Changing profile of prostatic abscess. J Braz Soc Urol 2008;34(2):164–70.
29. Vyas JB, Ganpule SA, Ganpule AP, et al. Transrectal ultrasound-guided aspiration in the management of prostatic abscess: A single-center experience. Indian J Radiol Imaging 2013;23(3):253–7.
30. Fabiani A, Filosa A, Maurelli V, et al. Diagnostic and therapeutic utility of transrectal ultrasound in urological office prostatic abscess management: a short report from a single urologic center. Arch Ital Urol Androl Organo Uff Soc Ital Ecogr Urol E Nefrol 2014;86(4):344–8.
31. Reddivari AKR, Mehta P. Prostatic Abscess. In: StatPearls. StatPearls Publishing; 2022. Available at: http://www.ncbi.nlm.nih.gov/books/NBK551663/. Accessed August 9, 2022.
32. Mateos JJ, Velasco M, Lomena F, et al. 111Indium labelled leukocyte scintigraphy in the detection of acute prostatitis. Nucl Med Commun 2002;23(11):1137–42.

33. Kim SH, Ha US, Yoon BI, et al. Microbiological and clinical characteristics in acute bacterial prostatitis according to lower urinary tract manipulation procedure. J Infect Chemother Off J Jpn Soc Chemother 2014;20(1):38–42.
34. Ramakrishnan K, Salinas RC. Prostatitis: acute and chronic. Prim Care 2010; 37(3):547–63, viii-ix.
35. Millán-Rodríguez F, Palou J, Bujons-Tur A, et al. Acute bacterial prostatitis: two different sub-categories according to a previous manipulation of the lower urinary tract. World J Urol 2006;24(1):45–50.
36. Nagy V, Kubej D. Acute bacterial prostatitis in humans: current microbiological spectrum, sensitivity to antibiotics and clinical findings. Urol Int 2012;89(4):445–50.
37. Chuang AY, Tsou MH, Chang SJ, et al. Mycobacterium abscessus granulomatous prostatitis. Am J Surg Pathol 2012;36(3):418–22.
38. Tamsel S, Killi R, Ertan Y, et al. A rare case of granulomatous prostatitis caused by Mycobacterium tuberculosis. J Clin Ultrasound JCU 2007;35(1):58–61.
39. Epstein DJ, Thompson LDR, Saleem A, et al. Fungal prostatitis due to endemic mycoses and Cryptococcus: A multicenter case series. Prostate 2020;80(12): 1006–11.
40. Larsen RA, Bozzette S, McCutchan JA, et al. Persistent Cryptococcus neoformans infection of the prostate after successful treatment of meningitis. California Collaborative Treatment Group. Ann Intern Med 1989;111(2):125–8.
41. Naber KG, Sörgel F. Antibiotic therapy–rationale and evidence for optimal drug concentrations in prostatic and seminal fluid and in prostatic tissue. Andrologia 2003;35(5):331–5.
42. Takasaki N, Ra S, Okada S, et al. [Transference of antibiotics into prostatic tissues: sampling method by transurethral resection for the measurement of the concentration of antibiotics in prostatic tissue]. Hinyokika Kiyo 1986;32(7):969–75.
43. Kwan ACF, Beahm NP. Fosfomycin for bacterial prostatitis: a review. Int J Antimicrob Agents 2020;56(4):106106.
44. Charalabopoulos K, Karachalios G, Baltogiannis D, et al. Penetration of Antimicrobial Agents into the Prostate. Chemotherapy 2003;49(6):269–79.
45. Wagenlehner FME, Weidner W, Naber KG. Therapy for prostatitis, with emphasis on bacterial prostatitis. Expert Opin Pharmacother 2007;8(11):1667–74.
46. Lipsky BA, Byren I, Hoey CT. Treatment of bacterial prostatitis. Clin Infect Dis Off Publ Infect Dis Soc Am 2010;50(12):1641–52.
47. Ludwig M, Schroeder-Printzen I, Schiefer HG, et al. Diagnosis and therapeutic management of 18 patients with prostatic abscess. Urology 1999;53(2):340–5.
48. Chou YH, Tiu CM, Liu JY, et al. Prostatic abscess: transrectal color Doppler ultrasonic diagnosis and minimally invasive therapeutic management. Ultrasound Med Biol 2004;30(6):719–24.
49. Yoon BI, Han DS, Ha US, et al. Clinical courses following acute bacterial prostatitis. Prostate Int 2013;1(2):89–93.
50. Ha US, Kim ME, Kim CS, et al. Acute bacterial prostatitis in Korea: clinical outcome, including symptoms, management, microbiology and course of disease. Int J Antimicrob Agents 2008;31(Suppl 1):S96–101.
51. Eliakim-Raz N, Babitch T, Shaw E, et al. Risk Factors for Treatment Failure and Mortality Among Hospitalized Patients With Complicated Urinary Tract Infection: A Multicenter Retrospective Cohort Study (RESCUING Study Group). Clin Infect Dis Off Publ Infect Dis Soc Am 2019;68(1):29–36.
52. Smithson A, Ramos J, Niño E, et al. Characteristics of febrile urinary tract infections in older male adults. BMC Geriatr 2019;19(1):334.

53. Ulleryd P, Zackrisson B, Aus G, et al. Selective urological evaluation in men with febrile urinary tract infection. BJU Int 2001;88(1):15–20.

54. Weidner W, Ludwig M. Diagnostic Management in Chronic Prostatitis. In: Weidner W, Madsen PO, Schiefer HG, editors. Prostatitis: etiopathology, diagnosis and therapy. Springer; 1994. p. 49–65.

55. Yoon BI, Kim S, Han DS, et al. Acute bacterial prostatitis: how to prevent and manage chronic infection? J Infect Chemother Off J Jpn Soc Chemother 2012; 18(4):444–50.

56. Zhao WP, Li YT, Chen J, et al. Prostatic calculi influence the antimicrobial efficacy in men with chronic bacterial prostatitis. Asian J Androl 2012;14(5):715–9.

57. Meares EM, Stamey TA. Bacteriologic localization patterns in bacterial prostatitis and urethritis. Invest Urol 1968;5(5):492–518.

58. McNaughton Collins M, Fowler FJ, Elliott DB, et al. Diagnosing and treating chronic prostatitis: do urologists use the four-glass test? Urology 2000;55(3): 403–7.

59. Nickel JC, Shoskes D, Wang Y, et al. How does the pre-massage and post-massage two-glass test compare to the Meares-Stamey four-glass test in men with chronic prostatitis/chronic pelvic pain syndrome? J Urol 2006;176(1):119–24.

60. Orland SM, Hanno PM, Wein AJ. Prostatitis, prostatosis, and prostatodynia. Urology 1985;25(5):439–59.

61. Jameson RM. Sexual activity and the variations of the white cell content of the prostatic secretion. Invest Urol 1967;5(3):297–302.

62. Budía A, Luis Palmero J, Broseta E, et al. Value of semen culture in the diagnosis of chronic bacterial prostatitis: a simplified method. Scand J Urol Nephrol 2006; 40(4):326–31.

63. Magri V, Wagenlehner FME, Montanari E, et al. Semen analysis in chronic bacterial prostatitis: diagnostic and therapeutic implications. Asian J Androl 2009; 11(4):461–77.

64. Heras-Cañas V, Gutiérrez-Soto B, Serrano-García ML, et al. [Chronic bacterial prostatitis. Clinical and microbiological study of 332 cases]. Med Clin (Barc) 2016;147(4):144–7.

65. Schaeffer AJ, Wu SC, Tennenberg AM, et al. Treatment of chronic bacterial prostatitis with levofloxacin and ciprofloxacin lowers serum prostate specific antigen. J Urol 2005;174(1):161–4.

66. Mutlu N, Mutlu B, Culha M, et al. The role of Chlamydia trachomatis in patients with non-bacterial prostatitis. Int J Clin Pract 1998;52(8):540–1.

67. Ostaszewska I, Zdrodowska-Stefanow B, Badyda J, et al. Chlamydia trachomatis: probable cause of prostatitis. Int J STD AIDS 1998;9(6):350–3.

68. Gümüş B, Sengil AZ, Solak M, et al. Evaluation of non-invasive clinical samples in chronic chlamydial prostatitis by using in situ hybridization. Scand J Urol Nephrol 1997;31(5):449–51.

69. Strohmaier WL, Bichler KH. Comparison of symptoms, morphological, microbiological and urodynamic findings in patients with chronic prostatitis/pelvic pain syndrome. Is it possible to differentiate separate categories? Urol Int 2000; 65(2):112–6.

70. Yu J, Fulcher AS, Turner MA, et al. Prostate cancer and its mimics at multiparametric prostate MRI. Br J Radiol 2014;87(1037):20130659.

71. Giannarini G, Mogorovich A, Valent F, et al. Prulifloxacin versus levofloxacin in the treatment of chronic bacterial prostatitis: a prospective, randomized, double-blind trial. J Chemother Florence Italy 2007;19(3):304–8.

72. Bundrick W, Heron SP, Ray P, et al. Levofloxacin versus ciprofloxacin in the treatment of chronic bacterial prostatitis: a randomized double-blind multicenter study. Urology 2003;62(3):537–41.
73. Naber KG, European Lomefloxacin Prostatitis Study Group. Lomefloxacin versus ciprofloxacin in the treatment of chronic bacterial prostatitis. Int J Antimicrob Agents 2002;20(1):18–27.
74. Perletti G, Marras E, Wagenlehner FME, et al. Antimicrobial therapy for chronic bacterial prostatitis. Cochrane Database Syst Rev 2013;8:CD009071.
75. Paglia M, Peterson J, Fisher AC, et al. Safety and efficacy of levofloxacin 750 mg for 2 weeks or 3 weeks compared with levofloxacin 500 mg for 4 weeks in treating chronic bacterial prostatitis. Curr Med Res Opin 2010;26(6):1433–41.
76. McGuire EJ, Lytton B. Bacterial prostatitis: treatment with trimethoprim-sulfamethoxazole. Urology 1976;7(5):499–500.
77. Meares EM. Long-term therapy of chronic bacterial prostatitis with trimethoprim-sulfamethoxazole. Can Med Assoc J 1975;112(13 Spec No):22–5.
78. Meares EM. Serum antibody titers in treatment with trimethoprim-sulfamethoxazole for chronic prostatitis. Urology 1978;11(2):142–6.
79. Paulson DF, White RD. Trimethoprium-sulfamethoxazole and minocycline- hydrochloride in the treatment of culture-proved bacterial prostatitis. J Urol 1978; 120(2):184–5.
80. Kurzer E, Kaplan S. Cost effectiveness model comparing trimethoprim sulfamethoxazole and ciprofloxacin for the treatment of chronic bacterial prostatitis. Eur Urol 2002;42(2):163–6.
81. Paulson DF, Zinner NR, Resnick MI, et al. Treatment of bacterial prostatitis. Comparison of cephalexin and minocycline. Urology 1986;27(4):379–87.
82. Skerk V, Schönwald S, Krhen I, et al. Comparative analysis of azithromycin and ciprofloxacin in the treatment of chronic prostatitis caused by Chlamydia trachomatis. Int J Antimicrob Agents 2003;21(5):457–62.
83. Grayson ML, Macesic N, Trevillyan J, et al. Fosfomycin for Treatment of Prostatitis: New Tricks for Old Dogs. Clin Infect Dis Soc Am 2015;61(7):1141–3.
84. Karaiskos I, Galani L, Sakka V, et al. Oral fosfomycin for the treatment of chronic bacterial prostatitis. J Antimicrob Chemother 2019;74(5):1430–7.
85. Los-Arcos I, Pigrau C, Rodríguez-Pardo D, et al. Long-Term Fosfomycin-Tromethamine Oral Therapy for Difficult-To-Treat Chronic Bacterial Prostatitis. Antimicrob Agents Chemother 2015;60(3):1854–8.
86. Hu WL, Zhong SZ, He HX. Treatment of chronic bacterial prostatitis with amikacin through anal submucosal injection. Asian J Androl 2002;4(3):163–7.
87. Rees J, Abrahams M, Doble A, et al. Prostatitis Expert Reference Group (PERG). Diagnosis and treatment of chronic bacterial prostatitis and chronic prostatitis/chronic pelvic pain syndrome: a consensus guideline. BJU Int 2015;116(4): 509–25.
88. Weidner W, Ludwig M, Brähler E, et al. Outcome of antibiotic therapy with ciprofloxacin in chronic bacterial prostatitis. Drugs 1999;58(Suppl 2):103–6.
89. Barbalias GA, Nikiforidis G, Liatsikos EN. Alpha-blockers for the treatment of chronic prostatitis in combination with antibiotics. J Urol 1998;159(3):883–7.
90. Schoeb DS, Schlager D, Boeker M, et al. Surgical therapy of prostatitis: a systematic review. World J Urol 2017;35(11):1659–68.
91. Naber KG, Roscher K, Botto H, et al. Oral levofloxacin 500 mg once daily in the treatment of chronic bacterial prostatitis. Int J Antimicrob Agents 2008;32(2): 145–53.